# Repairing and Reconstructing the Hand and Wrist

*Editor*

KEVIN C. CHUNG

# CLINICS IN PLASTIC SURGERY

www.plasticsurgery.theclinics.com

July 2019 • Volume 46 • Number 3

**ELSEVIER**

1600 John F. Kennedy Boulevard ● Suite 1800 ● Philadelphia, Pennsylvania, 19103-2899

http://www.theclinics.com

**CLINICS IN PLASTIC SURGERY Volume 46, Number 3**
**July 2019 ISSN 0094-1298, ISBN-13: 978-0-323-68235-0**

*Editor:* Jessica McCool
*Developmental Editor:* Meredith Madeira

*Clinics in Plastic Surgery* (ISSN 0094-1298) is published quarterly by Elsevier Inc., 360 Park Avenue South, New York, NY 10010-1710. Months of issue are January, April, July, and October. Business and Editorial Offices: 1600 John F. Kennedy Blvd., Suite 1800, Philadelphia, PA 19103-2899. Periodicals postage paid at New York, NY and additional mailing offices. Subscription prices are $543.00 per year for US individuals, $940.00 per year for US institutions, $100.00 per year for US students and residents, $607.00 per year for Canadian individuals, $1119.00 per year for Canadian institutions, $649.00 per year for international individuals, $1119.00 per year for international institutions, and $305.00 per year for Canadian and international students/residents. To receive student/resident rate, orders must be accompanied by name of affiliated institution, date of term, and the *signature* of program/residency coordinator on institution letterhead. Orders will be billed at individual rate until proof of status is received. Foreign air speed delivery is included in all *Clinics* subscription prices. All prices are subject to change without notice. **POSTMASTER:** Send address changes to *Clinics in Plastic Surgery*, Elsevier Health Sciences Division, Subscription Customer Service, 3251 Riverport Lane, Maryland Heights, MO 63043. **Customer Service: 1-800-654-2452 (US and Canada). From outside of the United States and Canada, call 314-447-8871. Fax: 314-447-8029. E-mail: JournalsCustomerService-usa@elsevier.com (for print support); JournalsOnlineSupport-usa@ elsevier.com (for online support).**

*Reprints.* For copies of 100 or more of articles in this publication, please contact the Commercial Reprints Department, Elsevier Inc., 360 Park Avenue South, New York, New York 10010-1710. Tel.: +1-212-633-3874; Fax: +1-212-633-3820; E-mail: reprints@elsevier.com.

*Clinics in Plastic Surgery* is covered in *Current Contents, EMBASE/Excerpta Medica, Science Citation Index, MEDLINE/ PubMed (Index Medicus), ASCA, and ISI/BIOMED.*

# Contributors

## EDITOR

**KEVIN C. CHUNG, MD, MS**
Chief of Hand Surgery, Michigan Medicine,
Director, University of Michigan
Comprehensive Hand Center, Charles B. G. de
Nancrede Professor of Surgery, Professor of
Plastic Surgery and Orthopaedic Surgery,
Assistant Dean for Faculty Affairs, Associate
Director of Global REACH, University of
Michigan Medical School, Ann Arbor,
Michigan, USA

## AUTHORS

**JOSHUA M. ADKINSON, MD**
Assistant Professor of Surgery, Division of
Plastic Surgery, Indiana University School
of Medicine, Indianapolis, Indiana,
USA

**ANDRE EU JIN CHEAH, MBBS, MMed, MBA**
Department of Hand and Reconstructive
Microsurgery, National University Health
System, Singapore

**ALPHONSUS K.S. CHONG, MBBS, FAMS**
Department of Hand and Reconstructive
Microsurgery, University Orthopaedics Hand
and Reconstructive Microsurgery Cluster,
National University Health System, Department
of Orthopaedic Surgery, Yong Loo Lin School
of Medicine, National University of Singapore,
Singapore

**BRIAN M. CHRISTIE, MD, MPH**
Resident, Division of Plastic Surgery,
Department of Surgery, University of
Wisconsin Hospital and Clinics, Madison,
Wisconsin, USA

**KEVIN C. CHUNG, MD, MS**
Chief of Hand Surgery, Michigan
Medicine, Director, University of Michigan
Comprehensive Hand Center, Charles B. G. de
Nancrede Professor of Surgery, Professor
of Plastic Surgery and Orthopaedic
Surgery, Assistant Dean for Faculty
Affairs, Associate Director of Global REACH,
University of Michigan Medical
School, Ann Arbor, Michigan,
USA

**SOUMEN DAS DE, MBBS (Hons), FRCSEd (Ortho), MPH**
Consultant, Department of Hand and
Reconstructive Microsurgery, National
University Health System, Singapore

**KYLE R. EBERLIN, MD**
Assistant Professor of Surgery, Division
of Plastic and Reconstructive Surgery,
Harvard Medical School, Massachusetts
General Hospital, Boston, Massachusetts,
USA

**KATE ELZINGA, MD**
Clinical Lecturer, Section of Plastic Surgery, University of Calgary, Foothills Medical Centre, Calgary, Alberta, Canada

**ANTHONY FOO, MD**
Consultant, Department of Hand and Reconstructive Microsurgery, National University Hospital, Singapore, Singapore

**MICHAEL B. GOTTSCHALK, MD**
Assistant Professor, Division of Upper Extremity Surgery, Department of Orthopaedic Surgery, Emory University, Atlanta, Georgia, USA

**YONG HU, MD**
Department of Hand and Foot Surgery, The Second Hospital of Shandong University, Jinan, People's Republic of China

**AMITABHA LAHIRI, MBBS, MS, MCh (Plast), FRCS (Edin), FAMS (Hand Surgery), MRes (Tissue Engineering)**
Senior Consultant, Department of Hand and Reconstructive Microsurgery, National University Hospital, Singapore, Singapore

**ELLEN Y. LEE, MD**
Associate Consultant, Department of Hand and Reconstructive Microsurgery, National University Health System, Singapore

**JANICE C.Y. LIAO, MBBS, MRCS**
Department of Hand and Reconstructive Microsurgery, University Orthopaedics Hand and Reconstructive Microsurgery Cluster, National University Health System, Singapore

**AYMERIC Y.T. LIM, FRCS**
Professor and Senior Consultant, Department of Hand and Reconstructive Microsurgery, National University Health System, Singapore

**JIN XI LIM, MBBS (Singapore), MMED Surgery (Singapore)**
Associate Consultant, Department of Hand and Reconstructive Microsurgery, University Orthopaedics, Hand and Reconstructive Microsurgery Cluster, National University Health System, Singapore

**SCOTT N. LOEWENSTEIN, MD**
Resident, Division of Plastic Surgery, Indiana University School of Medicine, Indianapolis, Indiana, USA

**PATRICIA MARTIN-PLAYA, MD**
Clinical Fellow, Department of Hand and Reconstructive Microsurgery, National University Hospital, Singapore, Singapore

**BRETT F. MICHELOTTI, MD**
Associate Professor, Division of Plastic Surgery, Department of Surgery, University of Wisconsin Hospital and Clinics, Madison, Wisconsin, USA

**SHIMPEI ONO, MD, PhD, FACS**
Department of Plastic, Reconstructive and Aesthetic Surgery, Nippon Medical School, Tokyo, Japan

**BRENT B. PICKRELL, MD**
Division of Plastic and Reconstructive Surgery, Harvard Medical School, Massachusetts General Hospital, Boston, Massachusetts, USA

**MARK E. PUHAINDRAN, MBBS, MMED (Surg)**
Head and Senior Consultant, Division of Musculoskeletal Oncology, Senior Consultant, Department of Hand and Reconstructive Microsurgery, National University Health System, National University Hospital, Singapore, Singapore

**PAYMON RAHGOZAR, MD**
Assistant Professor, Division of Plastic and Reconstructive Surgery, Department of Surgery, University of California, San Francisco Medical Center, San Francisco, California, USA

**SANDEEP JACOB SEBASTIN, MBBS, MRCS (UK), FAMS (Hand Surgery)**
Senior Consultant, Department of Hand and Reconstructive Microsurgery, National University Health System, Singapore

**SOPHIA A. STRIKE, MD**
Assistant Professor, Department of Orthopaedic Surgery, Johns Hopkins University School of Medicine, Johns Hopkins Outpatient Center, Baltimore, Maryland, USA

**AMIR H. TAGHINIA, MD, MPH, MBA**
Staff Surgeon, Department of Plastic and Oral Surgery, Boston Children's Hospital, Assistant Professor of Surgery, Harvard Medical School, Boston, Massachusetts, USA

**SIMON G. TALBOT, MD**
Associate Surgeon, Division of Plastic Surgery, Brigham and Women's Hospital, Associate Professor of Surgery, Harvard Medical School, Boston, Massachusetts, USA

**DAVID MENG KIAT TAN, MBBS (Singapore), MMED Surgery (Singapore)**
Assistant Professor, Department of Orthopaedic Surgery, Yong Loo Lin School of Medicine, National University of Singapore, Senior Consultant and Residency Director, Department of Hand and Reconstructive Microsurgery, University Orthopaedics, Hand and Reconstructive Microsurgery Cluster, National University Health System, Singapore

**RUTH EN SI TAN, MBBS**
Department of Hand and Reconstructive Microsurgery, National University Health System, Singapore

**JIN BO TANG, MD**
Professor, Chair, Department of Hand Surgery, The Hand Surgery Research Center, Affiliated Hospital of Nantong University, Nantong, Jiangsu, People's Republic of China

**WENDY Z.W. TEO, BA (Cantab), BM BCh (Oxon), LLM**
Department of Hand and Reconstructive Microsurgery, National University Health System, Singapore

**XIAOFEI TIAN, MD**
Department of Burns and Plastic Surgery, Children's Hospital, Chongqing Medical University, Chongqing, People's Republic of China

**ERIC R. WAGNER, MD, MS**
Assistant Professor, Division of Upper Extremity Surgery, Department of Orthopaedic Surgery, Emory University, Atlanta, Georgia, USA

**BIN WANG, MD, PhD**
Professor, Chief of Hand Surgery, Department of Plastic and Reconstructive Surgery, Shanghai 9th People's Hospital, Shanghai Jiaotong University School of Medicine, Shanghai, People's Republic of China

**ERIC D. WANG, MD**
Chief Resident, Division of Plastic and Reconstructive Surgery, Department of Surgery, University of California, San Francisco Medical Center, San Francisco, California, USA

**MICHIRO YAMAMOTO, MD, PhD**
Associate Professor, Department of Hand Surgery, Nagoya University Graduate School of Medicine, Nagoya, Aichi, Japan

**ALFRED P. YOON, MD**
Section of Plastic Surgery, Department of Surgery, Michigan Medicine, University of Michigan, Ann Arbor, Michigan, USA

# Contents

Tendinopathy and tendinitis are some of the most frequently encountered disorders in hand and upper extremity surgery. Patients often present with progressively increasing pain over a subacute or chronic period. In most cases it is a clinical diagnosis, with confirmation via advanced imaging. First-line treatment consists of conservative measures such as activity modification, splints, and injections. After a 3- to 6-month trial of nonoperative treatment, surgery usually involves decompression of the involved tendons and debridement of any inflammatory tissue. Patient and anatomic factors can affect the outcomes of both nonoperative and operative treatments.

Acute and chronic injuries to the finger extensor mechanism can result in swan neck and boutonniere deformities. Loss of coordination between the multiple, specialized components of the extensor mechanism results in tendon imbalances leading to altered interphalangeal joint flexion and extension forces. Treatments include corrective splinting and operative interventions. Swan neck deformities are functionally limiting. Surgical correction generally results in functional benefit. Boutonniere deformities are functional but aesthetically displeasing; proximal interphalangeal (PIP) joint flexion and the ability to make a fist are maintained. Surgical improvement can be attempted with caution. Attempts to improve PIP extension can impede flexion, resulting in a poor functional outcome.

"Stiff finger," defined as a finger with decreased range of motion in one or more joints, is commonly found after hand injury and is classified into flexion or extension deformities. Pathogenesis is due to dysfunction in one or more of the following anatomic components: (1) osseous and articular; (2) capsuloligamentous; (3) musculotendinous units; (4) soft tissue and fascia. Evaluation and treatment are based on accurate identification and correction of pathologic structures. The mainstay of treatment is directed hand therapy with exercises and splinting to mobilize stiff joints. Operative interventions are offered after gains from therapy have been exhausted.

Nerve sheath tumors of the upper extremity are among the common neoplastic pathologies encountered by hand surgeons. A majority of these tumors are benign schwannomas or neurofibromas and may be associated with neurofibromatosis. Clinical signs of malignant transformation include new onset of pain and rapid growth. Imaging characteristics, such as standardized uptake value greater than 4.0 on PET scan, may aid in the diagnosis of a malignant tumor. Surgical excision, often with intrafascicular dissection with nerve preservation, is recommended treatment of benign lesions. Wide surgical excision is recommended for malignant lesions.

Mutilating injuries include a wide and heterogeneous spectrum of clinical presentations, each being unique in terms of pattern of tissue damage, patient characteristics, and functional requirements. Understanding the principles of reconstruction of bone and soft tissues, a wide repertoire of surgical techniques, and the ability to plan the reconstructive journey leading to a functional hand are crucial. Management of these injuries involves several on-the-spot decisions by the surgeon. This article aims to equip the surgeon with the key principles and the bits of knowledge that are essential for effective planning and execution when dealing with such injuries.

The literature on surgical techniques and recent evidence in microsurgical digital and hand replantation is reviewed. Replantation should not be done routinely without considering postoperative functional outcomes. Achieving best outcomes is related to the success of microvascular anastomosis and to adequacy of bone fixation, tendon and nerve repair, and soft-tissue coverage. Replantation surgery has become a routine procedure. However, little is known about the decision-making process for digital and hand amputation. A study comparing the outcomes of digital and hand amputations treated with replantation or revision amputation is needed. Outcome assessment includes not only function but also patient-reported outcomes.

Hand infections can lead to debilitating and permanent disability, particularly if they are not treated promptly or properly. The unique anatomy of the hand, with its numerous enclosed and confined spaces, warrants special considerations. For instance, infections in deep spaces of the hand may require surgical drainage despite an appropriate course of antimicrobial treatment. Thorough history and examination are crucial in guiding further investigations and management, particularly because there are numerous mimickers of hand infections, such as gout and pseudogout.

Thin soft tissue covering extensor tendons make them prone to injury. The extensor mechanism achieves a delicate balance with the flexor system. Inappropriate management in the acute setting can lead to long-term deformity and dysfunction. Acute extensor tendon injuries are usually managed with splinting and/or primary repair of the tendon. In cases of tendon length loss, tendon graft or flap may be necessary for reconstruction. This article presents a series of cases illustrating the appropriate management of traumatic extensor tendon injuries.

Soft tissue defects of the hand commonly arise as a consequence of trauma or infection and after resection of tumors. Restoring a thin and pliable soft tissue envelope is critical to restoring mobility and optimizing functional outcomes. The appearance, color, and texture match as well as donor site issues are increasingly important aspects of hand reconstruction. This article discusses the principles of soft tissue reconstruction in the hand and presents a rational approach to clinical decision making to ensure optimal outcomes.

# Section II: Bone and Joint

Thumb carpometacarpal arthritis is a common condition treated by hand surgeons. This condition most frequently affects the elderly and postmenopausal women. Nonoperative treatment options include activity modification, orthoses, and injections. Although many patients can be treated conservatively, those with persistent and recalcitrant symptoms may benefit from surgical intervention. There are myriad surgical options, and the best option often depends on the patient's goals and functional demands, surgeon experience, and patient preference.

The management of phalangeal and metacarpal fractures continues to evolve. Nonoperative or less invasive techniques, limiting the need for soft tissue dissection and resultant stiffness, are being developed and becoming more popular. The competing forces of fracture stability to optimize healing and early mobilization to optimize function need careful balancing. As imaging, equipment, and techniques improve, hand surgeons can tailor individualized care to the unique needs of each patient.

Hand and wrist fractures are common in the pediatric population. Accurate diagnosis relies on the understanding of the physeal anatomy and carpal ossification. Treatment of these fractures is largely influenced by physeal biology and compliance with treatment. A majority have a favorable outcome with nonoperative treatment. Operative treatment should be considered in patients with clinical deformity, open fractures, and significant fracture displacement. Physeal-friendly surgical approaches and implants should be used to minimize the sequelae of physeal injury.

 Video content accompanies this article at http://www.plasticsurgery.theclinics.com.

Proximal interphalangeal joint (PIPJ) injuries are common and challenging to treat, involving a spectrum of conditions ranging from isolated ligamentous injuries to severe fracture dislocations. The main goal of treatment is to achieve a congruent, stable joint, which is key to achieving early range of motion and a favorable outcome. Injuries that do not compromise the stability of the joint may be treated nonsurgically, whereas those that render the joint unstable may be managed with one of many surgical strategies available. This article focuses on the current practices of treatment of injuries around the PIPJ.

 Video content accompanies this article at http://www.plasticsurgery.theclinics.com.

Carpal instability and distal radioulnar joint instability represent an important set of conditions responsible for pain and disability in the wrist. Either condition can occur as a result of ligamentous failure or loss of articular congruity from fractures or a combination of both. Instability itself is a clinical diagnosis supported by relevant imaging modalities. Carpal and distal radioulnar joint instability needs to be considered according to its stage and severity as well as other factors like etiology and chronicity to determine the optimal treatment option. This article summarizes the conditions most relevant to the practice of a hand surgeon, with emphasis divided equally between assessment and diagnosis, staging, and treatment. The 3 most common carpal instability conditions are outlined in this article together with a review on acute and chronic distal radioulnar joint instability.

Diagnosis and proper initial management of acute fractures of the carpal bones is critical because of the limited blood supply of many bones of the wrist and the role of the carpus in optimizing hand function. Pathology is correctly diagnosed by a focused history and examination. Injuries may be missed with a cursory examination and routine wrist radiographs. Together, fractures of the scaphoid and triquetrum make up nearly 90% of carpal bone fractures. Relative frequency, mechanism of injury, diagnosis, and management principles are covered for each of the bones of the wrist.

Numerous techniques are available for treating finger joint disorders such as osteoarthritis and inflammatory arthritis. Joint fusion and arthroplasty have different concepts but can improve hand function. Joint fusion is indicated in patients with painful finger joints with or without poor soft tissue condition. Implant arthroplasty is indicated for degenerative or inflammatory arthritis in elderly patients because implants may require future revision. Arthroplasty with an autologous osteochondral cartilage graft is an option for young patients with posttraumatic metacarpophalangeal or proximal interphalangeal joint osteoarthritis, whereas vascular joint transfers are rarely used. Surgeons must carefully check each patient's condition and treatment expectations.

Congenital hand difference is caused by abnormal embryonic development of the limb and represents one of the most prevalent congenital birth defects worldwide. Using the new classification system proposed by Oberg, Manske and Tonkin (OMT) and endorsed by the International Federation of Societies for Surgery of the Hand, congenital hand differences are classified into malformations, deformations, and dysplasias and syndromes. Malformations are subdivided into abnormal development of proximal-distal, radial-ulnar (anterior-posterior), dorsal-ventral, and unspecified axis. We introduce here the state-of-the-art surgical treatment for thumb duplication and syndactyly. The surgical principle, timing, procedures, and postsurgical management are described for each condition.

# CLINICS IN PLASTIC SURGERY

**THE CLINICS ARE AVAILABLE ONLINE!**
Access your subscription at:
www.theclinics.com

# Preface

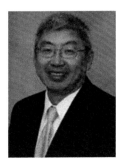

Kevin C. Chung, MD, MS
*Editor*

I am pleased to present this issue to you to share insights in treating common procedures for the hand and wrist. This issue is divided into soft tissue and bony reconstruction. The authors were selected for their expertise in providing proven treatment approaches for usual conditions faced by practitioners. My colleagues from the University of Singapore report their vast experience with soft tissue reconstruction and treating nerve compression syndrome. I am excited that Dr Jin Bo Tang, who is the world expert on flexor tendon repair, contributed his philosophy in repairing zone 2 flexor tendon injuries. Dr Shimpei Ono from Japan is a master in replantation surgery, who imparts his wisdom derived from the Japanese mastery of microsurgery. Other experts demystified challenging complex fractures of the hand and wrist, making treatment choices much clearer.

I asked the authors to present one treatment approach that had been proven to be effective in their practices, rather than sharing a number of techniques that may confuse the readers. Because of information overload in our hectic lives, this issue serves to present "just the facts" so that you can learn from the experts in an efficient and productive manner. I appreciate *Clinics in Plastic Surgery*'s invitation for me to assemble this issue for you. I am certain it will be a much-needed education companion to enhance the care of your patients.

Kevin C. Chung, MD, MS
Michigan Medicine
1500 E. Medical Center Drive
2130 Taubman Center, SPC 5340
Ann Arbor, MI 48109-5340, USA

*E-mail address:*
kecchung@med.umich.edu

Clin Plastic Surg 46 (2019) xiii
https://doi.org/10.1016/j.cps.2019.04.001
0094-1298/19/© 2019 Published by Elsevier Inc.

# Approach to Fingertip Injuries

Patricia Martin-Playa, MD, Anthony Foo, MD*

## KEYWORDS

- Fingertip injuries • Fingertip amputation • Nail bed injuries • Closed injuries • Psychosocial factors

## KEY POINTS

- Fingertip injuries are common and there is a wide spectrum of presentation.
- Restoration of a stable, pain-free, and normal looking fingertip is the main goal of treatment.
- Psychosocial factors are important considerations in the formulation of a treatment plan.

## INTRODUCTION

The fingertip comprises the nail complex and glabrous pulp, which are richly vascularized and innervated, built around the distal phalanx. Its dense innervation[1] and disproportionally large and intricate cortical representation[2] emphasize the importance of addressing psychological factors. Minor contusions can result in pain syndromes in some patients, whereas others adapt well to deformed fingertips, highlighting the nonlinear relationship between physical and psychological trauma.

## GOALS OF TREATMENT

The goals of treatment of any injured fingertip should be the restoration of a stable interface for object manipulation while looking as normal as possible. At the completion of treatment, the pulp should be stable and pain free, and the nail plate geometry should permit the manipulation of small objects.

## PLANNING TREATMENT

A focused history and physical examination is obtained to establish the most appropriate intervention for each patient. The characteristics of the injury determine the range of treatment, whereas psychosocial factors aid clinicians in selecting the most appropriate option. Psychosocial factors to be considered are occupation, hobbies, cultural norms, socioeconomic status, secondary motive, and clinician bias.[3–8]

## CLOSED INJURIES

The 3 main considerations for closed fingertip injuries are the nail plate, pulp, and bone. The size of the subungual hematoma is thought to correlate with the degree of the nail matrix injury, and an arbitrary figure of 50% is considered an indication for nail avulsion and matrix repair (**Fig. 1**) to facilitate anatomic healing.[9] An alternative approach, where nail trephination alone was performed regardless of the size of the hematoma, provided the nail plate was intact, yielded good pain relief with satisfactory nail plate regeneration.[10] The presence of a tuft fracture did not adversely affect the outcome in this series, in which patients with fractures received a splint to maintain the distal interphalangeal joint in extension for comfort.

## OPEN INJURIES WITHOUT TISSUE LOSS

Given the density of critical structures in the fingertip, it is prudent to exclude flexor tendon,

Disclosure Statement: The authors declare no potential conflicts of interest with respect to the research, authorship, and/or publication of this article.
Department of Hand and Reconstructive Microsurgery, National University Hospital, 1E Kent Ridge Road, Singapore 119228, Singapore
* Corresponding author.
E-mail address: tun.foo@gmail.com

Clin Plastic Surg 46 (2019) 275–283
https://doi.org/10.1016/j.cps.2019.02.001

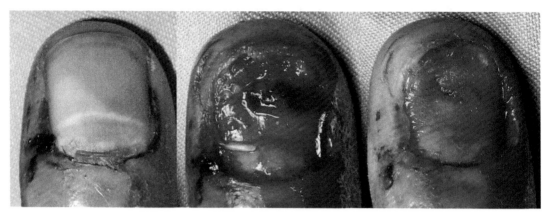

**Fig. 1.** A 75% hematoma with intact nail plate (*left*). Untidy laceration with interposed hematoma (*middle*). Laceration is evident after clearance of hematoma (*right*). Nail trephination is a viable alternative in this scenario.

digital nerve, or artery laceration in open injuries of the pulp (**Fig. 2**). Although distal digital nerve repair does not predict sensory recovery,[11,12] it is worth documenting and repairing neurotmetic injuries in clinical practice for which medicolegal risks are high. Nail matrix injuries are typically repaired with absorbable sutures to restore contour and surface for nail regeneration. Skin glue is an effective alternative to sutures for the repair of simple or complex lacerations and suitable for children in the emergency room setting.[13]

## OPEN INJURIES WITH TISSUE LOSS
### Healing by Secondary Intention

Pulp reconstruction after tissue loss receives disproportionate attention owing to the wide array of options for reconstruction, limited only by imagination. Before indulging our imagination, it is worth considering the possibility of healing through secondary intention, which can be surprisingly effective; its results may be aesthetically superior to graft or flap reconstruction, without incurring donor site morbidity.[14] Common indications for secondary intention healing are wounds without exposed bare bone or tendon, and a wound size of less than 1 cm$^2$. However, noncritical portion of exposed bone or tendon can be excised to facilitate healing. Wound vascularity rather than size is more important in considering treatment options; a small, well-vascularized wound (<1 cm$^2$) would almost certainly recover in a week or two, whereas larger wounds would take a few weeks more. Graft or flap reconstruction expedites the recovery process, while incurring potential donor morbidity. The principles of

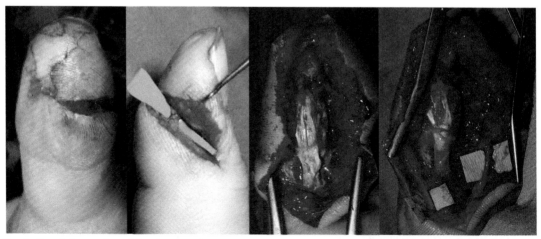

**Fig. 2.** Simple laceration of the thumb pulp resulted in transection of the digital nerve, which was repaired (*left*). Flexor tendon and digital nerves were found to be intact in a burst laceration of the pulp (*right*).

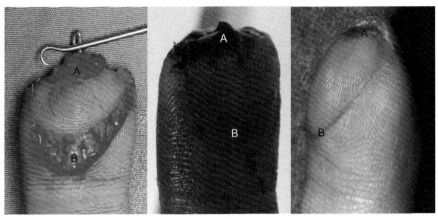

**Fig. 3.** Fingertip amputation treated with a modified local advancement flap (*left*). Residual defects (*A, B*) were allowed to heal by secondary intention (2 weeks, *middle*) with a satisfactory outcome (3 months, *right*).

secondary intention can be applied to reduce flap requirement, for example, using a smaller flap to cover only the critical portion, whereas residual defects are allowed to heal by secondary intention (**Fig. 3**).

## Composite Graft

The outcome of a composite graft is generally predictable in young children,[15] but outcomes were less predictable in adults.[16] In adults, we observed some degree of graft shrinkage and contour distortion with nail deformity (**Fig. 4**). As long as the patient understands the implications of the procedure, composite grafting is a good alternative with no donor morbidity.

## Skin Grafts

Moynihan[17] reported that the "condemnation of the use of Thiersch graft (split skin graft) has almost been unanimous," and this paradigm has been preserved and inherited by contemporary surgeons. It is worth noting that Moynihan stressed that a thin graft over a bony prominence was the cause of tenderness and sensitivity rather than the use of split thickness graft.[18,19] A full-thickness skin graft (FTSG) was applied with caution over exposed bone and tendon in the mid twentieth century, but contemporary investigators have shown that a FTSG can be reliably used in the context of exposed bone or tendon.[20] We use skin grafts judiciously for pulp reconstruction, and we note imperceptible differences between glabrous and nonglabrous graft in the long term, because the graft remodels according to stress to which it is exposed (**Fig. 5**). Donor site morbidity is prioritized over like-for-like reconstruction because there are limited donor sites for glabrous skin. The ulnar aspect of the hand has been described as a donor site, but we would avoid this area because it is often the surface on

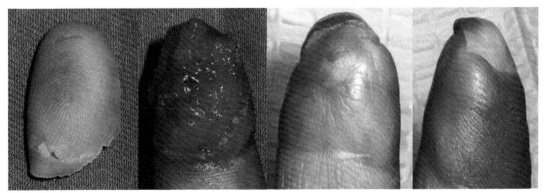

**Fig. 4.** Avulsion amputation of the pulp was replaced as a composite graft in an adult patient. Graft atrophy and fingertip contour and nail plate distortion observed 6 months later

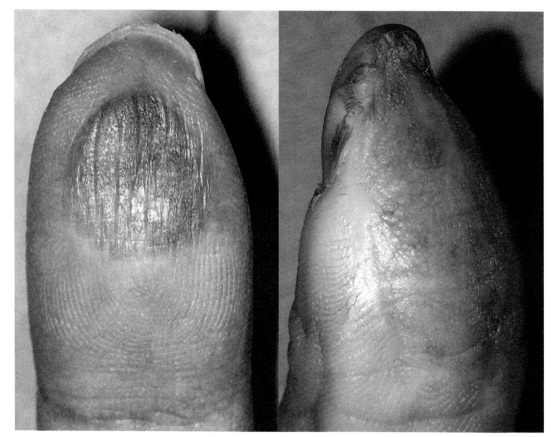

**Fig. 5.** Skin grafts remodel according to the stress imposed upon it. Glabrous remodeling of skin grafts noted in the long term at 3 years after split thickness skin graft (*left*), and 25 years after FTSG (*right*).

which the hand rests during activity. The palmar creases, midaxial skin, and dorsal joint creases provide FTSG that are up to 15 mm wide with minimal functional and cosmetic morbidity (**Fig. 6**).[21,22]

### Flap Reconstruction

Few topics excite hand surgeons as much as a discussion of the options for fingertip reconstruction. The majority of fingertip losses are adequately treated with VY advancement[23,24] and cross-finger flaps.[25] Island flaps extend the options for further refinement of reconstructive approach, while imposing greater technical demands. Surgical techniques on numerous flaps can be found in the works by these investigators.[26,27] These texts are by no means exhaustive, because new or modifications of known techniques are frequently reported in the literature.

Our flap selection process is based on the dichotomy of homodigital versus heterodigital options, followed by patient choice, and then surgeon expertise. Patients are shown a photo of

the anticipated outcome of the common flaps because their perception of the beautiful normal may vary. From a surgical perspective, we encourage younger colleagues to master VY advancement and cross-finger flaps before undertaking the various forms of neurovascular or vascular island flaps. We generally avoid heterodigital flaps to limit injury to a single digit, and similarly, cross-finger flaps are avoided in older patients owing to the higher risk of finger stiffness. VY flaps,[23,24] triangular,[28] or step-cut[29] neurovascular island flaps are our workhorses for fingertip reconstruction. Frequent contact areas such as radial aspect of index and middle fingers, and ulnar aspect of little finger are avoided as island flap donor sites to minimize scar sensitivity (**Fig. 7**). Dissection and mobilization of the neurovascular bundle up to the common digital artery bifurcation with or without adjacent arterial division is routinely performed to facilitate flap advancement of 15 to 20 mm. Proximal interphalangeal joint flexion is avoided, and postprocedure proximal interphalangeal joint mobilization is emphasized to minimize joint stiffness.

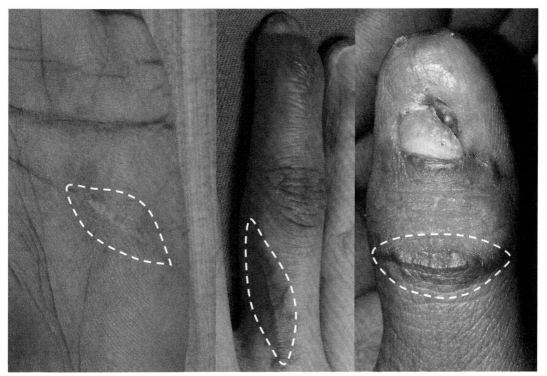

**Fig. 6.** FTSGs can be harvested from inconspicuous sites such as palmar crease (*left*), mid axial skin (*middle*), and dorsal digital crease (*right*) to optimize the appearance of the hand or digit.

Retrograde flow vascular island flaps[30,31] provide great flexibility for pulp reconstruction should collateral flow through palmar arches be well-preserved. The conventional technique requires FTSG to cover donor site along the mid axis of the proximal phalanx, whereas a modified approach we adopted could obviate the requirement to promote better donor site appearance (**Fig. 8**).

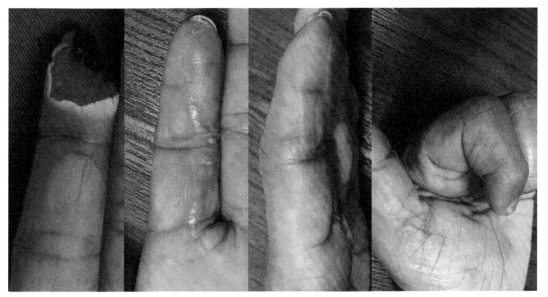

**Fig. 7.** Pulp loss of the left index finger was reconstructed with an ulnar-based triangular advancement flap to avoid sensitivity along the radial border of the index finger. Finger mobility exercise decreased joint stiffness.

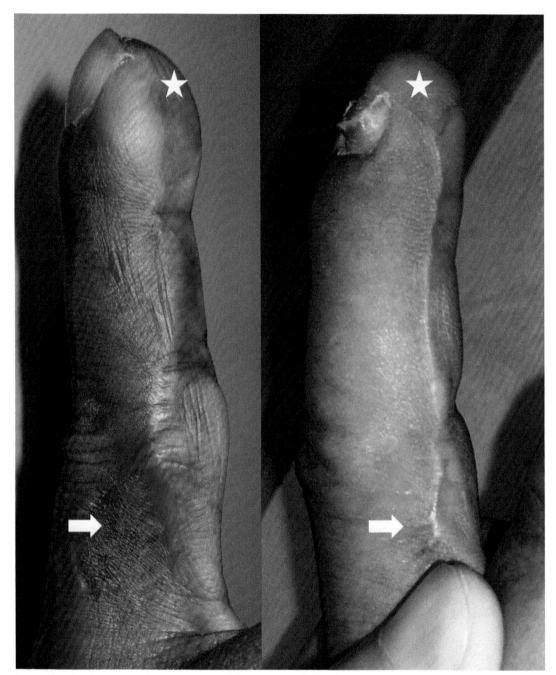

**Fig. 8.** Flap (*star*) and donor site (*arrow*) appearance with conventional (*left*) and modified (*right*) approaches, where the donor site was closed primarily rather than skin grafted to provide better appearance.

In our practice, we avoid heterodigital flaps to minimize cortical disorientation and donor site morbidity [32–34] for digital (eg, thumb) reconstruction. For thumb pulp reconstruction, we prefer either the locoregional flaps[33,35–37] or free toe pulp transfer. In the long term, there is no significant difference between the sensory perception of innervated and noninnervated flaps.[33]

## BONE LOSS

Bone loss and geometric distortion are concerns in oblique fingertip amputations. To minimize loss of bone support and fingertip length, a vascularized bone graft can be obtained as part of a VY flap[38] to reconstruct the fingertip while preserving length (**Fig. 9**).

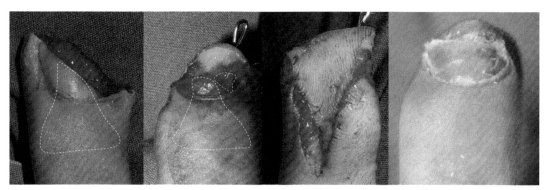

**Fig. 9.** Oblique amputation reconstructed with a osteocutaneous VY flap to reconstitute the nail complex contour (*bone outline in dashed line*). Satisfactory nail contour and normal looking fingertip after remodeling.

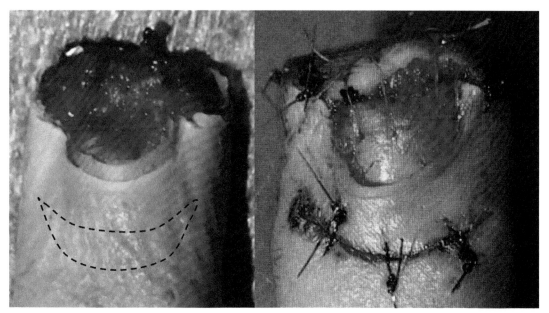

**Fig. 10.** A very short nail complex can be relatively lengthened by recessing the eponychium. A crescent area of skin is excised (*dashed lines*) and the eponychium is advanced proximally to expose more matrix.

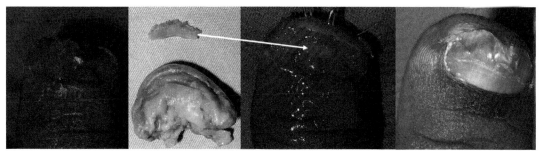

**Fig. 11.** Amputation injury with bone and matrix loss (*left*). Matrix graft obtained as spare parts from amputate (*middle*) replaced over VY advancement flap. Acceptable outcome achieved at 3 months (*right*).

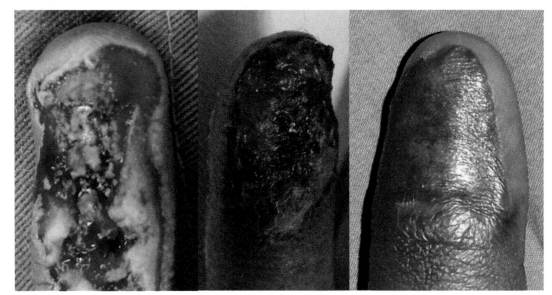

**Fig. 12.** Dorsal shaving injury resulting in loss of nail matrix (*left*), replaced by FTSG (intermediate stage, *middle*) and eventual satisfactory outcome (3 months, *right*).

## *Nail Complex Reconstruction*

In situations where residual nail complex is sparse, nailfold recession[39] could be considered to augment relative length of the nail plate (**Fig. 10**). Nail matrix graft from an amputated toe (**Fig. 11**) or a split thickness graft from the toes may be obtained to reconstruct missing matrix. In the complete loss of nail matrix, FTSG may be performed with satisfactory results. Of note is that the direct application of a graft on a bare distal phalanx cortex (**Fig. 12**) does not compromise graft nutrition.[40]

## SUMMARY

Fingertip injuries affect patients in numerous ways and outcomes are not always predictable. Each encounter calls for a considered evaluation of the functional and aesthetic expectations of patients, tailored to societal and cultural norms. The treatment goal of a pain-free and functional fingertip is weighed against the potential morbidity and expected outcome of the proposed procedure. The healing and remodeling trajectory of bone, pulp tissue, nail matrix, and grafts vary considerably. These variables are to be considered in the formulation of the overall treatment plan for fingertip injuries.

## REFERENCES

1. Mancini F, Chiara F, Ramirez JD, et al. A fovea for pain at the fingertips. Curr Biol 2013;23:496–500.

2. Roux FE, Djidjeli I. Functional architecture of the somatosensory homunculus detected by electrostimulation. J Physiol 2018;596(5):941–56.

3. Hustedt JW, Chung A, Bohl DD, et al. Evaluating the effect of comorbidities on the success, risk, and cost of digital replantation. J Hand Surg Am 2016;41(12):1145–52.

4. Payatakes AH, Nikolaos P, Fedorcik GG, et al. Current practice of microsurgery by members of the American society for surgery of the hand. J Hand Surg 2007;32A:541–7.

5. Shi Q, Sinden K, M JC, et al. A systematic review of prognostic factors for return to work following work-related traumatic injury. J Hand Ther 2014;27:55–62.

6. Peacock S, Patel S. Cultural influences on pain. Rev Pain 2008;1(2):6–9.

7. Steinberg F. The law of workers' compensation as it applies to hand injuries. Occup Med 1989;4(3):559–71.

8. Lee PW, Ho ES, Tsang AK, et al. Psychosocial adjustment of victims of occupational hand injuries. Soc Sci Med 1985;20(5):493–7.

9. Simon RR, Wolgin M. Subungual hematoma: association with occult laceration requiring repair. Am J Emerg Med 1987;5(4):302–4.

10. Seaberg DC, Angelos WJ, Paris PM. Treatment of subungual hematomas with nail trephination: a prospective study. Am J Emerg Med 1991;9(3):209–10.

11. Yamano Y. Replantation of the amputated distal part of the fingers. J Hand Surg Am 1985;10(2):211–8.

12. Dubert T, Houimli S, Valenti P, et al. Very distal finger amputations: replantation or "reposition-flap" repair? J Hand Surg Br 1997;22(3):353–8.

13. Yam A, Tan SH, Tan AB. A novel method of rapid nail bed repair using 2-octyl cyanoacrylate (Dermabond). Plast Reconstr Surg 2008;121(13):148e–9e.

14. Lee LP. A simple and efficient treatment for fingertip injuries. J Hand Surg Br 1995;20(1):63–71.

15. Butler DP, Murugesan L, Ruston J, et al. The outcomes of digital tip amputation replacement as a composite graft in a paediatric population. J Hand Surg Eur Vol 2016;41(2):164–70.

16. Chen SY, Wang CH, Fu JP, et al. Composite grafting for traumatic fingertip amputation in adults: technique reinforcement and experience in 31 digits. J Trauma 2011;70:148–53.

17. Moynihan FJ. Long-term results of split-skin grafting in finger-tip injuries. Br Med J 1961;2(5255):802–6.

18. Shepard GH. Treatment of nail bed avulsions with split-thickness nail bed grafts. J Hand Surg Am 1983;8(1):49–54.

19. Yong FC, Teoh LC. Nail bed reconstruction with split-thickness nail bed grafts. J Hand Surg Br 1992; 17(2):193–7.

20. Lee JH, Burn JS, Kang SY, et al. Full-thickness skin grafting with de-epithelization of the wound margin for finger defects with bone or tendon exposure. Arch Plast Surg 2015;42:334–40.

21. Tan RE, Ying CTQ, Sean LWH, et al. Well-camouflaged skin graft donor sites in the hand. Tech Hand Up Extrem Surg 2015;19(4):153–6.

22. Germann G, Rudolf KD, Levin SL, et al. Fingertip and thumb tip wounds: changing algorithms for sensation, aesthetics, and function. J Hand Surg Am 2017;42(4):274–84.

23. Atasoy E, Ioakimidis E, Kasdan ML, et al. Reconstruction of the amputated fingertip with a triangular volar flap. A new surgical procedure. J Bone Joint Surg Am 1970;52:921–6.

24. Tranquilli-Leali E. Ricostruzione dell'apice delle falangi ungueali mediante autoplastica volare peduncolata per scorrimento. Infort Traumatol Lav 1935; 1:186–93.

25. Gurdin M, Pangman WJ. The repair of surface defects of fingers by trans-digital flaps. Plast Reconstr Surg (1946) 1950;5(4):368–71.

26. Foucher G, Khouri RK. Digital reconstruction with island flaps. Clin Plast Surg 1997;24(1):1–32.

27. Rehim SA, Chung KC. Local flaps of the hand. Hand Clin 2014;30(2):137–51.

28. Venkataswami R, Subramanian N. Oblique triangular flap: a new method of repair for oblique amputations of the fingertip and thumb. Plast Reconstr Surg 1980;66(2):296–300.

29. Evans DM, Martin DL. Step-advancement island flap for fingertip reconstruction. Br J Plast Surg 1988; 41(2):105–11.

30. Lai CS, Lin SD, Yang CC. The reverse digital artery flap for fingertip reconstruction. Ann Plast Surg 1989;22(6):495–500.

31. Adani R, Busa R, Pancaldi G, et al. Reverse neurovascular homodigital island flap. Ann Plast Surg 1995;35(1):77–82.

32. Littler JW. The neurovascular pedicle method of distal transposition for reconstruction of the thumb. Plast Reconstr Surg (1946) 1953;12(5):303–19.

33. Woon CY, Lee JY, Teoh LC. Resurfacing hemipulp losses of the thumb: the cross finger flap revisited: indications, technical refinements, outcomes, and long-term neurosensory recovery. Ann Plast Surg 2008;61(4):385–91.

34. Teoh LC, Tay SC, Yong FC, et al. Heterodigical arterialized flaps for large finger wounds: results and indications. Plast Reconstr Surg 2003;111(6): 1905–13.

35. Pho RW. Local composite neurovascular island flap for skin cover in pulp loss of the thumb. J Hand Surg Am 1979;4(1):11–5.

36. Foucher G, Braun JB. A new island flap transfer from the dorsum of the index to the thumb. Plast Reconstr Surg 1979;63(3):344–9.

37. Brunelli F, Vigasio A, Valenti P, et al. Arterial anatomy and clinical application of the dorsoulnar flap of the thumb. J Hand Surg Am 1999;24(4):803–11.

38. Foo TL, Arul M. Osteocutaneous VY flap to preserve length in coronal oblique fingertip amputation. Hand Surg 2013;18(2):297–9.

39. Xing S, SHen Z, Jia W, et al. Aesthetic and functional results from nailfold recession following fingertip amputations. J Hand Surg Am 2015;40(1):1–7.

40. Puhaindran ME, Cordeiro PG, Disa JJ, et al. Full-thickness skin graft after nail complex resection for malignant tumors. Tech Hand Up Extrem Surg 2011;15(2):84–6.

# Nerve Compression in the Upper Limb

Ellen Y. Lee, MD*, Aymeric Y.T. Lim, FRCS

## KEYWORDS

- Nerve compression • Entrapment neuropathy • Carpal tunnel syndrome • Cubital tunnel syndrome
- Surgical release • Splinting

## KEY POINTS

- Nerve compression results in sensory and motor dysfunction. This dysfunction is initially progressive and follows the same pattern anywhere in the body.
- The same symptoms and signs are manifested in the distribution of the nerve affected.
- Nerves are compressed in fibro-osseous tunnels. Even though the symptom complex is known as compression neuropathy, the pathology also involves traction and adhesion.
- Anatomy is key to an organized examination that leads to an accurate clinical diagnosis.
- Management follows a set principle of multimodal nonsurgical treatment of patients with multiple levels of compression and surgical release of localized compression causing objective sensory and motor deficits.

 Video content accompanies this article at http://www.plasticsurgery.theclinics.com.

## INTRODUCTION

Nerve dysfunction is manifest in sensory and motor symptoms and signs. These follow the same pattern and only differ according to the distribution of the nerve. The dysfunction is caused by compression, stretching, or adhesions, although the compressive factor is the best recognized. Compressions occur in fibro-osseous tunnels that are well defined and give their names to well-known syndromes (**Table 1**). Outside these tunnels, nerve dysfunction may be caused by fibrous bands, space-occupying lesions, or accessory muscles (**Table 2**). Just as the symptomatology is predictable, the approach to management follows the same principles for any nerve.

## PATHOPHYSIOLOGY

Unyielding fibro-osseous tunnels occur at points of motion where the nerves cross over joints. Thus, the cause of nerve dysfunction is dynamic and involves traction and adhesion, in addition to compression. Histopathologic changes that occur with chronic compression are well described.[1] These changes are known to correspond to the patient's severity of symptoms and signs. The epineurium protects the nerve from compression and is most abundant at points where the nerve traverses joints. Resistance to stretch is afforded by the perineurium. Venous flow is blocked when a nerve is stretched by 8% of its resting length, and arterial ischemia is induced by stretching the nerve by 16%.[2]

Nowhere is it more evident that the pathology is not purely compression than in the carpal tunnel. In the normal population, the median nerve at the carpal tunnel inlet displays an arclike biphasic motion when making a fist. In the compression phase, the median nerve moves predominantly ulnar and volar as the fingers move from full extension to mid-flexion and is most deformed with the fingers

Disclosure Statement: The authors have nothing to disclose.
Department of Hand and Reconstructive Microsurgery, National University Health System, 1E Kent Ridge Road, NUHS Tower Block, Level 11, 119228, Singapore
* Corresponding author.
*E-mail address:* ellen_lee@nuhs.edu.sg

Clin Plastic Surg 46 (2019) 285–293
https://doi.org/10.1016/j.cps.2019.03.001
0094-1298/19/© 2019 The Authors. Published by Elsevier Inc. This is an open access article under the CC BY-NC-ND license (http://creativecommons.org/licenses/by-nc-nd/4.0/).

**Table 1**
**Common sites of nerve compression in the upper limb**

|  | Arm | Elbow | Forearm | Wrist | Hand |
|---|---|---|---|---|---|
| Median |  |  |  | Carpal tunnel |  |
| Ulnar |  | Cubital tunnel |  |  |  |
| Radial |  |  |  |  |  |

at mid-flexion position. This is followed by an escape phase wherein the median nerve slips ulnarly and dorsally as the fingers move from mid-flexion to full fist. This is accompanied by an increase in the nerve diameter, indicating relief of compression.[3] The gliding motion of the median nerve at the carpal tunnel inlet is significantly reduced in patients with carpal tunnel syndrome as a result of subsynovial edema or fibrosis[4,5] (Videos 1 and 2).

A proximal or distal point of compression can make the nerve more susceptible to dysfunction at another level due to compromised axoplasmic flow.[6,7] A systematic method of evaluation is necessary for patients presenting with multiple overlapping symptoms.

## CLINICAL ASSESSMENT

Peripheral nerves have autonomic, sensory, and motor functions. Autonomic and sensory deficits cause paresthesia, pain, or hypoesthesia along the distribution of the nerve. Motor deficits cause clumsiness, weakness, or paralysis of the involved muscles (**Fig. 1**). History is often insidious and begins with intermittent and nocturnal symptoms. Presence of predisposing conditions such as diabetes, hypothyroidism, connective tissue disorders, renal failure, recent or ongoing pregnancy, chronic alcoholism, vitamin deficiency or

hereditary neuropathy with liability to pressure palsies, and cervical radiculopathy should be documented. A check for occupational exposure to repetitive work or vibrating tools should be made. A standard functional assessment is made using Quick Disabilities of the Arm, Shoulder, and Hand (Q-DASH).

Examination is systematic regardless of the nerve involved and the location of the nerve entrapment. Understanding how the nerve is formed at the brachial plexus and the course it traverses to reach the hand is the key to an organized and complete examination. Remember to compare findings in both upper limbs and evaluate the entire length of the nerve, because multiple levels of entrapment are common.

- First, do a mindful observation for any skin changes and the presence of atrophy or abnormal posturing in the upper limb.
- Second, perform a sensory examination that is focused on differentiating nerve root compression with a dermatomal distribution of sensory deficit and a peripheral nerve compression with a localized deficit distal to the point of compression. This is most practically documented using the ten test[8] on an upper limb diagram. The test is consistent, reproducible, and does not require any special equipment.
- Manual muscle examination follows and this is organized following the order of innervation of muscles by the nerve. Any motor deficit is documented using the Medical Research Council grading system.
- Patients may present at an early stage when there are no objective sensory or motor deficits. Perform provocative tests that trigger the patient's symptoms by increasing the pressure or traction on the nerve.
- The hierarchical scratch collapse test helps in identifying the levels of compression on the affected nerve.[9]

**Table 2**
**Uncommon sites of nerve compression in the upper limb**

|  | Arm | Elbow | Forearm | Wrist | Hand |
|---|---|---|---|---|---|
| Median | Ligament of Struthers |  | Bicipital aponeurosis, 2 heads of PT, proximal arch of FDS, Gantzer muscle |  |  |
| Ulnar |  |  |  |  | Guyons canal |
| Radial |  |  | Radial tunnel/ganglion/ synovitis, SRN after exiting brachioradialis |  |  |

*Abbreviations:* FDS, flexor digitorum superficialis; PT, pronator teres; SRN, superficial radial nerve.

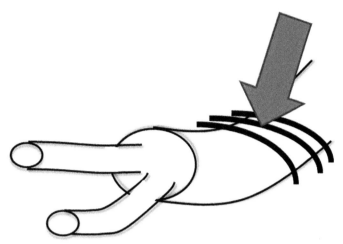

## Sensory

- Intermittent paresthesia at night / upon waking or activity induced
- Persistent paresthesia
- Objective sensory deficit

## Motor

- Clumsiness, subjective weakness
- Objective motor weakness
- Paralysis
- Atrophy

**Fig. 1.** Sensory and motor dysfunction in nerve compression.

Diagnosis is clinical, and grading for severity also follows a set progression (**Table 3**).

Electrodiagnostic tests are used as adjuncts to confirm levels of compression when considering multifocal neuropathy[10] or to document the severity of compression before surgery. High-resolution ultrasonography confirms the diagnosis by demonstrating swelling of the nerve proximal to the area of compression and establishes the presence of dynamic compression, nerve subluxation, or a mass causing compression.

**Table 3**
**Severity of entrapment neuropathy**

|  | Mild | Moderate | Severe |
|---|---|---|---|
| Sensory | Intermittent paresthesia | Persistent paresthesia, numbness, objective sensory deficit | Objective sensory deficit |
| Motor | None | Clumsiness, subjective weakness | Objective weakness, paralysis, atrophy |

## CARPAL TUNNEL SYNDROME

It was not until Phalen's landmark paper in 1966 that the diagnosis of median nerve compression at the wrist was well established. The history of carpal tunnel syndrome dates back to 1854, when Sir James Paget described symptoms of post-traumatic median nerve compression in the carpal tunnel. Dr. Herbert Galloway performed the first transverse carpal ligament release in 1924 for a patient whose wrist was crushed by a heavy falling window. This patient had a symptomatic neuroma of the palmar cutaneous branch of the median nerve and chronic pain after her surgery.[11] There was debate regarding the level of compression (cervical spine vs thoracic outlet vs carpal tunnel) in nontraumatic cases,[12] and Heathfield (1957) advised wrist splinting to confirm the site of compression.[13] In 1966, Dr. George Phalen published his 17-year experience with 654 hands in 439 patients, setting the foundation for how the condition today is managed today.[14]

A typical patient in Phalen's series was a woman aged 40 to 60 years presenting with chronic numbness and tingling in the median nerve distribution distal to the wrist and progressive clumsiness of the hand, often associated with a change to more strenuous manual labor. The patient is awakened by burning pain in the thumb, index, and long fingers that is relieved by vigorous shaking of the hand. Pain may be referred proximally, as high as the shoulder, but the sensory deficit is confined to the median nerve distribution. Dr. Phalen described clinical findings of sensory disturbance in the median nerve distribution (92%), thenar atrophy (41%), and the provocative tests (Tinel sign, wrist flexion test, and carpal compression test) that are used today. Surgery was recommended for patients with chronic symptoms at presentation, thenar atrophy, or recurrence after 3 to 4 steroid injections. In his series, only 40% of patients required surgery. The release of the transverse carpal ligament almost always relieved the patients' pain and numbness and improved thenar muscle power in 82% of hands with thenar atrophy. He had 2 complications; one had progression of thenar atrophy caused by incomplete distal release and another had recurrence of symptoms 3 years after the initial procedure caused by extensive scarring around the nerve.[14]

Carpal tunnel release under local anesthesia is currently the standard treatment of carpal tunnel syndrome. The choice of open, limited open, or endoscopic techniques has been addressed by many investigators through the years.[15–18] The most recent meta-analysis of 21 studies from 1992 to 2013 showed that patients treated endoscopically had earlier recovery of grip and pinch strength but this advantage was lost at 6 months. Patients treated endoscopically also had higher risk of nerve injury, lower risk of scar tenderness, earlier return to work, and similar risk of pillar pain and re-operation.[19] Both techniques are as effective in relieving symptoms and improving functional status; however, iatrogenic median nerve injury significantly worsens the patient's baseline function. We recommend a limited open approach for the release of idiopathic carpal tunnel syndrome (Video 3) because preservation of structures at risk (thenar motor branch, superficial palmar arch, common digital nerve to middle and ring fingers) is straightforward with this technique, and it does not add any additional equipment costs for the patient.

After surgery, the actual improvement in sleep disturbance was better than anticipated. Weakness improved the least. Improvement in other symptoms met patient's expectations.[20] Patients undergoing limited open carpal tunnel release returned to modified work at an average of 12 days and normal work duty at an average of 19 days. Patients with desk-bound jobs returned to work earlier than manual workers.[21]

Is there a role then for nonsurgical treatment of carpal tunnel syndrome? The natural history of carpal tunnel syndrome is not known. Theoretically, continued compression of the nerve will lead to progressive inflammation, fibrosis, demyelination, and ultimately axonal loss. However, a longitudinal study following 558 hands of 283 randomly selected industrial workers found 54% decrease in prevalence of carpal tunnel symptoms over a period of 11 years despite persistent slowing of maximum latency difference and 14 cm sensory latency in nerve conduction studies.[22] When a group of 36 patients who decided not to undergo surgery was compared with a matched group who underwent surgery, patient symptom scores and functional scores after 6 years follow-up improved significantly for both groups.[23] Patients who underwent surgery had significant symptom relief and improvement in function at 6 months after surgery that was sustained at 6 years. Patients who did not undergo surgery also had significant improvement in symptoms and function scores; however, their symptom score showed less improvement compared with the surgical group, whereas the improvement in function scores was comparable.

Accepted nonsurgical treatment of carpal tunnel syndrome include wrist splinting and steroid injections. Wrist splinting was effective for 15 months in two-thirds of patients without any of the 5 risk factors: age more than 50 years, symptom duration more than 10 months, constant paresthesia, stenosing flexor tenosynovitis, and a positive Phalen test result in less than 30 seconds. Sixty percent of patients with 1 factor, 83% with 2, and 93% of patients with 3 factors did not have relief by splinting.[24] A more recent study showed night splinting to be more effective than no treatment in improving symptom severity and functional status for at least 6 months.[25]

When combined with night splinting, steroid injection into the carpal tunnel has a short-term success rate of 80% that decreases to 22% at an average of 15 months.[26] In a more recent series, 22% (23/105 hands) were asymptomatic after 1 injection and continuous splinting for 3 weeks.[27] However, only 8% were asymptomatic after 1 year. Patients with mild symptoms, no sensory or motor deficit, and short duration of symptoms had the most satisfactory response to steroid injection and splinting.[26,27] Steroid injection is most useful for confirming the diagnosis of carpal tunnel syndrome. Patients who had a favorable response from steroid injection can expect a similar response from carpal tunnel release.

Recently, there is increasing interest in the effect of platelet-rich plasma (PRP) on nerve regeneration. Preclinical studies suggest the following mechanisms by which cell signaling molecules in PRP can modulate nerve regeneration[28]:

- Prevention of cell apoptosis and neuroprotection
- Stimulation of angiogenesis
- Modulation of inflammatory microenvironment
- Enhancement of axonal outgrowth and nerve guidance
- Dampening of both denervated muscle atrophy and scarring as a result of faster axonal sprouting

There are limited clinical studies showing the effect of PRP injection for carpal tunnel syndrome. The results of studies with a control group are summarized in **Table 4**. Three studies showed that PRP offers better symptom control and functional scores (improved visual analog scale [VAS], Boston Carpal Tunnel Questionnaire [BCTQ], Q-DASH scores) compared with night splint,[29] saline injection,[30] or triamcinolone injection[31] at 3 months after injection. One study compared PRP and wrist splinting with wrist splinting alone and found no significant difference in VAS and BCTQ scores.[32]

Overall, long-term randomized controlled trials are required to assess recurrence after PRP injection for carpal tunnel syndrome. Given the considerable increase in cost, PRP can be a viable alternative to steroid injection if its effects are positive in more patients and lasts significantly longer than steroid injection.

## CUBITAL TUNNEL SYNDROME

Cubital tunnel syndrome is the second most common compressive neuropathy in the upper limb. Its history also dates back to the 1807 when a 14-year-old girl presented to Dr. Henry Earle with a 3-year history of hypersensitivity and pain in the ulnar nerve distribution that prevented sleep. At one point, her pain was so severe that Mr. Earle (1816) transected her ulnar nerve above the medial epicondyle of the humerus. Intraoperatively, he noted that the epineurium of the ulnar nerve behind the medial condyle was firmer and thicker than normal. After surgery, the patient had permanent ulnar nerve deficit but was cured of her pain.[33] Approximately 70 years later, Photinos Panas (1878) tried a less aggressive approach by excising the ossified ligament that was found compressing the ulnar nerve at the elbow. He also described ulnar nerve palsies caused by repeated trauma and arthritic changes in the elbow that were treated with hydrotherapy, massage, and application of electrical current. Other

surgical treatments described during this era include deepening the epicondylar groove, elongation of the nerve by dissecting it out of its groove, and resection and repair of the nerve.[34,35] In 1898, Benjamin Curtis reported good outcome after anterior subcutaneous transposition of the ulnar nerve for ulnar neuritis after a bicondylar elbow fracture.[35]

As with carpal tunnel syndrome, there was discussion regarding the level of compression in non-trauma cases, whether it is caused by spinal cord disease or a cervical rib. To address this, Buzzard (1922) presented a case series to demonstrate the different clinical presentations of ulnar nerve neuritis at the level of the elbow. His series started with his own experience of pain in the ulnar nerve distribution after his elbow was hyperflexed and immobilized in a collar and cuff for a clavicle fracture. He goes on to describe cases brought about by repetitive strain on the elbow, prolonged immobilization while being bed bound, and those associated with a subluxing ulnar nerve or gout. For these, his recommended treatment was anterior transposition.[36]

In 1957, Geoffrey Osborne showed that, regardless of the type of elbow pathology, the nerve is being compressed against a band of fibrous tissue bridging the 2 heads of the flexor carpi ulnaris.[37] This fibrous band of transverse fibers compresses the nerve during elbow flexion, similar to the effect of the transverse carpal ligament in the wrist. In 1958, Feindel and Startford[38] described the role of an aponeurotic arch between the olecranon and the medial epicondyle compressing on the nerve in tardy ulnar nerve palsy. They called this arch the cubital tunnel, thus giving us the term "cubital tunnel syndrome." During this period, treatment options were simple decompression, anterior transposition: subcutaneous or submuscular, and medial epicondylectomy. The treatment options have remained so for more than 50 years and there is little consensus on the ideal procedure for this common problem. The last *Clinics in Plastic Surgery* update on upper limb entrapment neuropathy gave a comprehensive summary of the recent outcomes of these surgical procedures for cubital tunnel syndrome.[39] Comparing endoscopic versus open in situ decompression, in 2018, Buchanan and colleagues[40] found equivalent clinical outcome in terms of VAS and Bishop score. The endoscopic release cohort had lower rates of new-onset scar tenderness but higher rates of postoperative hematoma. The re-operation rates were not significantly different.

As with carpal tunnel syndrome, the natural history of idiopathic cubital tunnel syndrome is also not known. The closest available data are

**Table 4**
**Outcomes measured for platelet-rich plasma (PRP) injection for carpal tunnel syndrome compared with controls**

| | PRP | Control | Reference |
|---|---|---|---|
| VAS | (n = 26); improved compared with baseline; no significant difference versus control | 0.9% saline injection (n = 24); improved compared with baseline | Malahias et al,[30] 2018 (12 wk) |
| | PRP + wrist splint (n = 21); improved compared with baseline; no significant difference versus control | Wrist splint (n = 20); improved compared with baseline | Raeissadat et al,[32] 2018 (10 wk) |
| | (n = 30); significant reduction versus baseline and control | Wrist splint × 8 h (n = 30); overnight; improved compared with baseline | Wu et al,[29] 2017 (6 mo) |
| Q-DASH: score before versus 12 wk after injection >25% decrease | 76.9% (n = 26); significant improvement versus control | 33.3% (n = 24) | Malahias et al,[30] 2018 (12 wk) |
| BCTQ | PRP + wrist splint; improved compared with baseline; no significant difference versus control | Wrist splint; improved compared with baseline | Raeissadat et al,[32] 2018 (10 wk) |
| | Significant decrease versus baseline and control at 1 < 3 < 6 mo | Wrist splint × 8 h overnight; improved compared with baseline at 3 < 6 mo | Wu et al,[29] 2017 (6 mo) |
| | (n = 20); significant decrease versus baseline and control at 3 mo, not maintained at 6 mo | Triamcinolone 40 mg/1 mL (n = 20); significant decrease versus baseline at 3 mo, not maintained at 6 mo | Uzun et al,[31] 2017 (6 mo) |
| US measurement at carpal tunnel inlet | Mean 30% decrease in CSA; no significant difference versus control | Mean 17.3% decrease in CSA | Malahias et al,[30] 2018 (12 wk) |
| Finger pinch strength | Improved compared with baseline at 3 and 6 mo; no significant difference versus control | Improved compared with baseline at 6 mo | Wu et al,[29] 2017 (6 mo) |
| NCS | Median sensory nerve action potential peak latency and median compound muscle action potential onset latency; no significant difference | Median sensory nerve action potential peak latency and median compound muscle action potential onset latency; no significant difference | Raeissadat et al,[32] 2018 (10 wk) |
| | Sensory conduction velocity and distal motor latency; not significantly different from baseline | Sensory conduction velocity and distal motor latency; not significantly different from baseline | Wu et al,[29] 2017 (6 mo) |
| | Sensory conduction velocity and distal motor latency; not significantly different from baseline | Sensory conduction velocity and distal motor latency; not significantly different from baseline | Uzun et al,[31] 2017 (6 mo) |

(continued on next page)

**Table 4**
**(continued)**

|  | PRP | Control | Reference |
|---|---|---|---|
| Complications | None | None | Malahias et al,[30] 2018 (12 wk) |
|  | PRP + wrist splint (n = 21); 4, pruritus; 1, pain in fingers; 1, burning sensation | Wrist splint (n = 20); none | Raeissadat et al,[32] 2018 (10 wk) |
|  | None | None | Wu et al,[29] 2017 (6 mo) |
|  | None | None | Uzun et al,[31] 2017 (6 mo) |

*Abbreviations:* BCTQ, Boston Carpal Tunnel Questionnaire; CSA, cross-sectional area; NCS, nerve conduction study; Q-DASH, quick disabilities of the arm, shoulder, and hand; US, ultrasonography; VAS, visual analog scale.

those for cohorts of patients who did not undergo surgery. In a cohort of 30 patients with mild cubital tunnel syndrome, 90% were asymptomatic clinically and electrophysiologically at a mean follow-up of 22 months.[41] In a more recent cohort of 24 patients who underwent activity modification, 50% reported symptomatic improvement, of which 42% were symptom free at an average of 1 year.[42] In a larger cohort of 128 patients, 89% of patients with symptoms only, 67% of patients with abnormal sensorimotor thresholds, and 38% of patients with abnormal sensorimotor innervated density did not require surgery.[43]

Conservative treatment of cubital tunnel syndrome consists of mainly 3 techniques:

1. Activity modification: avoid flexing the elbow or resting the elbow on arm rests, stop triceps strengthening exercises;
2. Splint limiting elbow flexion to 45° to 70° or use of a night time towel orthosis to limit elbow flexion during sleep;
3. Use an elbow pad to prevent direct pressure on the nerve.

Compared with carpal tunnel syndrome, nonsurgical treatment of cubital tunnel syndrome is shown to be more effective in short-term studies. In 1985, Dimmond and Lister[44] followed up 73 patients treated with a splint for an average of 8 months and found an overall improvement of 86% compared with 50% in 31 patients treated surgically. Regarding the choice of nonsurgical treatment, activity modification alone worked just as well in patients with mild to moderate cubital tunnel syndrome compared with activity modification combined with nighttime use of an orthosis or nerve gliding exercises. Ninety percent of their 57 patients improved at 6 months. Two patients from each group did not improve and went on to have surgery.[45] Also unlike carpal tunnel syndrome, local steroid injection confers no additional benefit even

in the short term. In a randomized trial comparing ultrasound-guided steroid and lignocaine injection to the entry point of the cubital tunnel versus saline injection, 30% versus 28% of patients in both groups had a favorable outcome at 3 months after injection. Favorable outcome was defined as a subjective symptomatic improvement or complete recovery of symptoms. They did, however, find that the ulnar nerve cross-sectional area decreased significantly for those who had the steroid injection.[46] It seems that decreasing nerve inflammation alone does not address the clinical symptoms of idiopathic cubital tunnel syndrome. This confirms that entrapment neuropathy is not caused by compression alone.

Surgery is recommended for patients with objective sensory deficit of the ulnar 1.5 fingers, weakness that affects finger crossing, and intrinsic muscle atrophy. We perform an open in situ decompression for idiopathic cubital tunnel syndrome except when the ulnar nerve subluxes. An anterior subcutaneous transposition is performed for a subluxing ulnar nerve. Anterior transmuscular transposition is performed for recurrent cubital tunnel syndrome. Regardless of the choice of surgical procedure, it is crucial to observe the following principles in cubital tunnel surgery.

1. Preserve the medial antebrachial cutaneous nerves to avoid painful neuromas
2. Decompress all points of compression along the nerve.
3. Ensure there is no kinking of the nerve after transposition. Do not create new areas of compression.
4. Prevent destabilization of the nerve when performing a decompression.

## MULTIFOCAL NEUROPATHY

Multifocal neuropathy, formerly referred to as double-crush syndrome, is a condition wherein neuronal dysfunction occurs as a result of multiple synergistic pathologic processes that include mechanical and systemic causes. The actual incidence of multifocal neuropathy or double-crush syndrome is not known. The reported incidence ranges from less than 1% to 76%.[10] This condition should be considered in patients with more diffuse complaints, such as a patient referred for cubital tunnel syndrome complaining of medial forearm numbness. One must be suspicious and proceed with the systematic evaluation detailed earlier. Initial treatment is nonsurgical and should address each level of entrapment. Surgeons must collaborate with internists to correct or control the systemic conditions that contribute to nerve dysfunction.

## SUMMARY

Nerve compression occurs in fibro-osseous tunnels as the nerves cross joints. The pathology is traction and adhesion, aside from compression. This can occur at multiple sites along the course of the nerve. Regardless of the level, clinical assessment is standard, and a systematic approach to uncover all sites of compression is advised. Evolution of management for carpal tunnel and cubital tunnel syndrome has been reviewed with an emphasis on natural history and nonsurgical treatment, which are not commonly discussed. Treatment is multimodal and the systemic factors that contribute to nerve dysfunction should also be addressed.

## SUPPLEMENTARY DATA

Supplementary data related to this article can be found online at https://doi.org/10.1016/j.cps.2019.03.001.

## REFERENCES

1. MacKinnon SE, Novak CE. Compression neuropathies. In: Wolfe P, Kozin C, editors. Green's operative hand surgery. 7th edition. Philadelphia: Elsevier; 2017. p. 922.
2. Lundborg G, Rydevik B. Effects of stretching the tibial nerve of the rabbit: preliminary study of the intraneural circulation of the barrier function of the perineurium. J Bone Joint Surg Br 1973;55:390–401.
3. Goh CH, Lee BH, Lahiri A. Biphasic motion of the median nerve in the normal Asian population. Hand Surg 2015;20(1):73–80.
4. Liong K, Lahiri A, Lee S, et al. Mid-motion deformation of median nerve during finger flexion: a new insight into the dynamic aetiology of carpal tunnel syndrome. Hand Surg 2013;18:193–202.
5. Ettema AM, Zhao C, Amadio PC, et al. An K, Gliding characteristics of flexor tendon and tenosynovium in carpal tunnel syndrome: a pilot study. Clin Anat 2007;20:292299.
6. Upton AR, McComas AJ. The double crush in nerve entrapment syndromes. Lancet 1973;2:359–62.
7. Rempel D, Dahlin L, Lundborg G. Pathophysiology of nerve compression syndromes: response of peripheral nerves to loading. J Bone Joint Surg Am 1999;81(11):1600–10.
8. Strauch B, Lang A, Ferder M, et al. The ten test. Plast Reconstr Surg 1997;99(4):1074–8.
9. Davidge KM, Gontre G, Tang D, et al. The "hierarchical" Scratch Collapse Test for identifying multilevel ulnar nerve compression. Hand (N Y) 2015;10(3):388–95.
10. Cohen BH, Gaspar MP, Daniels AH, et al. Multifocal neuropathy: expanding the scope of double crush syndrome. J Hand Surg Am 2016;41(12):1171–5.
11. Amadio PC. The first carpal tunnel release? J Hand Surg Br 1995;20(1):40–1.
12. Kremer M, Gilliatt RW, Golding JS, et al. Acroparesthesia in the carpal-tunnel syndrome. Lancet 1953;265(6786):590–5.
13. Heathfield KW. Acroparaesthesiae and the carpal-tunnel syndrome. Lancet 1957;273(6997):663–6.
14. Phalen GS. The carpal-tunnel syndrome. Seventeen years' experience in diagnosis and treatment of six hundred fifty-four hands. J Bone Joint Surg Am 1966;48(2):211–28.
15. Hallock GG, Lutz DA. Prospective comparison of minimal incision "open" and two-portal endoscopic carpal tunnel release. Plast Reconstr Surg 1995;96(4):941–7.
16. Thoma A, Veltri K, Haines T, et al. A meta-analysis of randomized controlled trials comparing endoscopic and open carpal tunnel decompression. Plast Reconstr Surg 2004;114(5):1137–46.
17. Scholten RJ, Mink van der Molen A, Uitdehaag BM, et al. Surgical treatment options for carpal tunnel syndrome. Cochrane Database Syst Rev 2007;(4):CD003905.
18. Vasiliadis HS, Georgoulas P, Shrier I, et al. Endoscopic release for carpal tunnel syndrome. Cochrane Database Syst Rev 2014;(1):CD008265.
19. Sayegh ET, Strauch RJ. Open versus endoscopic carpal tunnel release: a meta-analysis of randomized controlled trials. Clin Orthop Relat Res 2015;473(3):1120–32.
20. Becker SJ, Makanji HS, Ring D. Expected and actual improvement of symptoms with carpal tunnel release. J Hand Surg Am 2012;37(7):1324–9.e1-5.
21. Cowan J, Makanji H, Mudgal C, et al. Determinants of return to work after carpal tunnel release. J Hand Surg Am 2012;37(1):18–27.
22. Nathan PA, Keniston RC, Myers LD, et al. Natural history of median nerve sensory conduction in industry: relationship to symptoms and carpal tunnel

syndrome in 558 hands over 11 years. Muscle Nerve 1998;21(6):711–21.

23. Pensy RA, Burke FD, Bradley MJ, et al. A 6-year outcome of patients who cancelled carpal tunnel surgery. J Hand Surg Eur Vol 2011;36(8):642–7.

24. Kaplan SJ, Glickel SZ, Eaton RG. Predictive factors in the non-surgical treatment of carpal tunnel syndrome. J Hand Surg Br 1990;15(1):106–8.

25. Premoselli S, Sioli P, Grossi A, et al. Neutral wrist splinting in carpal tunnel syndrome: a 3- and 6-months clinical and neurophysiologic follow-up evaluation of night-only splint therapy. Eura Medicophys 2006;42(2):121–6.

26. Gelberman RH, Aronson D, Weisman MH. Carpal-tunnel syndrome. Results of a prospective trial of steroid injection and splinting. J Bone Joint Surg Am 1980;62(7):1181–4.

27. Graham RG, Hudson DA, Solomons M, et al. A prospective study to assess the outcome of steroid injections and wrist splinting for the treatment of carpal tunnel syndrome. Plast Reconstr Surg 2004;113(2):550–6.

28. Sánchez M, Anitua E, Delgado D, et al. Platelet-rich plasma, a source of autologous growth factors and biomimetic scaffold for peripheral nerve regeneration. Expert Opin Biol Ther 2017;17(2):197–212.

29. Wu YT, Ho TY, Chou YC, et al. Six-month efficacy of platelet-rich plasma for carpal tunnel syndrome: a prospective randomized, single-blind controlled trial. Sci Rep 2017;7(1):94.

30. Malahias M-A, Nikolaou VS, Johnson EO, et al. Platelet-rich plasma ultrasound-guided injection in the treatment of carpal tunnel syndrome: a placebo-controlled clinical study. J Tissue Eng Regen Med 2018;12(3):e1480–8.

31. Uzun H, Bitik O, Uzun Ö, et al. Platelet-rich plasma versus corticosteroid injections for carpal tunnel syndrome. J Plast Surg Hand Surg 2017;51(5):301–5.

32. Raeissadat SA, Karimzadeh A, Hashemi M, et al. Safety and efficacy of platelet-rich plasma in treatment of carpal tunnel syndrome; a randomized controlled trial. BMC Musculoskelet Disord 2018;19(1):49.

33. Earle H. Cases and observations illustrating the influence of the nervous system, in regulating animal heat. Med Chir Trans 1816;7:173–94.

34. Bartels RH. History of the surgical treatment of ulnar nerve compression at the elbow. Neurosurgery 2001;49(2):391–9.

35. Eberlin KR, Marjoua Y, Jupiter JB. Compressive neuropathy of the ulnar nerve: a perspective on history and current controversies. J Hand Surg Am 2017;42(6):464–9.

36. Buzzard F. Some varieties of traumatic and toxic ulnar neuritis. Lancet 1922;1:317–9.

37. Osborne G. Ulnar neuritis. Postgrad Med J 1959;35:392–6.

38. Feindel W, Stratford J. The role of the cubital tunnel in tardy ulnar palsy. Can J Surg 1958;1(4):287–300.

39. Xing SG, Tang JB. Entrapment neuropathy of the wrist, forearm, and elbow. Clin Plast Surg 2014;41(3):561–88.

40. Buchanan PJ, Chieng LO, Hubbard ZS, et al. Endoscopic versus open in situ cubital tunnel release: a systematic review of the literature and meta-analysis of 655 patients. Plast Reconstr Surg 2018;141(3):679–84.

41. Eisen A, Danon J. The mild cubital tunnel syndrome. Its natural history and indications for surgical intervention. Neurology 1974;24(7):608–13.

42. Padua L, Aprile I, Caliandro P, et al. Natural history of ulnar entrapment at elbow. Clin Neurophysiol 2002;113(12):1980–4.

43. Dellon AL, Hament W, Gittelshon A. Nonoperative management of cubital tunnel syndrome: an 8-year prospective study. Neurology 1993;43(9):1673–7.

44. Dimond M, Lister G. Cubital tunnel syndrome treated by long-term splintage. Proceedings of the 1985 American Society for surgery of the hand annual meeting. J Hand Surg Am 1985;10:430.

45. Svernlöv B, Larsson M, Rehn K, et al. Conservative treatment of the cubital tunnel syndrome. J Hand Surg Eur Vol 2009;34(2):201–7.

46. Vanveen KE, Alblas KC, Alons IM, et al. Corticosteroid injection in patients with ulnar neuropathy at the elbow: a randomized, double-blind, placebo-controlled trial. Muscle Nerve 2015;52(3):380–5.

# Flexor Tendon Injuries

Jin Bo Tang, MD

## KEYWORDS

- Flexor tendon • Repair methods • Pulley release or venting • Early active motion
- Secondary surgeries

## KEY POINTS

- Zone 2 flexor tendon repairs have evolved greatly over the past 3 decades.
- The key developments in zone 2 repairs are (1) use of strong core suture, typically 4- or 6-strand repairs, (2) venting the critical annular pulley judiciously to avoid compression to the repaired tendon, (3) ensuring slightly tensional repair to prevent gapping at the repair site, (4) performing a digital extension-flexion test to ascertain quality surgical repair, and (5) early partial range active motion to ensure tendon gliding but not overloading the repair site.
- I prefer direct repair of the very distal flexor tendon or in making the distal junction of the grafted tendon. In zone 2 and proximal zone 1, I use a 6-strand repair method, the M-Tang repair, in repairing the flexor tendons.
- A few recent evolutions have been reported by surgeons, which hold promise to be adopted by other hand surgeons: (1) using a strong core suture-only repair method, (2) venting the A3 together with A4 pulleys in case of need to sacrifice clinically insignificant tendon bowstringing for gain of range of active motion of the finger, and (3) a wide-awake surgical setting for tendon repair or tenolysis.

## INTRODUCTION

Several recent articles have evaluated developments in flexor tendon repair and their contribution to progress toward reliable primary repair of the flexor tendons.[1–5] This article highlights the relevant anatomic and mechanical features, clinical methods, and essential elements in a reliable repair, then offers an overview of advancements in flexor tendon repair.

Zone 2 flexor tendon repairs have evolved greatly over the past 3 decades, and consequently, outcomes have changed dramatically since the last half of the twentieth century. Several major conceptual changes, and widespread use of some key surgical methods and postoperative motion protocols have helped to bring about the changes.[6–17] Current key practices include

Using strong core sutures, typically 4- or 6-strand repairs

Judicious venting of the critical annular pulley
Ensuring that a slight tension is created by the repair to prevent gapping
Performing digital extension-flexion tests to confirm the quality of the surgical repair
Early partial range active motion to ensure tendon gliding without overloading the repair

Having the patient wide awake without use of a tourniquet during surgery represents an important advancement, allowing active motion of the tendon during surgery.[11,12] Wide-awake surgery has also transformed how tenolysis and secondary tendon reconstruction are performed.

## ANATOMIC AND MECHANICAL KEY POINTS

A unique feature of the flexor tendon anatomy is the presence of segmental annular pulleys in the digital area, with the A2 pulley over the proximal two-thirds of the proximal phalanx being the

Disclosure Statement: The author has nothing to disclose.
Department of Hand Surgery, The Hand Surgery Research Center, Affiliated Hospital of Nantong University, 20 West Temple Road, Nantong 226001, Jiangsu, China
E-mail address: jinbotang@yahoo.com

Clin Plastic Surg 46 (2019) 295–306
https://doi.org/10.1016/j.cps.2019.02.003

largest and strongest, and the A4 pulley over the midpoint of the middle phalanx being the second largest (**Fig. 1**). The annular pulleys serve to prevent tendon bowstringing during digital flexion. Although the A3 and A1 pulleys also perform this function, their role is less critical than the A2 and A4. Loss of integrity of any one of the pulleys alone has no marked functional consequence, although anatomically, minor tendon bowstringing occurs at the site of the loss.

The middle and distal parts of the A2 pulley (1.5–1.7 cm long in adult middle finger) and the A4 pulley (about 0.5 cm long) are the narrowest and most constricting to the flexor tendons. These sites become compressive to the repaired tendons because of postoperative tendon swelling. These narrow pulley sites may be incised to allow the repaired tendons to glide more freely.

Several factors affect the strength of repaired tendon:

- The number of suture strands across the repair sites—strength is roughly proportional to the number of core sutures
- The tension of repairs—most relevant to gap formation and stiffness of repairs
- The core suture purchase
- The types of tendon-suture junction—locking or grasping

- The diameter of suture locks in the tendons—a small diameter of locks diminishes anchor power
- The suture calibers (diameter)
- The material properties of suture materials
- The curvature of tendon gliding paths—the repair strength decreases as tendon curvature increases
- The holding capacity of a tendon, affected by varying degrees of trauma and post-traumatic tissue softening

It must be realized that tendon curvature during finger flexion greatly affects the repair strength. A tendon under curvilinear tension is subjected to linear pulling and bending forces. Therefore, a repair in a tendon under a curvilinear load is weaker than that under a linear load; the repair strength decreases progressively as the curvature increases.[18,19] Therefore, the repair fails more easily in the flexed finger, and when the finger moves to approach full flexion, a bent tendon is particularly prone to fail. This is the mechanical basis of current partial active finger flexion protocols and 1 reason why a full fist should be avoided in the initial a few weeks after surgery (**Table 1**).

**Fig. 2** summarizes the breakdown of contributors of postoperative resistance to tendon gliding[20] that should be considered in planning

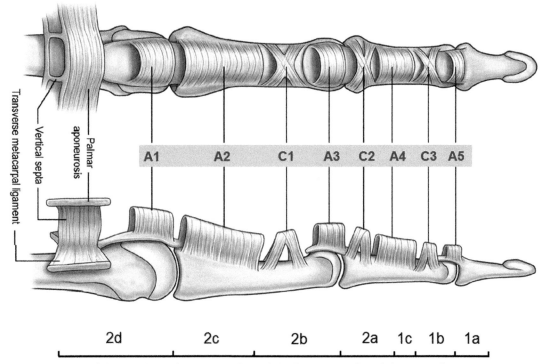

**Fig. 1.** Locations of the annular and cruciate pulleys of the fingers and the subdivisions of zone 1 and 2.

**Table 1**
**Resistance to tendon gliding during active finger flexion in initial weeks of tendon healing**

| Active Flexion | Resistance to Tendon Gliding | Healing Tendons during Active Motion |
|---|---|---|
| None to mild | Low | Not easily disrupted |
| Mild to moderate | Low or moderately high | Not easily disrupted |
| Moderate to full | Very high | Easy to disrupt; should avoid such motion |

and adjusting the active motion protocols. The safety margin of early active digital flexion can be enhanced by a strong surgical tendon repair or appropriately decompressing the tendon during surgery through releasing restricting pulleys, limiting the lengths of skin incisions, and minimizing the trauma to the tendon and sheath. After surgery, delicate adjustments in early active flexion to fit individual patients by a therapist or surgeon is also important.

## PRIMARY AND DELAYED PRIMARY REPAIR

Nowadays most lacerated flexor tendons in the hand and forearm are repaired on the same day of injury or a few days later. Primary repair indicates the end-to-end repair performed within 24 hours after tendon injury. When an experienced surgeon is not available on the day of injury, the repair can be deliberately delayed, and delayed primary repair is performed in a selective surgical setting. The delay usually has no adverse effects on outcomes, but in this period of delay, antibiotic use reduces the risk of infection of the wound. Delayed primary repair is the repair performed within 3 or even 4 weeks after injury. The end-to-end repair is often still possible 5 weeks after injury.

Zone 2 is the most complex and demanding and will be highlighted in the following section.

### Exposure and Finding Tendon Ends in Zone 2

The tendons are exposed through a Bruner skin incision of 1.5 to 2 cm (**Fig. 3**), which is usually sufficient to expose the tendons. The author and colleagues keep the skin incision as limited as possible to decrease edema of the digit and resistance to tendon gliding after surgery. Retraction of the proximal tendon stump is common, especially in delayed primary repair. If the proximal flexor digitorum profundus (FDP) tendon end has not retracted far proximally, flexion of the metacarpophalangeal (MCP) or proximal interphalangeal (PIP) joints can bring the proximal end into the incision site.

If the proximal FDP tendon end retracts to the palm, I do not extend the incision to the palm,

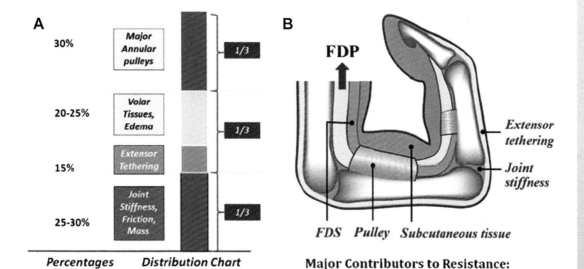

**Fig. 2.** The breakdown of contributors of postoperative resistance to tendon gliding. (*A*) Percentage contribution to the resistance. (*B*) Contributing factors. (*From* Wu YF, Tang JB. Tendon healing, edema, and resistance to flexor tendon gliding: clinical implications. Hand Clin 2013;29:167–78; with permission.)

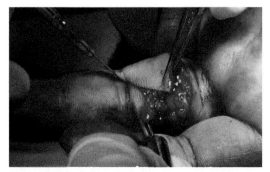

**Fig. 3.** A Bruner skin incision of 1.5 to 2 cm for exposure of the laceration site.

but instead make an additional incision in the distal palm. I can always find the retracted tendon end in the distal palm. From this small incision, the proximal tendon end is pushed distally within the synovial sheath bit by bit using 2 forceps (**Fig. 4**), like pushing a rope until the distal end is seen out of the distal opening in the sheath.

The forceps instrument is used to pull the exposed proximal end distally for about 1 cm. Then the finger is held in slight flexion; a 25-gauge needle is inserted at the base of the finger through the proximal tendon stump to hold the tendon during repair.

## Surgical Repair Techniques

The tendon tissue at the cut ends is often ragged and should be conservatively trimmed with a scissors. Basic requirements of a tendon repair in primary repair of a flexor tendon are sufficient strength, smooth tendon gliding surface with fewer suture exposures, prevention of gapping of the repair site under tension, and easy to perform. Different configurations of the repairs may produce good outcomes given all the requirements are meet. Surgeons in different centers use different multistrand repairs (**Fig. 5**).[21] I use the 6-strand M-Tang repair method in the repair in zone 2 (**Fig. 6**). I then add a simple running peripheral suture or add 3 or 4 separated stitches sparsely over the volar and lateral aspects of the repair site with 6-0 nylon.

## Methods of End-to-End Repair: Keys

There are 3 essential surgical keys of making a strong tendon repair. First, one must ensure core suture purchase of at least 0.7 to 1.0 cm to generate maximal holding power and a sufficiently large size (2 mm in diameter) of locks if a locking suture is used. Surgical repair strength decreases as the length of the purchase decreases. Tendon cut surfaces tend to soften after trauma. The repair

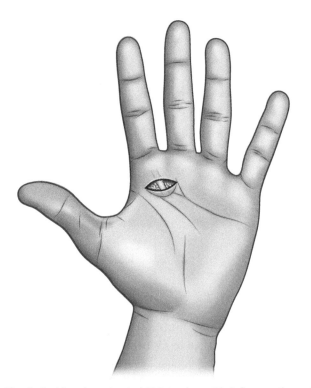

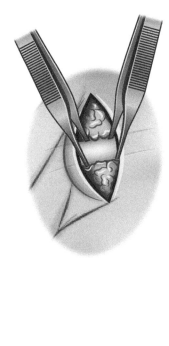

**Fig. 4.** Pushing the retracted FDP tendon with 2 forceps through a distal palm incision.

A

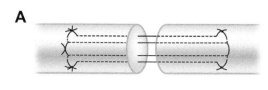

B

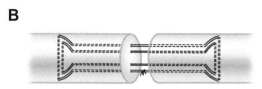

C

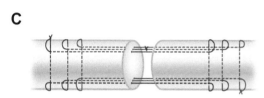

Fig. 5. Several multistrand core suture methods used by hand surgeons. (*A*) A 4-strand repair. (*B*) A 8-strand repair. (*C*) A 6-strand repair made from 3 groups (each in a different color) of the Kessler repair in asymmetric placement in 2 tendon stumps.

is at great risk of rupture if the suture purchase is short.

The second key in the repair is that certain tension across repair site should be maintained. To prevent gapping, it is important to ensure the repair has tension or a certain degree of bulkiness that results in 10% to 20% shortening of the tendon parts encompassed by core sutures, or a 20% to 30% increase in the diameter of junction site of the 2 tendon ends (**Fig. 7**).[22] A small amount of baseline tension would counteract the tension of the flexor muscles during resting or active motion. The repair site becomes more flattened once it is under the load of active digital flexion. Such degrees of bulkiness do not hamper tendon gliding with proper pulley venting.

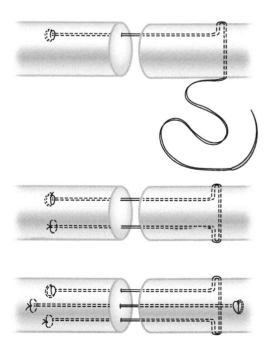

Fig. 6. The method of making a 6-strand M-Tang repair, which the author uses for the FDP and PFL repair.

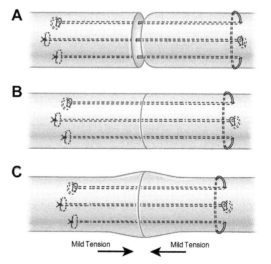

A

B

C

Mild Tension →   ← Mild Tension

Fig. 7. The appropriate tensioning of the repair site is a key to preventing gap formation (*A, B*) during active finger flexion. The recommended degree of bunching up is 20% to 30% (shown in *C*) increases in diameter of the tendons at the junction of the 2 tendon ends.

Finally, at least a 4-strand core suture is required; a 6-strand core suture is ideal. The caliber of suture used in adults is either 4-0 or 3-0.

Locking suture-junction in the tendon is not a must, although locking anchors are slightly more secure. If the locks are incorporated, the locking circles of the suture in the tendon should be of a sufficient size (approximately 2 mm in diameter).

Peripheral sutures mainly serve to tidy up the repaired tendon stumps. Most surgeons now choose to insert only simple or sparse peripheral stitches. Some surgeons even do not supplement peripheral stitches when multistrand core sutures have been used.[23,24] In the presence of a strong multistrand core repair that has been tensioned over the repair site, peripheral sutures become less important than previously thought.

I do not usually repair the flexor digitorum superficialis (FDS) tendon unless the FDS injury is partial or the wound is very clean. I do not repair the FDS tendon during delayed primary repair or if the injury is in the area of the A2 pulley (zone 2C).

### Venting of the Critical Pulleys

It was previously believed that the A2 and A4 pulleys were sacrosanct and should not be divided. One of the important improvements in tendon repair in recent decades is the understanding that clinically significant bowstringing does not occur when the A2 pulley is released up to two-thirds of its length and that the A4 pulley can be entirely released, given the integrity of the other critical pulleys.[13,15] A part of the synovial sheath including cruciate pulleys can be released together with the annular pulleys. The method of release is a longitudinal cut through the midline with a scissors.

However, no more than 1.5 to 2 cm total of the pulleys with the synovial sheath should be released.[13] A pulley release does not need to be lengthy, because in the proximal part of a finger of an average adult, the flexor tendons glide only 1.5 to 2 cm with full digital extension and flexion. This judicious pulley venting permits unimpeded gliding of a strong but slightly bunched or edematous tendon repair site during early active tendon motion after surgery.

I have observed that judicious venting or division of the A4 pulley does not lead to clinically significant bowstringing, although anatomically there is minor tendon bowstringing that leads to no clinical consequence. The same is true of division of up to two-thirds of the A2 pulley.

### Performing Digital Extension-Flexion Test: Methods

After repairing the tendon and venting of pulleys, I always verify the quality of the repair and adequate venting through a digital extension-flexion test.[14,22] The repaired finger is held at full extension to confirm that no gaps are seen between the 2 cut ends. Next, the finger is moderately flexed to make sure the repaired tendon moves smoothly. Finally, the finger is further pushed to marked flexion to confirm that the repair site does not bunch against the pulleys and that venting of the pulley is adequate.

Under local anesthesia with sedation, brachial plexus blocks, or general anesthesia, the previously mentioned test is performed with the surgeon's hand holding the repaired finger to obtain passive finger motion. The wide-awake local anesthesia without a tourniquet approach offers a major advantage of the wide-awake surgery,[25] as the patient can actively move the tendon to ascertain repair quality.

If gapping is found between tendon ends, the repair is too loose and should be revised with additional core or peripheral sutures. If the pulley is found to block smooth tendon gliding, it should be further released. However, such additional release should be progressive, 1 to 2 mm at a time, with repeated digital extension-flexion tests, to ensure the release is just enough to let the repair site glide smoothly, rather than making 1 lengthy additional cut.

## POSTOPERATIVE ACTIVE MOTION PROTOCOLS

I use a dorsal splint extending from the distal forearm to the fingertips for postoperative protection. Some other surgeons use an even shorter splint.[16] The exact wrist position is unimportant. The wrist can be in neutral, mild flexion, or mild extension, as long as the patient is comfortable. The splint should be slightly flexed at the MCP joint, usually for 30° to 40°, and be straight beyond this joint. The wrist position for splinting should avoid marked flexion (which is uncomfortable) or marked extension (which adds a lot of tension to the repaired tendon).

There is no need to start motion or therapy in the first 3 or 4 days after surgery, which also avoids pain and discomfort.[1] From day 4 or 5, the patient should perform at least a few sessions of digital motion exercises. In each session, to lessen resistance of joint stiffness, full passive finger motion—usually 20 to 40 repetitions—should be performed before active digital flexion. Then active digital flexion should proceed gradually. In the first 3 to 4 weeks, only one-half to two-thirds active motion range should be the goal. Extreme digital flexion should be avoided, because marked finger flexion would overload the repaired tendons, risking repair disruption (**Fig. 8**). Most patients have marked swelling at this time; a full range of active motion of the operated finger is difficult to achieve. Aiming for full active flexion of the finger is both unnecessary and unrealistic. However, full passive finger flexion and extension should always be performed to make the hand and finger as supple as possible.

From the end of week 3 or 4, a full range of active flexion is the goal. Some patients who have difficulty with full active flexion at week 4 or 5 may gradually achieve full flexion in later weeks. However, exercise to reduce joint stiffness and prevent extension lag should always be performed for eventual recovery of active finger flexion. The splint protection can be removed at the end of week 5 or 6, but therapy usually should persist for a few weeks to get rid of often seen remaining stiffness of the distal interphalangeal (DIP) joint, with or with nighttime splint protection. After week 6, I sometimes urge patients to wear a splint only when they go outside, which prevents unintentional use or injury.

## MORE RECENT EVOLUTION OF METHODS

The major conceptual changes in repairing flexor tendons are summarized in **Table 2**. Although most of the advancements have already been discussed, here I summarize the changes over the last 5 to 6 years.

### Placing the Knots Between the Two Tendon Ends May Not Favor the Repair

The modified Kessler repair was popular, but for zone 2 flexor tendon repair, this repair is now seldom used. It has also been realized that the original Kessler repair with knots over the tendon surface is actually slightly better than the modified version in terms of preventing gapping.[26] Most current multistrand repairs have knots over the tendon surface, and no adverse clinical consequences have been noted with these repairs (**Fig. 9**). It is now believed that placement of the knots between tendon ends is not beneficial or unimportant.[26–28]

### Asymmetric Suture Configurations May be Preferable to Symmetric Designs

Recent investigations have revealed that asymmetry in the configuration of sutures attaching 2 tendon stumps is better than symmetric suture placement.[29,30] Asymmetric placement likely

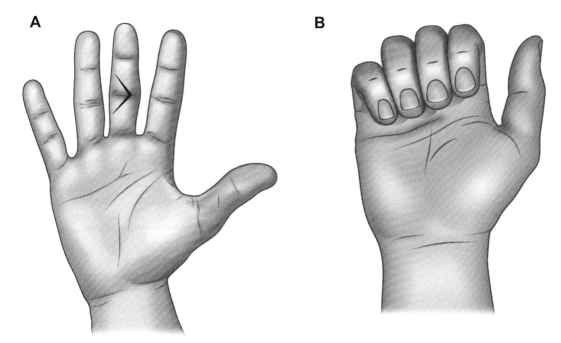

**A**    **B**

**Fig. 8.** Partial range active motion in the initial 2 to 3 weeks after surgery. Full fist or marked active finger flexion should be avoided to prevent repair rupture. (*A*) Active flexion starts from full extension. (*B*) Active flexion upto two-thirds of flexion arc is shown.

**Table 2**
**The major conceptual changes in repairing flexor tendons over the past 3 decades**

| Subjects | 1980s and 1990s | 2010s |
|---|---|---|
| **Surgical techniques** | | |
| Tendon repair: zone 2 | 2-strand suture | Multistrand suture (4 or 6 strands) |
| A2 pulley | Should not be violated | Can be partially vented if needed |
| A4 pulley | Should not be violated | Can be entirely vented if needed |
| Synovial sheath | Closure recommended | Do not need to repair the sheath |
| Suture purchase of repair | Not been stressed | Should be more than 0.7–1 cm |
| Tension across repair site | Not been discussed | An essential key of surgical repair |
| Extension-flexor test | None | A common quality check point |
| Wide-awake surgery | Not incorporated | A better approach of tendon repair |
| **After surgery** | | |
| Wrist position in protection | Wrist flexion stressed | Flexible, from mild flexion to extension |
| Starting motion within 4 d | Common | Unnecessary; no motion is better |
| Active flexion: first 2–3 weeks | Not popular | Popular |
| Avoid extreme flexion | None | A key to ensure safety of active flexion |
| Place-and-hold motion | Popular | Not a useful or efficient exercise |
| Out-of-splint motion | None | Advocated for reliable patients |

favors gap resistance, and this design can be found in some popular suture configurations.

## A Tensioned Slightly Bunched Repair is Better Than a Flat Tension-Free Repair

A flat, tension-free repair should be avoided. A tensioned slightly bunched repair favors gap resistance and does not hamper tendon gliding as the narrow pulleys are released.

## Slightly Extended Pulley Venting to Benefit Finger Flexion Outweighs the Drawbacks of Minor Tendon Bowstringing

The author and colleagues tend to be conservative in deciding the length of pulley release. The allowable length may be slightly longer than what was proposed originally, in particular, if such a release greatly favors gliding of the repaired tendon, and the bowstringing caused by slightly extended release is noticeable but still mild. This practice appears especially beneficial at the PIP joint area. Such extended release from the A4 to A3 pulleys (including the sheath between them), if needed, may favor tendon gliding at the cost of mild bowstringing at the PIP joint, which actually does not affect normal function of the finger.[23,24,31–34]

## Peripheral Suture is Unnecessary When a Strong Core Suture (a 6-Strand Repair) is Used

This is a recent observation. A few surgeons have reported not adding peripheral sutures when a

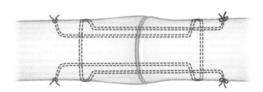

**Fig. 9.** A tendon repair showing most of the recognized points for making a reliable repair: sufficient lengths of suture purchase, no knots between the tendon ends, tension across repair site, slightly bunching up at the junction of the 2 tendon ends, and asymmetry of the suture strands in 2 tendon ends.

strong 6-strand repair is made with tension; no repair ruptures were reported.[23,24]

## Wide-Awake Surgery Allows Effective Testing of Tendon Gliding

This is a major development in flexor tendon repair. With active participation by the patient during surgery, the extension-flexion test provides the best validation of a successful repair. Surgeons can even educate the patient about postoperative motion during the procedure.[34–37]

## Tendon-to-Bone Junction Can be Achieved Without Conventional Pull-Out Suture

As explained previously, a strong direct repair has replaced the pullout suture in my practice. The fact is that the terminal tendon just proximal to its insertion to the distal phalanx is distal to the DIP joint, which does not require motion. Adhesions are allowed to develop to help strengthen the repair. Therefore, as much as possible, suture strands can be used to achieve a strong and usually somewhat bulky repair, which favors both healing and strength.

## Limiting the Length of Incision Decreases Gliding Resistance to the Tendon

A surgical incision less than 2 cm long is recommended to allow exploration of the wound site and expose the tendon in the finger or thumb. Such a short incision decreases postoperative edema and resistance to tendon gliding. Making a lengthy Bruner incision increases edema. If the tendon is retracted proximally to the palm, an additional incision is made, rather than extending the incision from the finger to the palm.

## Wrist Positioning is Unimportant, and a Short Splint is Safe

It is now understood that if the tendon repair is strong, the wrist does not have to be placed in a specific position. This allows considerable freedom in wrist positioning.

## Out-of-Splint Exercise is Safe

In my own practice, I have found out-of-splint motion to be safe for compliant patients; in fact, it is actually more efficient. Splinting mainly serves to protect the patient from getting hurt or unintentional hand use. For this reason, the splint should be worn only between exercise sessions and at night.

## OUTCOMES

When they followed an updated protocol, young or junior hand surgeons were able to obtain reliably good outcomes with few or no repair ruptures.[22] Surgeons from other units have reported zero ruptures in case series of more than 50 tendons.[23,38,39] Repair rupture appears to no longer be a major concern if all modern guidelines are carefully followed. Rupture occurs only in patients who actively use the fingers in the first few weeks after surgery, although there are rare instances (estimated to be <1%) of unexplained ruptures of ordinarily reliable repairs.[22] However, although cases of tenolysis have dropped considerably,[40] adhesions remain a concern, and severe tissue damage always poses the risk of developing dense adhesions.

## REPAIR IN OTHER ZONES AND THUMB FLEXOR TENDONS
### Zone 1

When the FDP tendon is cut in distal zone 1, pullout sutures through the dorsal nail have been a common treatment, but I no longer use them. I prefer direct repair using several strong core sutures (ie, up to 10 or 12-strand core suture repair). The direct repair connects the proximal stump to the remnant of the distal stump and tissues such as periosteum adjacent to the tendon insertion on the distal phalanx (**Fig. 10**). The methods of proximal zone 1 repairs and zone 2 are similar.

### Zones 3, 4, and 5

The FDP tendons in zone 3 are repaired similarly as in zone 2. The repairs are easier because of lack of sheath over the tendon. The injuries in the carpal tunnel area (zone 4) are rare and are often accompanied by lacerations in the median nerve and arteries. The transverse carpal ligament has to be opened to facilitate repairs. Zone 5 injuries often involve multiple tendons with neurovascular injury. Repair of the FDS and FDP tendons is preferred, and early postoperative motion is advised.

### Thumb Flexor Tendon

The FPL tendon repairs follow the same methods of repairs of the FDP tendon in fingers. The surgical incision should usually be less than 2 cm. The oblique pulley has to be vented to allow performing the repair. I use the 6-strand M-Tang repair for all FPL tendons (**Fig. 11**).[22,41] The proximal tendon frequently retracts into the thenar muscles, which can be retrieved through an incision in thenar muscles or the carpal tunnel.

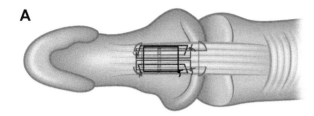
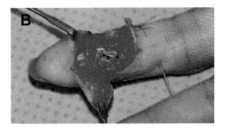

**Fig. 10.** (*A*) The method of a strong direct repair for repairing the tendon cut at or close to tendon-bone insertion of the finger. (*B*) An operative picture of this repair.

## TENOLYSIS, PULLEYS, TENDON GRAFTING, AND STAGED RECONSTRUCTION
### Tenolysis

It is estimated that about 10% to 20% of the patients still need tenolysis after primary or delayed primary repair. Tenolysis is best performed in a wide-awake setting without a tourniquet. The patient should move actively during the procedure to demonstrate ample active tendon motion. I perform wide-awake tenolysis whenever possible. The patient is asked to forcefully flex the finger and wrist to break any remaining adhesions after surgical release of adhesions.

### Tendon Grafting and Staged Reconstruction

Although I follow established methods and principles for these procedures, I use direct repair of the grafted tendon to the residual stump of the distal FDP tendon when making a distal junction. For that purpose, I retain the distal stump for 1 cm (or slightly less) when removing the FDP tendons. Starting the end of week 1 after surgery, I instruct the patients to perform a full range of passive motion and less-aggressive active flexion of the finger that underwent surgery.

## SUMMARY OF ADVANCEMENTS FOR ACHIEVING IDEAL REPAIR OUTCOMES

Zone 2 flexor tendon repairs have evolved greatly over the past 3 decades, including several key developments:

Use of strong core sutures, typically 4- or 6-strand repairs
Judicious venting of the critical annular pulley
Ensuring that some tension is created by the repair to prevent gapping
Performing digital extension-flexion tests to confirm the quality of the surgical repair
Early partial-range active motion to ensure tendon gliding without overloading the repair

Direct repair of the terminal FDP tendon or in making the distal junction of the grafted tendon is my preference. A few recent changes reported by surgeons hold the promise of wider adoption:

Using strong core-suture-only repair
Venting the A3 together with A4 pulleys if greater range of motion of the finger is needed
Using a wide-awake setting for tendon repair, including grafting

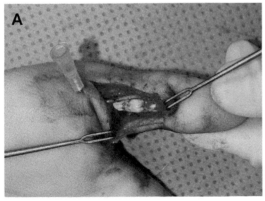
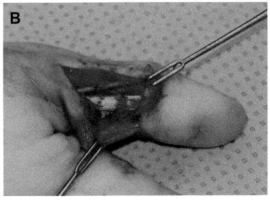

**Fig. 11.** The M-Tang repair for an FPL tendon cut. (*A*) After completion of repair, before taking the temporary needle fixation away, the tendon is seen slightly bunched up. (*B*) After the needle fixation is taken away, the tendon is flatter. No gapping was seen at thumb extension.

# REFERENCES

1. Tang JB. New developments are improving flexor tendon repair. Plast Reconstr Surg 2018;141: 1427–37.
2. Giesen T, Calcagni M, Elliot D. Primary flexor tendon repair with early active motion: experience in Europe. Hand Clin 2017;33:465–72.
3. Wong JK, Peck F. Improving results of flexor tendon repair and rehabilitation. Plast Reconstr Surg 2014; 134:913e–25e.
4. Elliot D, Giesen T. Primary flexor tendon surgery: the search for a perfect result. Hand Clin 2013;29:191–206.
5. Tang JB. Recent evolutions in flexor tendon repairs and rehabilitation. J Hand Surg Eur Vol 2018;43: 469–73.
6. Wu YF, Tang JB. Recent developments in flexor tendon repair techniques and factors influencing strength of the tendon repair. J Hand Surg Eur Vol 2014;39:6–19.
7. Wu YF, Tang JB. Effects of tension across the tendon repair site on tendon gap and ultimate strength. J Hand Surg Am 2012;37:906–12.
8. Savage R. In vitro studies of a new method of flexor tendon repair. J Hand Surg Br 1985;10:135–41.
9. Tang JB. The double sheath system and tendon gliding in zone 2C. J Hand Surg Br 1995;20:281–5.
10. Lalonde DH. Conceptual origins, current practice, and views of wide awake hand surgery. J Hand Surg Eur Vol 2017;42:886–95.
11. Lalonde DH, Martin AL. Wide-awake flexor tendon repair and early tendon mobilization in zones 1 and 2. Hand Clin 2013;29:207–13.
12. Tang JB. Clinical outcomes associated with flexor tendon repair. Hand Clin 2005;21:199–210.
13. Tang JB. Indications, methods, postoperative motion and outcome evaluation of primary flexor tendon repairs in Zone 2. J Hand Surg Eur Vol 2007;32: 118–29.
14. Tang JB. Outcomes and evaluation of flexor tendon repair. Hand Clin 2013;29:251–9.
15. Kwai Ben I, Elliot D. "Venting" or partial lateral release of the A2 and A4 pulleys after repair of zone 2 flexor tendon injuries. J Hand Surg Br 1998;23:649–54.
16. Tang JB. Release of the A4 pulley to facilitate zone II flexor tendon repair. J Hand Surg Am 2014;39: 2300–7.
17. Howell JW, Peck F. Rehabilitation of flexor and extensor tendon injuries in the hand: current updates. Injury 2013;44:397–402.
18. Tang JB, Xu Y, Wang B. Repair strength of tendons of varying gliding curvature: a study in a curvilinear model. J Hand Surg Am 2003;28:243–9.
19. Tang JB, Cao Y, Xie RG. Effects of tension direction on strength of tendon repair. J Hand Surg Am 2001; 26:1105–10.
20. Wu YF, Tang JB. Tendon healing, edema, and resistance to flexor tendon gliding: clinical implications. Hand Clin 2013;29:167–78.
21. Tang JB, Amadio PC, Boyer MI, et al. Current practice of primary flexor tendon repair: a global view. Hand Clin 2013;29:179–89.
22. Tang JB, Zhou X, Pan ZJ, et al. Strong digital flexor tendon repair, extension-flexion test, and early active flexion: experience in 300 tendons. Hand Clin 2017;33:455–63.
23. Giesen T, Sirotakova M, Copsey AJ, et al. Flexor pollicis longus primary repair: further experience with the Tang technique and controlled active mobilization. J Hand Surg Eur Vol 2009;34:758–61.
24. Giesen T, Reissner L, Besmens I, et al. Flexor tendon repair in the hand with the M-Tang technique (without peripheral sutures), pulley division, and early active motion. J Hand Surg Eur Vol 2018;43: 474–9.
25. Tang JB. Wide-awake primary flexor tendon repair, tenolysis and tendon transfer. Clin Orthop Surg 2015;7:275–81.
26. Chang MK, Wong YR, Tay SC. Biomechanical comparison of modified Lim/Tsai tendon repairs with intra- and extra-tendinous knots. J Hand Surg Eur Vol 2018;43:919–24.
27. Chang MK, Wong YR, Tay SC. Biomechanical comparison of the Lim/Tsai tendon repair with a modified method using a single looped suture. J Hand Surg Eur Vol 2017;42:915–9.
28. Chen J, Wu YF, Xing SG, et al. Suture knots between tendon stumps may not benefit tendon repairs. J Hand Surg Eur Vol 2018;43:1005–6.
29. Wu YF, Tang JB. The effect of asymmetric core suture purchase on gap resistance of tendon repair in linear cyclic loading. J Hand Surg Am 2014;39: 910–8.
30. Kozono N, Okada T, Takeuchi N, et al. A biomechanical comparison between asymmetric Pennington technique and conventional core suture techniques: 6-strand flexor tendon repair. J Hand Surg Am 2018;43:79.e1–8.
31. Moriya K, Yoshizu T, Tsubokawa N, et al. Outcomes of release of the entire A4 pulley after flexor tendon repairs in zone 2A followed by early active mobilization. J Hand Surg Eur Vol 2016;41:400–5.
32. Moriya K, Yoshizu T, Tsubokawa N, et al. Clinical results of releasing the entire A2 pulley after flexor tendon repair in zone 2C. J Hand Surg Eur Vol 2016;41:822–8.
33. Moriya K, Yoshizu T, Tsubokawa N, et al. Outcomes of flexor tendon repairs in zone 2 subzones with early active mobilization. J Hand Surg Eur Vol 2017;42:896–902.
34. Reissner L, Zechmann-Mueller N, Klein HJ, et al. Sonographic study of repair, gapping and tendon bowstringing after primary flexor digitorum

profundus repair in zone 2. J Hand Surg Eur Vol 2018;43(5):480–6.

35. Lalonde DH. Wide-awake flexor tendon repair. Plast Reconstr Surg 2009;123:623–5.

36. Higgins A, Lalonde DH, Bell M, et al. Avoiding flexor tendon repair rupture with intraoperative total active movement examination. Plast Reconstr Surg 2010; 126:941–5.

37. Tang JB, Gong KT, Zhu L, et al. Performing hand surgery under local anesthesia without a tourniquet in China. Hand Clin 2017;33:415–24.

38. Zhou X, Li XR, Qing J, et al. Outcomes of the six-strand M-Tang repair for zone 2 primary flexor tendon repair in 54 fingers. J Hand Surg Eur Vol 2017;42:462–8.

39. Pan ZJ, Xu YF, Pan L, et al. Zone 2 flexor tendon repairs using a tensioned strong core suture, sparse peripheral stitches and early active motion: results in 60 fingers. J Hand Surg Eur Vol 2019;44:361–6.

40. Moriya K, Yoshizu T, Tsubokawa N, et al. Incidence of tenolysis and features of adhesions in the digital flexor tendons after multi-strand repair and early active motion. J Hand Surg Eur Vol 2019;44:354–60.

41. Pan ZJ, Qin J, Zhou X, et al. Robust thumb flexor tendon repairs with a six-strand M-Tang method, pulley venting, and early active motion. J Hand Surg Eur Vol 2017;42:909–14.

# Tendon Transfers for Peripheral Nerve Palsies

Scott N. Loewenstein, MD, Joshua M. Adkinson, MD*

## KEYWORDS

• Radial neuropathy • Ulnar neuropathy • Median neuropathy • Tendon transfer • Peripheral nerve

## KEY POINTS

- Upper extremity peripheral nerve injuries may lead to incomplete recovery and persistent functional impairment.
- Tendon transfers offer the potential for restoration of function.
- The three most common ulnar nerve palsy-related deficits corrected by tendon transfers include claw hand, weak power grip, and weak pinch.
- Opponensplasty can restore function of the thumb after median nerve palsy.
- The loss of wrist, finger, and thumb extension after radial nerve palsy is reliably treated with tendon transfers.

## INTRODUCTION

Recovery after peripheral nerve injury varies and is often incomplete. Poor prognostic factors include older age, proximal nerve injury, surgeon inexperience, concomitant bone or soft tissue injury, poor quality nerve repair, and delay in repair.[1] Tendon transfers remain the standard when primary nerve repair does not, or is not expected to, achieve adequate restoration of function. Injured or repaired nerves are assessed by serial examinations and most peripheral nerves recover at a rate of 1 mm per day. If there are no signs of reinnervation after nerve repair or the timing since nerve injury would not allow for adequate muscle recovery, tendon transfers may be indicated. The decision to perform an early tendon transfer at the time of nerve repair or before expected reinnervation is considered on a case-by-case basis.

A successful tendon transfer relies on osseous stability with supple joints, pliable soft tissue free of scar (especially if tendon grafting is planned), an expendable donor with adequate excursion and power to restore lost function, and a donor with a direct line of pull that is synergistic with the function of the muscle to be restored.[2,3] Risks of tendon transfer surgery include extensive surgical dissection, postoperative immobilization (with risk for stiffness), potential for scar formation that may restrict tendon excursion, loss of muscle strength, rupture or attenuation of the transfer, and potential inadequacy of muscle-tendon balance.[2] We perform an end-to-side tendon repair when there is some chance for native nerve recovery; otherwise, we recommend a Pulvertaft weave or running mattress suture. Appropriate tensioning of a tendon transfer may be difficult to assess intraoperatively and follows the classic recommendations for joint positioning.

## ULNAR NERVE PALSY

Three main functional deficits predominate in low ulnar palsy: ulnar claw, difficulties with grip, and weakened pinch (**Table 1**). We do not routinely correct the small finger abduction deformity (ie, Wartenberg sign), although techniques exist to address this rare complaint.[4,5] High ulnar palsy

---

Disclosure Statement: The authors have no financial interest in commercial ventures related to this article.
Division of Plastic Surgery, Indiana University School of Medicine, 545 Barnhill Drive, Emerson Hall, Suite 232, Indianapolis, IN 46202, USA
* Corresponding author.
E-mail address: jadkinso@iu.edu

Clin Plastic Surg 46 (2019) 307–315
https://doi.org/10.1016/j.cps.2019.02.004

**Table 1**
**Functional deficits in ulnar nerve palsy**

| Deficit | Cause |
| --- | --- |
| Claw hand | Occurs because of paralysis of the intrinsic finger flexors. |
| | At the MCPJ the extrinsic extensors are normally balanced by intrinsic flexors, but without the innervation of the intrinsic flexors, the balance favors hyperextension at the MCPJ. |
| | The pull of the extrinsic extensors results in volar plate laxity over time, and MCPJ hyperextension develops. Hyperextension of MCPJ increases the tension of flexor tendons, and combined with loss of the normal extension force of the intrinsic at the PIPJ and DIPJs, PIPJ and DIPJ flexion results. |
| | Clawing tends to affect the ulnar fingers more than the radial fingers because the index and middle are median-innervated. |
| | In combined median and ulnar nerve palsies, all fingers are affected. |
| Grip difficulties Weakened grip Asynchronous finger flexion | Weakened grip occurs because of paralysis of the intrinsic muscles, which participate in power grip as the intrinsics initiate MCPJ flexion. |
| | Patients also frequently endorse asynchronous finger flexion, whereby finger tips come into contact into the palm immediately after flexion, which leads to pushing objects away from the hand. In ulnar nerve palsy, this occurs because the remaining extrinsic flexors cause a distal to proximal sequence of finger flexion; there is a loss of initial MCPJ flexion during grip that typically occurs because of intrinsic activation. |

(continued on next page)

**Table 1**
**(continued)**

| Deficit | Cause |
| --- | --- |
| Weakened pinch | Power (thumb-index) pinch is decreased by 80%[7] ulnar palsy. This results from paralysis of ulnar-innervated AdP, half of FPB, and the FDI. |
| | Half of the FPB is at least partially median-innervated, which may allow for maintenance of pinch in ulnar nerve palsy. |
| Wartenberg sign | Abduction deformity of the small finger (ie, Wartenberg sign) is caused by unopposed abduction by EDM with a loss of the abducting force from the third palmar interosseous. |

*Abbreviations:* AdP, adductor pollicis muscle; DIPJ, distal interphalangeal joint; EDM, extensor digiti minimi muscle; FDI, first dorsal interosseous muscle; FPB, flexor pollicis brevis muscle; MCPJ, metacarpophalangeal joint; PIPJ, proximal interphalangeal joint.

rarely leads to a claw deformity because the paralyzed flexor digitorum profundus muscle (FDP)$_{ring}$ and FDP$_{small}$ do not pull the digits into flexion (**Fig. 1**). We consider early tendon transfer for patients with a poor prognosis for recovery (eg, high ulnar nerve injuries).[1]

## Correction of Ulnar Claw and Asynchronous Finger Flexion

In claw hand, inability of the extrinsic finger extensors to extend the proximal interphalangeal joint (PIPJ) and distal interphalangeal joint (DIPJ) results from the hyperextended posture of the

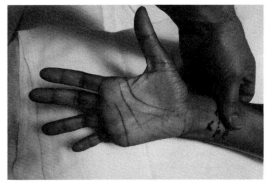

**Fig. 1.** Claw hand posture.

metacarpophalangeal joint (MCPJ).[6] The Bouvier test distinguishes patients who have full active interphalangeal joint (IPJ) extension with the MCPJ placed in flexion and only need MCPJ flexion ("simple claw") from patients who need both MCPJ flexion and PIPJ extension ("complex claw").[7]

### Flexor digitorum superficialis muscle (Zancolli) lasso for simple claw deformity

The surgical treatment of patients with a simple claw is straightforward, but does not address flexion asynchrony or result in an increase in grip strength.[8] The goal of surgery is to induce MCPJ flexion or, at a minimum, prevent MCPJ hyperextension so that the IPJs can fully extended.

Numerous procedures have been described to address a simple claw deformity, including dorsal bone blocking at the MCPJ,[9] capsular plication or advancement,[10] and tenodesis.[11] MCPJ arthrodesis is typically reserved for combined high ulnar and median nerve injuries where a dynamic tendon transfer donor is unavailable.

We prefer an FDS (Zancolli) lasso procedure for simple clawing.[12] The FDS$_{ring}$ and FDS$_{small}$ are divided distal to A1 pulley, looped around the pulley, and sutured back onto itself. In high ulnar injuries, the FDS$_{ring}$ and FDS$_{small}$ cannot be sacrificed so the FDS$_{long}$ is split into two slips and used for the small finger and ring finger in a similar fashion.

### Flexor digitorum superficialis muscle (modified Stiles-Bunnell) transfer for complex claw deformity

A deficit of IPJ extension during Bouvier testing is caused by attenuation of the central slip or lateral band volar subluxation from long-standing claw deformity.[7] In these cases, dynamic procedures to produce simultaneous MCPJ flexion and IPJ extension are indicated. Many techniques are described and vary based on donor motor unit, route, and insertion site (**Table 2**).

Our procedure of choice for complex clawing in low ulnar nerve palsy is the modified Stiles-Bunnell technique. The FDS$_{ring}$ is divided just proximal to the PIPJ and split longitudinally into two slips, each of which is sewn into the radial lateral bands of the small finger and ring finger.[13] In high ulnar palsies, the FDS$_{long}$ is split into three or four slips to correct all affected digits,[14] because the FDS$_{ring}$ is not expendable (**Fig. 2**). Excellent results have been obtained with this procedure, evidenced by correction of the asynchronous flexion in up to 93% of patients.[15]

There is significant risk for donor finger morbidity when using an FDS transfer. Swan-

**Table 2**
**Tendon transfers for correcting ulnar claw**

| Classification | Examples |
|---|---|
| **Donor motor unit** | |
| Flexor | FDS |
| | PL |
| Extensor | ECRL |
| | ECRB |
| | BR |
| **Route** | |
| Volar | Volar to the carpus through the carpal canal and then volar to deep transverse intermetacarpal ligament |
| Dorsal | Dorsal to the carpus through the intermetacarpal spaces, then volar to the deep transverse intermetacarpal ligaments (usually through the lumbrical canal) |
| **Insertion site** | |
| Pulley system | A1 |
| | A2 |
| | Both A1 and proximal A2 pulleys |
| Extensor apparatus | Lateral band |
| Bone fixation | Phalanx |

*Abbreviations:* BR, brachioradialis muscle; ECRB, extensor carpi radialis brevis muscle; ECRL, extensor carpi radialis longus muscle; PL, palmaris longus muscle.

neck deformity occurs in 15%, isolated DIP flexion posturing in 29%, and PIP flexion contracture in 26%.[16] The risk for postoperative IPJ hyperextension is mitigated by either dividing FDS proximal to the decussation (which maintains some restraint against hyperextension) or by using a remaining slip of FDS as a tenodesis across the PIPJ. Using FDS to correct clawing does not improve grip strength[7]; this requires the addition of donor motor units.

### Extensor carpi radialis longus muscle or extensor carpi radialis brevis muscle (Brand) transfer to correct complex ulnar claw

The Brand technique for complex clawing uses extensor carpi radialis longus muscle (ECRL) or extensor carpi radialis brevis muscle (ECRB) to provide both MCPJ flexion and IPJ extension. The extensor is harvested at the wrist, extended with a tendon graft, and routed either through the carpal tunnel or dorsally across the wrist and then passed volar to the deep transverse

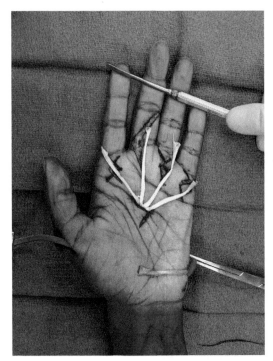

**Fig. 2.** FDS tendon divided into four slips for correction of clawing.

metacarpal ligament. It is secured distally to the lumbricals tendons and/or lateral bands.[17]

Activation of this tendon transfer is not intuitive and re-education is more difficult with ECRL than with the FDS transfer. For example, when routed dorsally, extension of the wrist slackens the graft, so the patient must be taught to prevent wrist extension while contracting their wrist extensor. Passing the transfer through the carpal tunnel weakens wrist extension, which consequently weakens grip. The volar route can also lead to crowding of carpal tunnel and may put the median nerve at risk of compression.[17]

### Comparative outcomes

Ozkan and colleagues[18] reviewed outcomes for tendon transfers to correct clawing in ulnar nerve palsy. They found the postoperative improvement in grip strength for the Stiles-Bunnell four-tailed procedure (7% improvement) was minimal, and ECRL four-tailed procedure (15% improvement) and the Zancolli lasso procedure (16% improvement) were modest. With long-standing paralysis, the Stiles-Bunnell four-tailed procedure most successfully corrected clawing. Conversely, Brand[17] reported that the wrist extensors better corrected ulnar clawing, as compared with FDS transfers. In 861 fingers assessed at an average of 2 years after ECRL or ECRB transfer, hand opening was

rated as excellent in 50% and good in 34% compared with 31% excellent and 42% good in the 564 fingers after FDS transfer.[15]

### Restoration of pinch

Reconstructing pinch involves restoring thumb adduction, restoring index finger abduction, or both (**Table 3**). In our experience, restoring thumb adduction with an adductorplasty is sufficient to restore adequate pinch function in most patients. Importantly, the vector of pull must parallel the fibers of the adductor pollicis muscle (AdP) and have adequate strength to restore appropriate function.[19]

### Flexor digitorum superficialis muscle (Littler) transfer to restore pinch

The Littler FDS transfer is a classic technique used to correct pinch after an ulnar nerve injury. The $FDS_{ring}$[13] or $FDS_{long}$[19] is harvested between the A1 and A2 pulley.[20] It is passed deep to the flexor tendons of the index and long fingers, parallel and superficial to the transverse fibers of AdP, and secured to the AdP tendon or the thumb proximal phalanx.[13] The $FDS_{ring}$ variation of this technique is contraindicated in high ulnar palsy because the transfer would sacrifice the only remaining extrinsic flexor to ring finger. Hamlin and Littler[21] report that key pinch strength in 22 patients improved from an average of 30% of uninjured side to 71% of uninjured side after FDS transfer.

| Table 3 Tendon transfers for correction of key pinch in ulnar palsy | |
|---|---|
| Deficiency | Donor |
| Index finger abduction | ECRL<br>FDS<br>EIP<br>EPB<br>PL<br>APL |
| Thumb adduction | $FDS_{ring}$<br>$FDS_{long}$<br>ECRB<br>BR<br>ECRL<br>EDM<br>FPB<br>EIP |

*Abbreviations:* APL, abductor pollicis longus muscle; BR, brachioradialis muscle; EDM, extensor digiti minimi muscle; EIP, extensor indicis proprius; EPB, extensor pollicis brevis muscle; FPB, flexor pollicis brevis muscle; PL, palmaris longus muscle.

*Extensor carpi radialis brevis muscle (Smith)
transfer to restore pinch*
The Smith ECRB transfer is an alternative to correct key pinch. The ECRB is extended by a free tendon graft passed through the second[19] or third[22] intermetacarpal space, tunneled deep to the flexor tendons but superficial to the AdP, and inserted into the AdP tendon (**Fig. 3**). Smith[23] noted that 14 of 15 patients reported significant improvements in their ability to use the thumb for pinch and grasp. For those that improved, key pinch force on the affected side doubled postoperatively.[7]

## LOW MEDIAN NERVE PALSY

Low median nerve palsy results in the loss of thumb opposition, because the median nerve innervates the thenar muscles and contributes 70% to 74% of thumb abduction strength.[24] Median nerve injuries tend to have better outcomes with primary repair than other peripheral nerve injuries.[1] For example, Jensen[25] found that 55% recovered opposition following neurorrhaphy alone, with opponensplasty indicated in only 14% of patients.

### *Opponensplasty*

There are many techniques described for opponensplasty that vary based on insertion site and donor motor unit (**Table 4**). The four most common transfers include the extensor indicis proprius (EIP)

(Burkhalter) transfer, the FDS (Bunnell) transfer, the palmaris longus muscle (PL) (Camitz) transfer, and the abductor digiti minimi muscle (ADM) (Huber) transfer.

### *Extensor indicis proprius (Burkhalter) opponensplasty*
In the EIP opponensplasty, first described by Burkhalter, the EIP is redirected around the ulnar wrist (superficial to extensor carpi ulnaris muscle and just proximal to pisiform) and woven into abductor pollicis brevis muscle (APB) under maximal tension. It is used in low median, high median, or combined median and ulnar nerve palsy. Burkhalter and coworkers[26] reported that at least 88% of patients achieved at least 75% of contralateral thumb function. Opposition to the tip of at least the small or ring finger is achieved in greater than 80% of patients.[27,28]

### *Flexor digitorum superficialis muscle (Bunnell) transfer*
In the FDS (Bunnell) transfer, the $FDS_{ring}$ is incised distally, the flexor carpi ulnaris muscle (FCU) tendon split longitudinally to fashion a pulley at[29] or distal[30] to the pisiform, and $FDS_{ring}$ is passed through this pulley and sutured to the APB insertion (**Fig. 4**). Alternatively, Guyon canal[31] or the transverse carpal ligament[32] is used as a pulley, but some propose that these routes may not achieve true thumb opposition.[29] This transfer has limited application because the FDS tendon

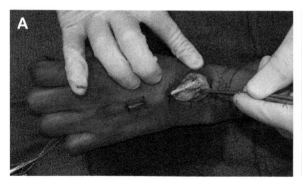

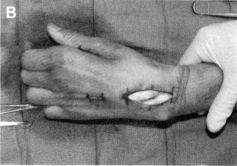

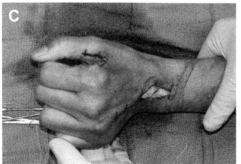

Fig. 3. (*A*) ECRB tendon extended with a PL graft. (*B*) Adducted posture of the thumb with wrist flexed. (*C*) Abducted posture of the thumb with wrist extended.

**Table 4**
**Opponensplasty for median nerve palsy**

| Classification | Examples |
| --- | --- |
| Insertion site | Proximal phalanx dorsoulnar base |
| | First metacarpal radiodorsal ridge |
| | FPB and opponens pollicis |
| | APB |
| | EPL |
| | Combined EPL and AdP |
| | EPB |
| Donor motor unit | EIP (Burkhalter) |
| | FDS (Bunnell) |
| | PL (Camitz) |
| | ADM (Huber) |
| | ECU (Phalen and Miller) |
| | EDM |
| | ECRL or ECRB |
| | FCU |
| | APL |
| | BR |

*Abbreviations:* APL, abductor pollicis longus muscle; BR, brachioradialis muscle; ECU, extensor carpi ulnaris muscle; EDM, extensor digiti minimi muscle; EPL, extensor pollicis longus muscle; FPB, flexor pollicis brevis muscle; PL, palmaris longus muscle.

is commonly disrupted in post-traumatic low median nerve palsy.

### Palmaris longus muscle (Camitz) transfer
The PL transfer is most useful for restoring thumb function in patients with advanced carpal tunnel syndrome.[33] It is one of the weakest opposition transfers, but has a low complication rate.

### Abductor digiti minimi muscle (Huber) transfer
The ADM transfer is a useful option for restoration of opposition in patients with combined median and radial nerve palsy, where other preferred options are unavailable. This transfer has found greater utility in treating congenital thumb hypoplasia, where it offers opposition and thenar eminence augmentation.

### Comparative outcomes
Extensor lag of the index finger is a potential complication of the EIP opponensplasty and FDS transfer risks formation of a swan-neck deformity and digital flexion contracture.[26] The FDS opponensplasty, however, is stronger and has greater donor tendon length.[34] In one study, 75% of patients undergoing the FDS transfer were satisfied, compared with only 57% of patients receiving the EIP transfer.[35] In another study, 85% of patients undergoing an EIP transfer were able to oppose to the ring or small finger, compared with only 30% of patients after FDS transfer.[36]

## HIGH MEDIAN NERVE PALSY

In addition to the loss of opposition, high median nerve palsy leads to loss of extrinsic finger flexion. High median nerve palsy has been shown to cause a 36% decrease in pinch strength and a 43% decrease in grip strength. Pronation is also weakened to 65% the unaffected side.[37] These injuries are rare, representing approximately 0.1% of all upper extremity peripheral nerve injuries.[38] Because of the poor recovery of function with high median nerve injuries, early tendon transfer should be considered. As with high ulnar nerve injuries, nerve transfers show promise, but are outside the scope of this article.

In addition to opponensplasty, we recommend brachioradialis muscle (BR) to Flexor pollicis longus to restore thumb IPJ flexion. An ECRB transfer is an alternative for restoration of thumb flexion; to preserve active wrist extension, this transfer should not be combined with ECRL transfer. Flexion of the index and long fingers is lost in high median nerve palsy and is restored through ECRL to $FDP_{index}$ and $FDP_{long}$ transfer.

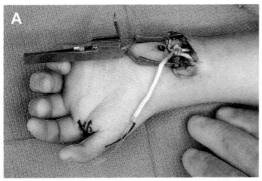 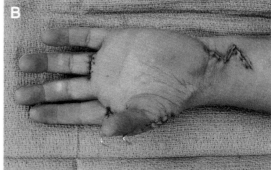

**Fig. 4.** (*A*) FDS opponensplasty before tendon insertion. (*B*) After tendon routing into the APB insertion.

**Table 5**
**Tendon transfers for radial nerve palsy**

| Function | Transfer |
| --- | --- |
| Wrist extension | PT to ECRB and/or ECRL |
| | FDS to ECRB and/or ECRL |
| Finger extension | FCU and/or FCR to EDC |
| | FDS to EDC |
| Thumb extension | FDS$_{small}$ to EPL |
| | FDS$_{ring}$ to EPL |
| | PL to EPL |
| | BR to EPL |
| | FCR to EPL |
| | FDS to EPL ± EIP |
| | FCR to APL and EPB |

*Abbreviations:* APL, abductor pollicis longus muscle; ECU, extensor carpi ulnaris muscle; EPB, extensor pollicis brevis muscle; EPL, extensor pollicis longus muscle; FCR, flexor carpi radialis muscle.

Alternatively, side-to-side tenorrhaphy of the FDP$_{ring}$ and FDP$_{small}$ to the FDP$_{index}$ and FDP$_{long}$ may be used. Unlike the ECRL transfer for digital flexion, tenorrhaphy can only restore composite, but not independent, digital flexion. As such, tenorrhaphy is only indicated in combined median and radial nerve palsies.

## RADIAL NERVE PALSY

Radial nerve palsy results in an inability to extend the wrist, extend the fingers at the MCPJs, and radially abduct the thumb. Grip strength is substantially weakened in radial nerve palsy because of an inability to stabilize the wrist to transmit the power of the flexors, and an early tendon transfer to restore wrist extension should be considered. Bevin[39] found only 66% of patients with a high radial nerve injury and primary nerve repair without tendon transfers achieved results good enough to return to work, but 100% patients who underwent tendon transfers without nerve repair were able to return to work.

### Wrist Extension

Wrist extension is typically restored by pronator teres muscle (PT) transfer to ECRB,[40] ECRL,[41] or both (**Table 5**).[42] This transfer markedly improves grip and overall hand function. Dabas and colleagues[43] found that the PT to ECRB transfer resulted in a 48% increase in grip strength and a 90% increase in key pinch strength at 6 months postoperatively. If the PT is transferred to both ECRL and ECRB, pathologic radial deviation of the wrist may occur (>70% of patients), whereas insertion into ECRB only rarely causes radial

deviation of the wrist (10% of patients).[44] An alternative for restoring wrist extension is transfer of FDS$_{long}$ and FDS$_{ring}$ to the radial wrist extensors.[45]

### Finger Extension

Finger extension is restored by transferring FCU[40] or flexor carpi radialis muscle (FCR)[46] to the extensor digitorum communis muscle (EDC). Wrist flexors are commonly used as donor motor units because they function synergistically with digital extension. The FCU transfer can restore greater than 50% of contralateral unaffected finger extension power.[47] The FCR transfer restores 79% of contralateral unaffected power grip, compared with only 49% with the FCU transfer.[48] Some studies have found greater loss of wrist range of motion[44,49] when FCU is transferred compared with FCR, whereas other studies have shown no difference.[48,50]

We prefer to transfer FCR to EDC around the radial border of the forearm to restore finger extension because unlike the FCU that has muscle attachment along the ulna, FCR harvest is much easier with no bone attachment and does not require a long forearm incision (**Fig. 5**). We do not include extensor digiti minimi muscle as a recipient in this transfer because it may result in excessive abduction of the small finger, but rather attach to the small finger EDC.[51]

### Thumb Extension

Thumb extension is restored independently from digital extension. Various donor tendons to restore thumb extension have been described, including FDS$_{small}$,[51] FDS$_{ring}$,[42] PL,[46,51] BR,[51] and FCR.[51] Our preferred donor to restore thumb extension in radial nerve palsy is PL. The PL tendon is transferred around the radial side of the forearm and sutured end-to-end to the extensor pollicis longus muscle. To create a straight line of pull, the

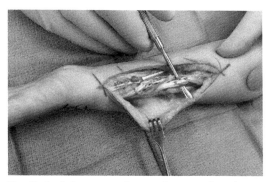

**Fig. 5.** Radial nerve palsy tendon transfers (PT to ECRB, FCR to EDC, PL to EPL). Instrument on the PT transfer.

extensor pollicis longus muscle tendon is divided at the musculotendinous junction and withdrawn out of the third extensor compartment. It is then transferred subcutaneously to the PL donor tendon in the forearm.[40] This technique can produce simultaneous thumb interphalangeal and MCP extension along with abduction of thumb metacarpal.[40] The FDS is an alternative option for restoring finger and thumb extension.[42]

## REFERENCES

1. Ruijs AC, Jaquet JB, Kalmijn S, et al. Median and ulnar nerve injuries: a meta-analysis of predictors of motor and sensory recovery after modern microsurgical nerve repair. Plast Reconstr Surg 2005;116(2): 484–94 [discussion: 495–6].

2. Giuffre JL, Bishop AT, Spinner RJ, et al. The best of tendon and nerve transfers in the upper extremity. Plast Reconstr Surg 2015;135(3):617e–30e.

3. Sammer DM, Chung KC. Tendon transfers: part I. Principles of transfer and transfers for radial nerve palsy. Plast Reconstr Surg 2009;123(5):169e–77e.

4. Blacker GJ, Lister GD, Kleinert HE. The abducted little finger in low ulnar nerve palsy. J Hand Surg Am 1976;1(3):190–6.

5. Chung MS, Baek GH, Oh JH, et al. Extensor indicis proprius transfer for the abducted small finger. J Hand Surg Am 2008;33(3):392–7.

6. Fowler S. Extensor apparatus of the digits. J Bone Joint Surg 1949;31B(3):477.

7. Hastings H 2nd, Davidson S. Tendon transfers for ulnar nerve palsy. Evaluation of results and practical treatment considerations. Hand Clin 1988;4(2): 167–78.

8. Sapienza A, Green S. Correction of the claw hand. Hand Clin 2012;28(1):53–66.

9. Mikhail IK. Bone block operation for clawhand. Surg Gynecol Obstet 1964;118:1077–9.

10. Leddy JP, Stark HH, Ashworth CR, et al. Capsulodesis and pulley advancement for the correction of claw-finger deformity. J Bone Joint Surg Am 1972; 54(7):1465–71.

11. Parkes A. Paralytic claw fingers: a graft tenodesis operation. Hand 1973;5(3):192–9.

12. Zancolli E. Intrinsic paralysis of the ulnar nerve: physiopathology of the claw hand. In: Zancolli E, editor. Structural and dynamic bases of hand surgery. 2nd edition. Philadelphia: JB Lippincott; 1979. p. 159–206.

13. Littler JW. Tendon transfers and arthrodeses in combined median and ulnar nerve paralysis. J Bone Joint Surg Am 1949;31A(2):225–34.

14. Riordan DC. Tendon transfers in hand surgery. J Hand Surg Am 1983;8(5 Pt 2):748–53.

15. Brand PW. Paralytic claw hand; with special reference to paralysis in leprosy and treatment by the sublimis transfer of Stiles and Bunnell. J Bone Joint Surg Br 1958;40-B(4):618–32.

16. Brandsma JW, Ottenhoff-De Jonge MW. Flexor digitorum superficialis tendon transfer for intrinsic replacement. Long-term results and the effect on donor fingers. J Hand Surg Br 1992;17(6):625–8.

17. Brand PW. Tendon grafting: illustrated by a new operation for intrinsic paralysis of the fingers. J Bone Joint Surg 1961;43:444–53.

18. Ozkan T, Ozer K, Gulgonen A. Three tendon transfer methods in reconstruction of ulnar nerve palsy. J Hand Surg Am 2003;28(1):35–43.

19. Cook S, Gaston RG, Lourie GM. Ulnar nerve tendon transfers for pinch. Hand Clin 2016;32(3):369–76.

20. North ER, Littler JW. Transferring the flexor superficialis tendon: technical considerations in the prevention of proximal interphalangeal joint disability. J Hand Surg Am 1980;5(5):498–501.

21. Hamlin C, Littler JW. Restoration of power pinch. J Hand Surg Am 1980;5(4):396–401.

22. Omer GE Jr. Reconstruction of a balanced thumb through tendon transfers. Clin Orthop Relat Res 1985;(195):104–16.

23. Smith RJ. Extensor carpi radialis brevis tendon transfer for thumb adduction: a study of power pinch. J Hand Surg Am 1983;8(1):4–15.

24. Boatright JR, Kiebzak GM. The effects of low median nerve block on thumb abduction strength. J Hand Surg Am 1997;22(5):849–52.

25. Jensen EG. Restoration of opposition of the thumb. Hand 1978;10(2):161–7.

26. Burkhalter W, Christensen R, Brown P. Extensor indicis proprius opponensplasty. J Bone Joint Surg Am 1973;55:725–32.

27. Anderson GA, Lee V, Sundararaj GD. Extensor indicis proprius opponensplasty. J Hand Surg Br 1991; 16(3):334–8.

28. Al-Qattan MM. Extensor indicis proprius opponensplasty for isolated traumatic low median nerve palsy: a case series. Can J Plast Surg 2012;20(4): 255–7.

29. Bunnell S. Opposition of the thumb. J Bone Joint Surg 1938;20:269–84.

30. Sakellarides HT. Modified pulley for opponens tendon transfer. J Bone Joint Surg Am 1970;52(1): 178–9.

31. Brand P. Tendon transfers in the forearm. In: Flynn JE, editor. Hand surgery. 2nd edition. Baltimore (MD): Williams & Wilkins; 1975. p. 189–200.

32. Snow JW, Fink GH. Use of a transverse carpal ligament window for the pulley in tendon transfers for median nerve palsy. Plast Reconstr Surg 1971; 48(3):238–40.

33. Terrono AL, Rose JH, Mulroy J, et al. Camitz palmaris longus abductorplasty for severe thenar atrophy secondary to carpal tunnel syndrome. J Hand Surg Am 1993;18(2):204–6.

34. Cooney WP, Linscheid RL, An KN. Opposition of the thumb: an anatomic and biomechanical study of tendon transfers. J Hand Surg Am 1984;9(6): 777–86.

35. Patond K, Betal B, Gautam V. Results of thumb correction in leprosy using different techniques. Indian J Lepr 1999;71(2):155–66.

36. Anderson GA, Lee V, Sundararaj GD. Opponensplasty by extensor indicis and flexor digitorum superficialis tendon transfer. J Hand Surg Br 1992; 17(6):611–4.

37. Bertelli JA, Soldado F, Lehn VL, et al. Reappraisal of clinical deficits following high median nerve injuries. J Hand Surg Am 2016;41(1):13–9.

38. Boswick JA Jr, Stromberg WB Jr. Isolated injury to the median nerve above the elbow. A review of thirteen cases. J Bone Joint Surg Am 1967;49(4): 653–8.

39. Bevin AG. Early tendon transfer for radial nerve transection. Hand 1976;8(2):134–6.

40. Riordan DC. Radial nerve paralysis. Orthop Clin North Am 1974;5(2):283–7.

41. Bik P. Tendon transfers for the radial nerve palsy. ONA J 1978;5(2):42.

42. Boyes JH. Tendon transfers for radial palsy. Bull Hosp Joint Dis 1960;21:97–105.

43. Dabas V, Suri T, Surapuraju PK, et al. Functional restoration after early tendon transfer in high radial nerve paralysis. J Hand Surg Eur Vol 2011;36(2): 135–40.

44. Tsuge K. Tendon transfers for radial nerve palsy. Aust N Z J Surg 1980;50(3):267–72.

45. Deiler S, Wiedemann E, Stock W, et al. Clinical experiences in tendon transfers for radial nerve palsy by a new method of Wiedemann. Orthopade 1997; 26(8):684–9.

46. Starr CL. Army experiences with tendon transference. JBJS 1922;4(1):3–21.

47. Moberg E, Nachemson A. Tendon transfers for defective long extensors of the wrist and fingers. Acta Chir Scand 1967;133(1):31–4.

48. Skoll PJ, Hudson DA, de Jager W, et al. Long-term results of tendon transfers for radial nerve palsy in patients with limited rehabilitation. Ann Plast Surg 2000;45(2):122–6.

49. Ropars M, Dreano T, Siret P, et al. Long-term results of tendon transfers in radial and posterior interosseous nerve paralysis. J Hand Surg Br 2006;31(5):502–6.

50. Raskin KB, Wilgis EF. Flexor carpi ulnaris transfer for radial nerve palsy: functional testing of long-term results. J Hand Surg Am 1995;20(5):737–42.

51. Beasley RW. Tendon transfers for radial nerve palsy. Orthop Clin North Am 1970;1(2):439–45.

# Tendinopathies of the Forearm, Wrist, and Hand

Eric R. Wagner, MD, MS*, Michael B. Gottschalk, MD

## KEYWORDS

• Tendinitis • Tenosynovitis • Tendinopathy • Trigger finger • De Quervain

## KEY POINTS

• Tendinitis and tendinopathy are often clinical diagnoses in the hand, wrist, and forearm with specific physical examination findings and common presentations.
• The first-line treatment of any hand, wrist, or forearm tendinitis or tendinopathy is nonoperative, including injections, splints, and activity modification.
• Surgery for tendinitis or tendinopathy of the hand, wrist, or forearm usually involves decompression of the pulley or retinaculum, with other procedures specific to each pathologic situation.
• There are many considerations for failure of nonoperative and operative treatment, including patient and anatomic factors.

## INTRODUCTION

Nonacute tendon disorders constitute one of the most common encountered complaints evaluated and treated by hand surgeons.[1] Most chronic tendon disorders of the hand, wrist, and distal forearm are associated with inflammatory, mechanical, or degenerative processes. The exact causes are often unknown. Many of these tendon disorders can be successfully treated nonoperatively with activity modification, splints, and/or corticosteroid injections. However, in refractory cases surgical intervention is often successful in relieving the patient's symptoms. Many factors to be considered in each separate pathologic process have been shown to affect the outcomes of nonoperative and operative management.

This review focuses on 7 of the most common chronic tendon disorders of the hand, wrist, and forearm, summarizing their presentation, potential etiology, important considerations, nonoperative and operative treatment, and factors affecting the outcomes of these treatments.

## TRIGGER FINGER

Trigger finger is the most common tendon disorder in the upper extremity, occurring in approximately 2% of the general population.[1] It is thought to occur as the result of friction between the tendon and A1 pulley, leading to thickening and inflammation of the pulley and tendon.[2] Although there are no known causes attributed directly to this pathologic process, the incidence is higher in females and in patients with diabetes mellitus (DM) or rheumatoid arthritis,[3–5] with one study noting up to a 20% incidence in patients with DM.[6] Of note, histopathologic analyses of trigger-finger specimens demonstrate a striking absence of inflammation.[1,7] Many patients who develop trigger finger also have or eventually develop concomitant carpal tunnel syndrome.[8–12] The diagnosis is made clinically, with pain localized to the A1 pulley, triggering or locking of the digit in flexion, and often a painful nodule.

The first step in the treatment of all patients should be conservative measures, including corticosteroid injections,[13–17] either into the tendon

Disclosure Statement: The authors have nothing to disclose that is relevant to this publication.
Division of Upper Extremity Surgery, Department of Orthopaedic Surgery, Emory University, 59 Executive Park South, Atlanta, GA 30329, USA
* Corresponding author.
E-mail address: Eric.r.wagner@emory.edu

sheath,[18,19] superficial to the sheath,[19,20] or distal to the annular pulley,[21] as well as splinting and activity modification. Splints immobilize the metacarpophalangeal (MCP) and/or proximal (PIP) and distal interphalangeal (DIP) joints (**Fig. 1**), with success rates from 36% to 93%.[22–24] The efficacy of corticosteroids is between 50% and 90%,[13–17] with potentially improved success rates in extrasheath injections.[20] A systematic review of 297 digits demonstrated injection to have 57% overall efficacy,[25] whereas a Cochrane review showed its superiority over lidocaine alone or a placebo.[26] Furthermore, A1 pulley thickness on ultrasonography decreases over 3 to 4 weeks after corticosteroid injection.[19,27] The number of corticosteroid injections that patients should receive is controversial; a second injection can increase the response rate from 57% to 86%,[14] but more than 2 injections is the least cost-effective strategy given the high failure rate.[16] A higher symptom recurrence rate has been demonstrated in patients with DM,[15,28] younger age,[15] involvement of other digits,[15] history of other tendinopathies,[15] and metabolic syndrome.[29]

The standard surgical treatment of trigger finger is open release through either a transverse, oblique, or Bruner-type incision (**Fig. 2**). The main risk of this procedure is iatrogenic damage to the volar digital nerves. After dissection through skin and subcutaneous adipose tissue, the A1 pulley is visualized and digital nerves are protected. The pulley is then completely released. Overall, the outcome of trigger-finger release is successful in 72% to 100%, with major complications occurring in less than 3% of patients.[14,17,30–33] One analysis of 254 trigger fingers had complete resolution of symptomatic triggering in 100%, with full motion regained in 249 of 254 fingers after open release.[34]

Factors associated with worse outcomes after release include longer duration of preoperative symptoms,[35] PIP flexion contracture,[35] male sex,[31] and use of sedation.[31] Many surgeons prefer to perform the wide-awake local anesthesia with no tourniquet (WALANT) technique to allow the

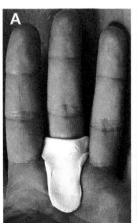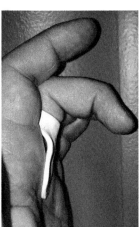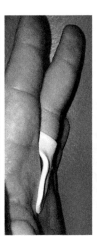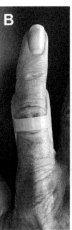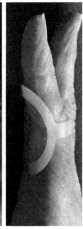

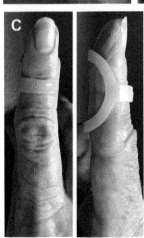

**Fig. 1.** Splint options for trigger finger. The initial steps of trigger-finger treatment may involve the use of an MCP (*A*), PIP (*B*), or DIP (*C*) extension blocking splint.

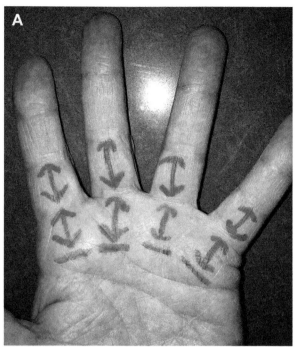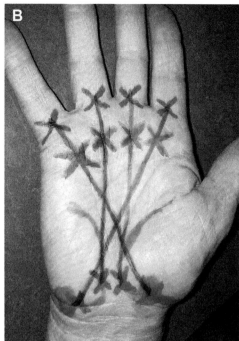

**Fig. 2.** Open and percutaneous trigger-finger release. (*A*) Open release of the A1 pulley is often performed through a transverse incision directly over the MCP joint on the volar surface. Localization of the incision on the volar surface can be performed by either a finger breadth proximal to the most proximal finger crease or slightly less than the distance between the proximal and middle finger creases. (*B*) Percutaneous release landmarks include: (1) Index line from midpoint of digit to radial border of pisiform; (2) middle and ring line from midpoint of digit to radial (middle) and ulnar (ring) borders of intersection of thenar-hypothenar eminence; (3) little line from midpoint of digit to scaphoid tubercle.

patient to move the finger to confirm complete relief of the triggering, a method that is more cost-effective.[36] Special considerations should be taken for children, because the trigger finger (except trigger thumb) may be caused by anatomic variants, such as abnormal flexor digitorum superficialis insertion.[37] Further special consideration should be given to patients with recurrent trigger fingers, DM, and rheumatoid arthritis,[3] in whom the underlying etiology might arise from flexor digitorum profundus (FDP) entrapment at flexor digitorum superficialis (FDS) decussation.[38] This condition is treated with release of one slip of the FDS or splitting the FDS at the decussation to provide more room for the FDP.[38]

Although percutaneous trigger-finger release was described in 1958,[39] it has recently gained popularity because of its similar efficacy to the open procedure, without an increase in complications.[14,32,40–42] In a meta-analysis of 2100 percutaneous releases, there was a 94% success rate with only 4 major complications.[43] This technique is usually performed using an 18-gauge needle; however, special knifes or procedure-specific blades can also be used.[44] When performing this procedure, it is critical to know the surface anatomic landmarks (see **Fig. 2**). One useful technical tip is to perform the procedure with the MCP joint hyperextended over towels to bring the digital nerves dorsally away from the pulley.[3]

## DE QUERVAIN TENOSYNOVITIS

Irritation of the first dorsal extensor compartment tendons associated with pain underlies de Quervain tenosynovitis. The mechanism underlying this condition is mechanical irritation of the extensor pollicis brevis (EPB) and abductor pollicis longus (APL) rubbing against the narrow fibroosseous sheath overlying the first compartment.[2] However, similar to trigger finger, an absence of inflammation has been noted on histopathologic evaluation of specimens from patients with de Quervain tenosynovitis.[1,45] The incidence is higher in females,[46] particularly those post partum, and in patients who perform activities with repeated ulnar deviation, such as hammering or skiing. Most patients present with pain localized just proximal to the radial styloid over the first compartment with occasional palpable inflammation of the retinaculum (**Fig. 3**). The Finkelstein test (**Fig. 4**),[47] performed by adducting and pronating the thumb

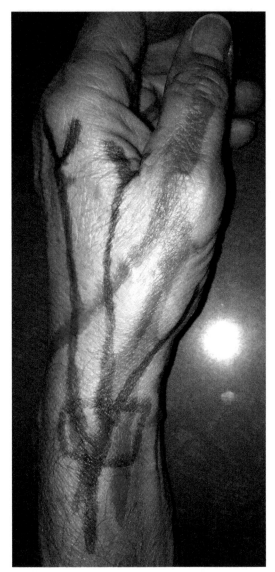

**Fig. 3.** De Quervain disease. The first compartment containing the EPB and AbPL is in close proximity to the SBRN.

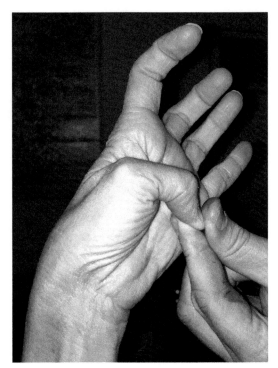

**Fig. 4.** Finkelstein test, performed by adducting and pronating the thumb over the palm, reproducing pain localized to the first dorsal compartment.

over the palm, is positive. The basis for this examination was demonstrated by Kutsumi and colleagues,[48] where in 15 cadavers the EPB tendon had a greater bulk and tethering effect when the thumb was flexed and adducted in comparison with other tendons, including the APL.

The first step in treating patients with de Quervain disease is corticosteroid injections into the first dorsal compartment, forearm-based thumb spica splinting, and activity modification to avoid repetitive stress of the irritated tendons. Injections have efficacy rates of between 62% and 93%,[17,49] whereas the efficacy of splints is controversial. In a series of 249 patients, Lane and colleagues[50]

demonstrated complete (76%) or partial (7%) relief of symptoms in 83% of patients after corticosteroid injection. In an analysis of 7 trials, Richie and Briner[51] found that 83% of patients with de Quervain tenosynovitis were successfully treated with injection alone, compared with 64% with splint and injection, or 14% with splint alone. A Cochrane review of a comparative trial found similar results, with a 100% efficacy associated with a corticosteroid injection compared with 0% efficacy with splint alone.[52] Injection with or without splinting should be attempted for 3 to 6 months to allow adequate time to bring down the tendon irritation and associated inflammation. One possible physical examination finding that potentially predicts failure of nonoperative management was described by Alexander and colleagues[53] to diagnose a separate EPB compartment.

The main surgical approach for de Quervain disease is open decompression, with excellent outcomes demonstrated at long-term follow-up.[54] The first dorsal extensor retinaculum is visualized and decompressed through a longitudinal incision. The superficial branch of the radial nerve (SBRN) is at risk during the approach, and must be visualized and protected to avoid painful neuromas. Special consideration should note the common anatomic anomalies encountered, including a septum dividing the first compartment, separate EPB sub-compartment, and multiple slips of the APL tendon.[55] One additional consideration intraoperatively involves EPB and APL tendon subluxation during ulnar deviation after surgical decompression. If this occurs, lengthening and reconstruction of the retinaculum can be performed, followed by splinting in radial deviation for 4 to 6 weeks. In addition, endoscopic first compartment release[56] and APL slip excision[57] have shown promise, possibly decreasing pain and enhancing functional outcomes.[58]

## EXTENSOR COMPARTMENT ULNARIS TENDINITIS

Ulnar-sided wrist pain has a wide differential diagnosis, with one of the more common being extensor carpi ulnaris (ECU) tendinitis. The ECU is at risk for tendinitis in part because of its anatomy. The ECU travels through the sixth dorsal extensor compartment with the distal ulnar groove within its own separate fibro-osseous subsheath. During forearm pronation the tendon is straight, but angles 30° during supination (**Fig. 5**). The ECU pressure and strain is greatest during supination[59] and wrist flexion,[60] whereas the tendon is primarily stabilized by the distal 50% of its subsheath.[60] Furthermore, it is predisposed to irritation given its many functions, including its role as a dynamic distal radioulnar joint (DRUJ) stabilizer,[61,62] carpal pronation that potentially stabilizes the lunotriquetral joint,[63] and wrist extensor in supination.[64] The tendinopathy is thought to result from repetitive loading and contraction of the ECU with the forearm in supination,[59] such as tennis players with Western grip[65] and two-handed backhand hitting strokes.[66]

Patients at risk for ECU tendinopathies often participate in "ball-and-stick" sports such as tennis, golf, and hockey. Patients have a gradual onset of pain with or without a vague history of an injury.[66] Patients present with pain localized to the sixth dorsal compartment, worse with forearm supination and wrist flexion. Occasionally

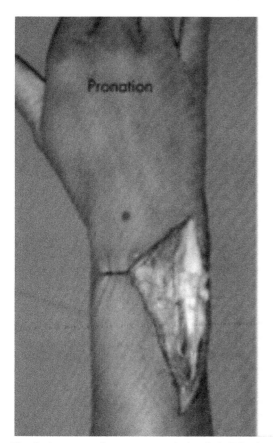
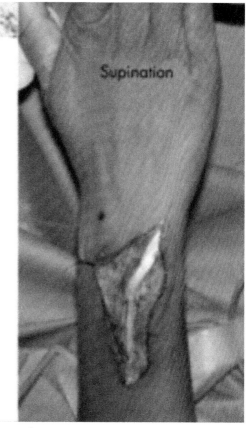

**Fig. 5.** Anatomy of extensor carpi ulnaris (ECU). The ECU is straight in pronation, but curves at a 30° angle in supination, creating increased pressure and tension on the tendon and its subsheath. (*From* Montalvan B, Parier J, Brasseur JL, et al. Extensor carpi ulnaris injuries in tennis players: a study of 28 cases. Br J Sports Med 2006;40:426; with permission.)

they will report dysesthesias in the superficial branch of the ulnar nerve (SBUN). On examination, patients report pain with resisted wrist extension and ulnar deviation, or forced supination, wrist flexion, and ulnar deviation. When examining the patient it is important to differentiate between intra-articular pathology, such as a triangular fibrocartilage complex (TFCC) injury, and extra-articular ECU disorder, as well as ECU tendinitis from ECU subluxation. The synergy test (**Fig. 6**)[67] is helpful in differentiating ECU from intra-articular TFCC injury. This test is performed with the elbow flexed 90° and full forearm supination, whereby resisted thumb abduction produces isometric ECU contraction. In the original description by Ruland and Hogan,[67] 10 of 11 patients with isolated ECU tendinitis had a positive test, whereas 21 of 21 without ECU tendinitis had a negative test. Other tests for ECU disorder include the ice cream scoop test[68] and carpal supination test.[59] ECU subluxation should be noted in any of these provocative maneuvers and compared with the opposite wrist. Ulnar impaction syndrome, another common cause of ulnar-sided wrist pain, can be ruled out on plain radiographs. MRI will often demonstrate edema and tenosynovial thickening in the sixth compartment on gadolinium-enhanced T1-weighted sequences.[69] MRI has been shown to have a sensitivity of 57% and specificity of 88% in diagnosing ECU tendinopathy.[70] Dynamic ultrasound can be used to rule out ECU subluxation.[71] Of note, it is important to examine the opposite wrist, as in one study of 26 asymptomatic tennis players, 92% had ECU tendinosis and 73% had dynamic ECU instability on ultrasonography.[71]

The initial treatment of ECU tendinitis is nonoperative management consisting of activity modification, anti-inflammatory medications, splinting, corticosteroid injection, and gradual return to sport. The splints are ideally positioned in extension and ulnar deviation with the forearm in either neutral or pronation. The splint duration varies in the successful case series in the literature from

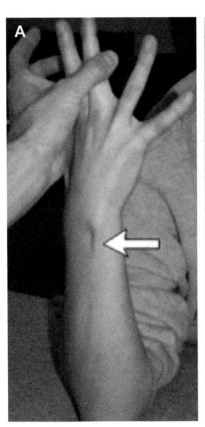
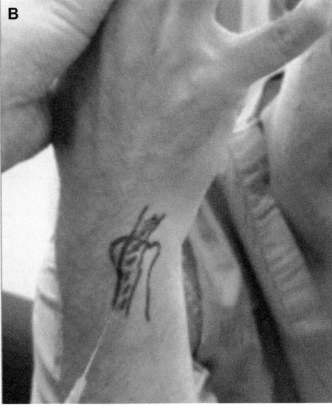

**Fig. 6.** Synergy and diagnostic lidocaine injection tests. (*A*) The synergy test is helpful in differentiating ECU from intra-articular TFCC disability. This test is performed with the elbow flexed 90° and full forearm supination, because resisted thumb abduction produces isometric ECU contraction. (*B*) A diagnostic lidocaine injection in the ECU subsheath can be used to differentiate ECU disorder from other sources of ulnar-sided wrist pain. The subluxing ECU tendon is visualized by the *arrow*. (*From* Ruland RT, Hogan CJ. The ECU synergy test: an aid to diagnose ECU tendinitis. J Hand Surg Am 2008;33:1777–82; with permission.)

4 to 6 weeks[66] to 3 months.[72] The literature has produced variable results on nonoperative management with splints and corticosteroids.[66,72–74] However, it should be noted that greater than 3 corticosteroid injections has been attributed to a risk of ECU tendon rupture in tennis players.[66] Special considerations for tennis players include modifying their swing to a single backhand stroke,[66] using an Eastern grip,[65] using hybrid or gut strings,[65] using a lighter and shorter racquet, and playing on grass courts.

Failure of nonoperative management of ECU tendinitis for at least 6 to 12 weeks often requires surgical intervention tailored to the pathologic situation. One option involves a sixth compartment release, either alone or concomitantly with a subsheath repair and/or excision of the fifth/sixth compartment septum.[75] The sixth compartment is approached via a longitudinal incision over the ECU, taking care to protect the SBUN branches. After compartment release a tenosynovectomy might also be performed in cases of advanced tenosynovitis,[76] and debridement might be required for tendinopathy. Repair of the sixth compartment retinaculum is controversial, with good outcomes reported both with[76] and without[73,77] repair. An accessory ECU[78] is a common cause of failure of nonoperative management (**Fig. 7**). In one series of 43 patients with ECU tendinitis, 40 were successfully treated nonoperatively, whereas 2 of the 3 who failed nonoperative management had an accessory slip of the ECU treated successfully with sixth compartment release and slip excision.[72]

When evaluating a patient with suspected ECU disorder, it is important to consider and/or rule out the other possible causes of ulnar-sided wrist pain, including TFCC disorder, ulnar styloid nonunion, DRUJ disorder, and lunotriquetral (LT) injuries. This is not only critical to confirm the diagnosis, but many cases of ECU have other concomitant disorder that may affect the outcomes of treatment. In a study of 15 patients with ECU tendinitis treated with synovectomy, of the 5 who did not achieve good/excellent results, 4 had a concomitant scapholunate or LT injury and 1 had an ulnar styloid nonunion.[76] One effective strategy to diagnose isolated ECU tendinopathy is a diagnostic injection into the ECU subsheath with lidocaine.[67]

## FOURTH AND FIFTH COMPARTMENT TENOSYNOVITIS

The fourth compartment containing the extensor digitorum communis (EDC) and the fifth compartment containing the extensor digiti minimi (EDM) can also be associated with tenosynovitis.[79] Multiple causes are potentially associated with this condition, with the most common being inflammatory arthritis, although it has also been associated with noninflammatory processes such as wrist arthritis, stiffness, or trauma.[79,80] For example, a prior distal radius fracture, osteophytes from radiocarpal or DRUJ arthritis, or limited motion might alter tendon mechanics, inducing inflammation in the EDC or EDM.

Patients present with pain and swelling localized to the fourth or fifth compartments, with limited wrist extension. Pain is worse with resisted wrist or finger extension. In certain cases an inflammatory mass of thickened synovium will move as the tendons move during finger flexion and extension, known as the "tuck sign."[81] MRI will often demonstrate tenosynovitis in the fourth or fifth compartment.

The initial treatment of tenosynovitis of the fourth or fifth extensor compartments should include activity modification, anti-inflammatory medications, and splints. Splints should immobilize the wrist at minimum, with MCP immobilization if tolerated by the patients. Corticosteroid injections into either compartment can also be considered. Failure of at least 3 to 6 months of nonoperative management may require tenosynovectomy.[79]

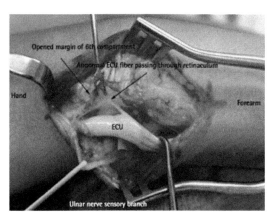

**Fig. 7.** Accessory ECU slip, which can predispose the patient to fail nonoperative management and ultimately requires surgical excision. (*From* Eo S, Bahk S, Jones NF. Wrist pain due to abnormal extensor carpi ulnaris tendon. Arch Plast Surg 2016;43:389–90; with permission.)

## INTERSECTION SYNDROME

Tenosynovitis of the second dorsal compartment as the first dorsal compartment crosses over is a rare clinical entity first described by Velpeau and later termed intersection syndrome by Dobyns and colleagues.[82] Over the years the syndrome has been given other names such as "peritendinitis crepitans," "APL bursitis," "crossover tendinitis," "bugaboo forearm," and "crossover syndrome."[83] The pathophysiology, although not well understood, is an entity distinct from that of de Quervain tenosynovitis. The intersection of the first and second compartment is proximal in the forearm and is located at an average of 4 cm proximal to the Lister tubercle, forming an angle of 60°.[84,85] The clinical entity is defined as pain with wrist flexion or extension with associated swelling over the mid-forearm at this level. This overuse syndrome is often seen in patients who perform repetitive wrist motions as seen in rowing, weightlifting, canoeing, and skiing. In addition, historical reports often called these patients "squeakers" given the audible crepitus that can be heard in some patients that is pathognomonic for the condition.[82] More recently, diagnostic ultrasonography and MRI have demonstrated changes around the first and second compartments. These findings include effusions within the sheaths of the second and/or first compartment, as well as peritendinous edema.[84,85]

Once a formal diagnosis has been confirmed, initial treatment is often conservative and includes rest, ice, oral anti-inflammatories, bracing with a thumb spica splint, and corticosteroid injections. Once patients have failed these nonoperative measures, a surgical release centered over the intersection of the 2 compartments and carried proximally by releasing the first and second compartment fascia has demonstrated good results.[86] Grundberg and Reagan[86] reviewed the results of 13 patients who underwent surgery for intersection syndrome. At an average of 10 months' follow-up, all patients were able to return to their employment. The investigators noted swelling within the sheaths of the APL and EPB, but more consistent edema within the extensor carpi radialis (ECR) longus and ECR brevis sheath. It is their opinion that release of the second compartment provided ultimate relief for the patient.

## EXTENSOR POLLICIS LONGUS TENOSYNOVITIS

Extensor pollicis longus (EPL) tenosynovitis is a rare clinical entity outside of the rheumatoid hand.[81,87,88] Described in the literature by mostly case reports, the etiology is vague but is most commonly associated after sustaining nondisplaced distal radius fractures. When a history of trauma is lacking, the history is often remarkable for pain over the third compartment and pain with passive flexion of the interphalangeal joint of the thumb. MRI may provide a false negative given the acute angle the tendon takes after the Lister tubercle, but ultrasonography is able to provide a more dynamic examination and has been proved superior in diagnosing this rare clinical entity.

Although nonoperative measures can be used, such as with intersection syndrome, experts often recommend decompression of the third compartment with or without transposition. McMahon and Posner[87] have recommended decompression with repair of the retinaculum to prevent bowstringing, whereas Huang and Strauch[81] recommended decompression and transposition of the tendon. In patients whose diagnosis was made late and an attritional rupture identified, a tendon transfer of the extensor indicis proprius to the EPL has garnered excellent results.

## FLEXOR CARPI RADIALIS TENDINITIS

Flexor carpi radialis (FCR) tendinitis was first described in 1930 by Winterstein.[89] A rare clinical entity, it is encountered most commonly in patients with concomitant wrist conditions such as ganglion cysts and scaphotrapeziotrapezoidal arthritis.[89–93] Patients complain of pain over the volar aspect of the wrist with associated resisted wrist flexion. MRI often demonstrates increased fluid signal with enhancement surrounding the FCR tendon sheath.[92] The diagnosis is often confirmed with a lidocaine injection into the FCR sheath.

In patients who have significant relief with the injection but have failed the conservative measures described earlier, a tenosynovectomy and release of the tendon sheath has provided excellent results. The anatomy and technique as described by Gabel and Bishop[90,91] showed a high correlation in those patients with concomitant wrist disorder, which may also need to be addressed at the time of a surgery.

## SUMMARY

Tendinitis or tendinopathy of the upper extremity is a common disorder treated by hand surgeons. The diagnosis is usually clinical, whereas management starts with nonoperative modalities, such as activity modification, corticosteroid injections, and splinting. Operative treatment of these conditions is generally successful after the failure of conservative measures. In each condition there are multiple factors that affect the outcomes of nonoperative and operative management.

## REFERENCES

1. McAuliffe JA. Tendon disorders of the hand and wrist. J Hand Surg Am 2010;35(5):846–53 [quiz: 853].

2. Farnebo S, Chang J. Practical management of tendon disorders in the hand. Plast Reconstr Surg 2013;132(5):841e–53e.

3. Adams JE, Habbu R. Tendinopathies of the hand and wrist. J Am Acad Orthop Surg 2015;23(12): 741–50.

4. Koh S, Nakamura S, Hattori T, et al. Trigger digits in diabetes: their incidence and characteristics. J Hand Surg Eur Vol 2010;35(4):302–5.

5. Sungpet A, Suphachatwong C, Kawinwonggowit V. Trigger digit and BMI. J Med Assoc Thai 1999; 82(10):1025–7.

6. Fitzgibbons PG, Weiss AP. Hand manifestations of diabetes mellitus. J Hand Surg Am 2008;33(5):771–5.

7. Sbernardori MC, Bandiera P. Histopathology of the A1 pulley in adult trigger fingers. J Hand Surg Eur Vol 2007;32(5):556–9.

8. Grandizio LC, Beck JD, Rutter MR, et al. The incidence of trigger digit after carpal tunnel release in diabetic and nondiabetic patients. J Hand Surg Am 2014;39(2):280–5.

9. Hayashi M, Uchiyama S, Toriumi H, et al. Carpal tunnel syndrome and development of trigger digit. J Clin Neurosci 2005;12(1):39–41.

10. Hombal JW, Owen R. Carpal tunnel decompression and trigger digits. Hand 1970;2(2):192–6.

11. Lin FY, Manrique OJ, Lin CL, et al. Incidence of trigger digits following carpal tunnel release: a nationwide, population-based retrospective cohort study. Medicine (Baltimore) 2017;96(27):e7355.

12. Wessel LE, Fufa DT, Boyer MI, et al. Epidemiology of carpal tunnel syndrome in patients with single versus multiple trigger digits. J Hand Surg Am 2013;38(1):49–55.

13. Dala-Ali BM, Nakhdjevani A, Lloyd MA, et al. The efficacy of steroid injection in the treatment of trigger finger. Clin Orthop Surg 2012;4(4):263–8.

14. Sato ES, Gomes Dos Santos JB, Belloti JC, et al. Treatment of trigger finger: randomized clinical trial comparing the methods of corticosteroid injection, percutaneous release and open surgery. Rheumatology (Oxford) 2012;51(1):93–9.

15. Rozental TD, Zurakowski D, Blazar PE. Trigger finger: prognostic indicators of recurrence following corticosteroid injection. J Bone Joint Surg Am 2008; 90(8):1665–72.

16. Korrigan CL, Stanwix MG. Using evidence to minimize the cost of trigger finger care. J Hand Surg Am 2009;34(6):997–1005.

17. Huisstede BM, Gladdines S, Randsdorp MS, et al. Effectiveness of conservative, surgical, and postsurgical interventions for trigger finger, Dupuytren disease, and De Quervain disease: a systematic review. Arch Phys Med Rehabil 2018;99(8): 1635–49.e21.

18. Jianmongkol S, Kosuwon W, Thammaroj T. Intra-tendon sheath injection for trigger finger: the randomized controlled trial. Hand Surg 2007;12(2): 79–82.

19. Shinomiya R, Sunagawa T, Nakashima Y, et al. Impact of corticosteroid injection site on the treatment success rate of trigger finger: a prospective study comparing ultrasound-guided true intra-sheath and true extra-sheath injections. Ultrasound Med Biol 2016;42(9):2203–8.

20. Taras JS, Raphael JS, Pan WT, et al. Corticosteroid injections for trigger digits: is intrasheath injection necessary? J Hand Surg Am 1998;23(4):717–22.

21. Pataradool K, Buranapuntaruk T. Proximal phalanx injection for trigger finger: randomized controlled trial. Hand Surg 2011;16(3):313–7.

22. Rodgers JA, McCarthy JA, Tiedeman JJ. Functional distal interphalangeal joint splinting for trigger finger in laborers: a review and cadaver investigation. Orthopedics 1998;21(3):305–9 [discussion: 309–10].

23. Valdes K. A retrospective review to determine the long-term efficacy of orthotic devices for trigger finger. J Hand Ther 2012;25(1):89–95 [quiz: 96].

24. Colbourn J, Heath N, Manary S, et al. Effectiveness of splinting for the treatment of trigger finger. J Hand Ther 2008;21(4):336–43.

25. Fleisch SB, Spindler KP, Lee DH. Corticosteroid injections in the treatment of trigger finger: a level I and II systematic review. J Am Acad Orthop Surg 2007;15(3):166–71.

26. Peters-Veluthamaningal C, van der Windt DA, Winters JC, et al. Corticosteroid injection for trigger finger in adults. Cochrane Database Syst Rev 2009;(1):CD005617.

27. Miyamoto H, Miura T, Isayama H, et al. Stiffness of the first annular pulley in normal and trigger fingers. J Hand Surg Am 2011;36(9):1486–91.

28. Baumgarten KM, Gerlach D, Boyer MI. Corticosteroid injection in diabetic patients with trigger finger. A prospective, randomized, controlled double-blinded study. J Bone Joint Surg Am 2007;89(12): 2604–11.

29. Roh YH, Lee BK, Kim JK, et al. Effect of metabolic syndrome on the outcome of corticosteroid injection for trigger finger: matched case-control study. J Hand Surg Am 2016;41(10):e331–5.

30. Will R, Lubahn J. Complications of open trigger finger release. J Hand Surg Am 2010;35(4):594–6.

31. Everding NG, Bishop GB, Belyea CM, et al. Risk factors for complications of open trigger finger release. Hand (N Y) 2015;10(2):297–300.

32. Dierks U, Hoffmann R, Meek MF. Open versus percutaneous release of the A1-pulley for stenosing tendovaginitis: a prospective randomized trial. Tech Hand Up Extrem Surg 2008;12(3):183–7.

33. Salim N, Abdullah S, Sapuan J, et al. Outcome of corticosteroid injection versus physiotherapy in the treatment of mild trigger fingers. J Hand Surg Eur Vol 2012;37(1):27–34.

34. Lange-Riess D, Schuh R, Honle W, et al. Long-term results of surgical release of trigger finger and trigger thumb in adults. Arch Orthop Trauma Surg 2009;129(12):1617–9.

35. Baek JH, Chung DW, Lee JH. Factors causing prolonged postoperative symptoms despite absence of complications after a1 pulley release for trigger finger. J Hand Surg Am 2018. https://doi.org/10.1016/j.jhsa.2018.06.023.

36. Codding JL, Bhat SB, Ilyas AM. An economic analysis of MAC versus WALANT: a trigger finger release surgery case study. Hand (N Y) 2017;12(4):348–51.

37. Bae DS, Sodha S, Waters PM. Surgical treatment of the pediatric trigger finger. J Hand Surg Am 2007;32(7):1043–7.

38. Le Viet D, Tsionos I, Boulouednine M, et al. Trigger finger treatment by ulnar superficialis slip resection (U.S.S.R.). J Hand Surg Br 2004;29(4):368–73.

39. Lorthioir J Jr. Surgical treatment of trigger-finger by a subcutaneous method. J Bone Joint Surg Am 1958;40-A(4):793–5.

40. Wang J, Zhao JG, Liang CC. Percutaneous release, open surgery, or corticosteroid injection, which is the best treatment method for trigger digits? Clin Orthop Relat Res 2013;471(6):1879–86.

41. Gilberts EC, Beekman WH, Stevens HJ, et al. Prospective randomized trial of open versus percutaneous surgery for trigger digits. J Hand Surg Am 2001;26(3):497–500.

42. Bamroongshawgasame T. A comparison of open and percutaneous pulley release in trigger digits. J Med Assoc Thai 2010;93(2):199–204.

43. Zhao JG, Kan SL, Zhao L, et al. Percutaneous first annular pulley release for trigger digits: a systematic review and meta-analysis of current evidence. J Hand Surg Am 2014;39(11):2192–202.

44. Chao M, Wu S, Yan T. The effect of miniscalpel-needle versus steroid injection for trigger thumb release. J Hand Surg Eur Vol 2009;34(4):522–5.

45. Clarke MT, Lyall HA, Grant JW, et al. The histopathology of de Quervain's disease. J Hand Surg Br 1998;23(6):732–4.

46. Wolf JM, Sturdivant RX, Owens BD. Incidence of de Quervain's tenosynovitis in a young, active population. J Hand Surg Am 2009;34(1):112–5.

47. Finkelstein H. Stenosing tendovaginitis at the radial styloid process. J Bone Joint Surg 1930;12:509–40.

48. Kutsumi K, Amadio PC, Zhao C, et al. Finkelstein's test: a biomechanical analysis. J Hand Surg Am 2005;30(1):130–5.

49. Ilyas AM. Nonsurgical treatment for de Quervain's tenosynovitis. J Hand Surg Am 2009;34(5):928–9.

50. Lane LB, Boretz RS, Stuchin SA. Treatment of de Quervain's disease:role of conservative management. J Hand Surg Br 2001;26(3):258–60.

51. Richie CA 3rd, Briner WW Jr. Corticosteroid injection for treatment of de Quervain's tenosynovitis: a pooled quantitative literature evaluation. J Am Board Fam Pract 2003;16(2):102–6.

52. Peters-Veluthamaningal C, van der Windt DA, Winters JC, et al. Corticosteroid injection for de Quervain's tenosynovitis. Cochrane Database Syst Rev 2009;(3):CD005616.

53. Alexander RD, Catalano LW, Barron OA, et al. The extensor pollicis brevis entrapment test in the treatment of de Quervain's disease. J Hand Surg Am 2002;27(5):813–6.

54. Scheller A, Schuh R, Honle W, et al. Long-term results of surgical release of de Quervain's stenosing tenosynovitis. Int Orthop 2009;33(5):1301–3.

55. Kulthanan T, Chareonwat B. Variations in abductor pollicis longus and extensor pollicis brevis tendons in the Quervain syndrome: a surgical and anatomical study. Scand J Plast Reconstr Surg Hand Surg 2007;41(1):36–8.

56. Kang HJ, Hahn SB, Kim SH, et al. Does endoscopic release of the first extensor compartment have benefits over open release in de Quervain's disease? J Plast Reconstr Aesthet Surg 2011;64(10):1306–11.

57. Okada M, Kutz JE. Excision of aberrant abductor pollicis longus tendon slips for decompression of de Quervain's disease. J Hand Surg Eur Vol 2011;36(5):379–82.

58. Kang HJ, Koh IH, Jang JW, et al. Endoscopic versus open release in patients with de Quervain's tenosynovitis: a randomised trial. Bone Joint J 2013;95-B(7):947–51.

59. Kataoka T, Moritomo H, Omori S, et al. Pressure and tendon strain in the sixth extensor compartment of the wrist during simulated provocative maneuvers for diagnosing extensor carpi ulnaris tendinitis. J Orthop Sci 2015;20(6):993–8.

60. Ghatan AC, Puri SG, Morse KW, et al. Relative contribution of the subsheath to extensor carpi ulnaris tendon stability: implications for surgical reconstruction and rehabilitation. J Hand Surg Am 2016;41(2):225–32.

61. Spinner M, Kaplan EB. Extensor carpi ulnaris. Its relationship to the stability of the distal radio-ulnar joint. Clin Orthop Relat Res 1970;68:124–9.

62. Iida A, Omokawa S, Moritomo H, et al. Biomechanical study of the extensor carpi ulnaris as a dynamic wrist stabilizer. J Hand Surg Am 2012;37(12):2456–61.

63. Salva-Coll G, Garcia-Elias M, Leon-Lopez MM, et al. Role of the extensor carpi ulnaris and its sheath on dynamic carpal stability. J Hand Surg Eur Vol 2012;37(6):544–8.

64. Horii E, An KN, Linscheid RL. Excursion of prime wrist tendons. J Hand Surg Am 1993;18(1):83–90.

65. Tagliafico AS, Ameri P, Michaud J, et al. Wrist injuries in nonprofessional tennis players: relationships with different grips. Am J Sports Med 2009;37(4):760–7.

66. Montalvan B, Parier J, Brasseur JL, et al. Extensor carpi ulnaris injuries in tennis players: a study of 28 cases. Br J Sports Med 2006;40(5):424–9 [discussion: 429].

67. Ruland RT, Hogan CJ. The ECU synergy test: an aid to diagnose ECU tendonitis. J Hand Surg Am 2008; 33(10):1777–82.

68. Ng CY, Hayton MJ. Ice cream scoop test: a novel clinical test to diagnose extensor carpi ulnaris instability. J Hand Surg Eur Vol 2013;38(5):569–70.

69. Jeantroux J, Becce F, Guerini H, et al. Athletic injuries of the extensor carpi ulnaris subsheath: MRI findings and utility of gadolinium-enhanced fat-saturated T1-weighted sequences with wrist pronation and supination. Eur Radiol 2011;21(1):160–6.

70. Kuntz MT, Janssen SJ, Ring D. Incidental signal changes in the extensor carpi ulnaris on MRI. Hand (N Y) 2015;10(4):750–5.

71. Sole JS, Wisniewski SJ, Newcomer KL, et al. Sonographic evaluation of the extensor carpi ulnaris in asymptomatic tennis players. PM R 2015;7(3): 255–63.

72. Futami T, Itoman M. Extensor carpi ulnaris syndrome. Findings in 43 patients. Acta Orthop Scand 1995;66(6):538–9.

73. Nachinolcar UG, Khanolkar KB. Stenosing tenovaginitis of extensor carpi ulnaris: brief report. J Bone Joint Surg Br 1988;70(5):842.

74. Kollitz KM, Iorio ML, Huang JI. Assessment and treatment of extensor carpi ulnaris tendon pathology: a critical analysis review. JBJS Rev 2015;3(6). https://doi.org/10.2106/JBJS.RVW.N.00070.

75. Hajj AA, Wood MB. Stenosing tenosynovitis of the extensor carpi ulnaris. J Hand Surg Am 1986; 11(4):519–20.

76. Allende C, Le Viet D. Extensor carpi ulnaris problems at the wrist—classification, surgical treatment and results. J Hand Surg Br 2005;30(3):265–72.

77. Kip PC, Peimer CA. Release of the sixth dorsal compartment. J Hand Surg Am 1994;19(4):599–601.

78. Eo S, Bahk S, Jones NF. Wrist pain due to abnormal extensor carpi ulnaris tendon. Arch Plast Surg 2016; 43(4):389–90.

79. Cooper HJ, Shevchuk MM, Li X, et al. Proliferative extensor tenosynovitis of the wrist in the absence of rheumatoid arthritis. J Hand Surg Am 2009; 34(10):1827–31.

80. Drury BJ. Traumatic tendovaginitis of the fifth dorsal compartment of the wrist. Arch Surg 1960;80:554–6.

81. Huang HW, Strauch RJ. Extensor pollicis longus tenosynovitis: a case report and review of the literature. J Hand Surg Am 2000;25(3):577–9.

82. Dobyns JH, Sim FH, Linscheid RL. Sports stress syndromes of the hand and wrist. Am J Sports Med 1978;6(5):236–54.

83. Balakatounis K, Angoules AG, Angoules NA, et al. Synthesis of evidence for the treatment of intersection syndrome. World J Orthop 2017;8(8):619–23.

84. Draghi F, Bortolotto C. Intersection syndrome: ultrasound imaging. Skeletal Radiol 2014;43(3):283–7.

85. Lee RP, Hatem SF, Recht MP. Extended MRI findings of intersection syndrome. Skeletal Radiol 2009; 38(2):157–63.

86. Grundberg AB, Reagan DS. Pathologic anatomy of the forearm: intersection syndrome. J Hand Surg Am 1985;10(2):299–302.

87. McMahon MS, Posner MA. Triggering of the thumb due to stenosing tenosynovitis of the extensor pollicis longus: a case report. J Hand Surg 1994;19(4): 623–5.

88. Kardashian G, Vara AD, Miller SJ, et al. Stenosing synovitis of the extensor pollicis longus tendon. J Hand Surg 2011;36(6):1035–8.

89. Brink PR, Franssen BB, Disseldorp DJ. A simple blind tenolysis for flexor carpi radialis tendinopathy. Hand (N Y) 2015;10(2):323–7.

90. Bishop AT, Gabel G, Carmichael SW. Flexor carpi radialis tendinitis. Part I: operative anatomy. J Bone Joint Surg Am 1994;76(7):1009–14.

91. Gabel G, Bishop AT, Wood MB. Flexor carpi radialis tendinitis. Part II: results of operative treatment. J Bone Joint Surg Am 1994;76(7):1015–8.

92. Parellada AJ, Morrison WB, Reiter SB, et al. Flexor carpi radialis tendinopathy: spectrum of imaging findings and association with triscaphe arthritis. Skeletal Radiol 2006;35(8):572–8.

93. Weeks PM. A cause of wrist pain: non-specific tenosynovitis involving the flexor carpi radialis. Plast Reconstr Surg 1978;62(2):263–6.

# Managing Swan Neck and Boutonniere Deformities

Kate Elzinga, MD[a],*, Kevin C. Chung, MD, MS[b]

## KEYWORDS

- Boutonniere deformity • Swan neck deformity • Extensor tendon mechanism
- Extensor tendon tenotomy • Mallet finger • Oblique retinacular ligament

## KEY POINTS

- The extensor mechanism of the finger is an intricate, highly coordinated structure formed by extrinsic and intrinsic muscles and retinacular ligaments. A disruption in any of its components can lead to pathologic flexion or extension deformities at the interphalangeal joints.
- Corrective splinting is generally the first line of treatment of swan neck and boutonniere deformities of the fingers.
- Surgical intervention aims at rebalancing the extensor tendon forces across the proximal and distal interphalangeal joints. To be successful, joints must be supple and free of arthritis.
- Complete correction of swan neck and boutonniere deformities is difficult to achieve, but the function and esthetics of the interphalangeal joints of the fingers can be greatly improved with splinting and operative interventions.

## INTRODUCTION

The extensor mechanism of the finger is a complex, intricate, highly coordinated structure formed by extrinsic and intrinsic muscles and retinacular ligaments (**Fig. 1**). Swan neck and boutonniere finger deformities result from extensor tendon imbalances. They can present acutely, most commonly in the setting of trauma (sharp laceration, blunt avulsion, burns) or as a progressive deformity (secondary to arthritis). Swan neck deformities are more common than boutonniere deformities.

A swan neck deformity presents with hyperextension at the proximal interphalangeal joint (PIP) and flexion at the distal interphalangeal joint (DIP). The PIP hyperextension impairs the patient's ability to make a fist. Surgical correction can be pursued to restore the patient's hand function.

A boutonniere deformity is defined by flexion at the PIP and hyperextension at the DIP. Grasp and fist are preserved and the patient typically retains good hand function, but the deformity can be aesthetically displeasing. Surgical improvement should only be attempted with caution after thorough patient education. Improving PIP extension can impede PIP flexion, resulting in a poor functional outcome.

Before any tendon rebalancing to correct a swan neck or boutonniere deformity, passive range of motion must be optimized. Hand therapy is important for all patients with these injuries. Corrective splinting, range of motion exercises, and education are essential elements of the patient's care.

Radiographs are taken to ensure that there is no arthritic change present in patients who will be

Disclosure Statement: The authors have nothing to disclose.
[a] Section of Plastic Surgery, University of Calgary, Foothills Medical Centre, Room 382, 1403 - 29 Street Northwest, Calgary, Alberta T2N 2T9, Canada; [b] Section of Plastic Surgery, The University of Michigan Medical School, The University of Michigan Health System, 1500 East Medical Center Drive, 2130 Taubman Center, SPC 5340, Ann Arbor, MI 48109-0340, USA
* Corresponding author.
*E-mail address:* kate.elzinga@ahs.ca

Clin Plastic Surg 46 (2019) 329–337
https://doi.org/10.1016/j.cps.2019.02.006

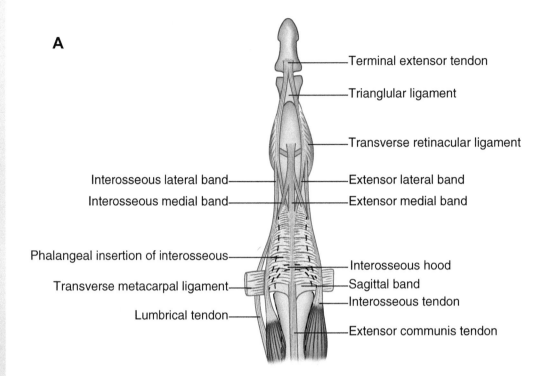

**A**

Terminal extensor tendon

Trianglular ligament

Transverse retinacular ligament

Interosseous lateral band

Extensor lateral band

Interosseous medial band

Extensor medial band

Phalangeal insertion of interosseous

Interosseous hood

Transverse metacarpal ligament

Sagittal band

Interosseous tendon

Lumbrical tendon

Extensor communis tendon

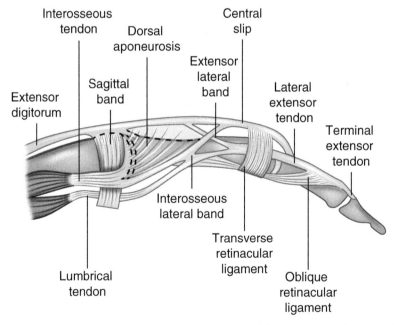

**B**

Interosseous tendon

Central slip

Dorsal aponeurosis

Extensor lateral band

Sagittal band

Lateral extensor tendon

Extensor digitorum

Terminal extensor tendon

Interosseous lateral band

Lumbrical tendon

Transverse retinacular ligament

Oblique retinacular ligament

**Fig. 1.** The extensor tendon mechanism, shown here from a posterior (*A*) and lateral (*B*) view, is formed by extrinsic (extensor digitorum communis) and intrinsic (lumbrical and dorsal interosseous) muscles and retinacular (spiral oblique and transverse retinacular) ligaments. It permits extension through the interphalangeal joints.

undergoing soft tissue reconstructive procedures. When there are signs of arthritis, arthroplasty and arthrodesis are preferred treatments.

## ANATOMY

The extensor mechanism of the finger is formed by extrinsic muscles (extensor digitorum communis) and intrinsic muscles (lumbrical and the dorsal interosseous muscles). As it passes over the dorsal proximal phalanx, the extensor digitorum communis trifurcates into a single central slip and 2 lateral bands (radial and ulnar). The central slip inserts onto the dorsal base of the middle phalanx and is responsible for PIP extension. The lateral bands join the lumbrical and dorsal interosseous muscles to form the conjoint lateral bands. The conjoint lateral bands travel distally and insert onto the dorsal base of the distal phalanx, providing DIP extension.

The triangular ligament is located over the distal proximal phalanx. It counteracts the pull of the oblique retinacular ligament (ORL). It functions to maintain the conjoint lateral bands dorsally over the proximal phalanx. An injury to the triangular ligament can result in lateral and volar subluxation of the distal conjoint lateral bands to cause a swan neck deformity.

The retinacular ligaments, the ORL, and the transverse retinacular ligament coordinate the motion of the extensor mechanism by facilitating simultaneous PIP and DIP flexion and simultaneous PIP and DIP extension.

The ORL travels volar to the axis of the PIP and dorsal to the axis of the DIP. It is functionally present in 40% to 50% of the population.[1] It originates from the volar middle third of the proximal phalanx and the flexor sheath, travels deep to the transverse retinacular ligament dorsally, and inserts on the lateral terminal extensor tendon distally.[2]

When the PIP flexes, the ORL is relaxed, permitting DIP flexion. When the PIP extends, the ORL tightens, and the DIP extends.

The transverse retinacular ligament begins from the lateral flexor tendon sheath at the PIP and terminates at the lateral border of the conjoint lateral bands. When the PIP flexes, it pulls the lateral bands volarly over the PIP. With PIP extension, it limits the dorsal translation of the lateral bands (**Fig. 2**).

## SWAN NECK RECONSTRUCTION

Swan neck deformities can arise from pathology at the metacarpophalangeal (MCP) joint, PIP, or DIP. Causes include volar MCP subluxation, a lax PIP volar plate, a flexor digitorum superficialis

laceration, intrinsic muscle contracture, or a mallet finger. Treatment is aimed at the cause of the deformity.

Chronic mallet injuries are the most common cause of a swan neck deformity. The extensor tendon disruption at the DIP leads to DIP flexion and PIP hyperextension as the lateral bands migrate volarly. Swan neck deformities are first treated with splinting. The DIP is splinted in extension (neutral to 10° of hyperextension), and the PIP is splinted in a dorsal blocking splint with 40° to 60° of flexion.[3] The splint is worn full time for 8 weeks and then weaned off during the day over the following 6 weeks. It is worn at night for 3 months.

If nonoperative measures fail, surgical treatment options for a chronic mallet injury include[4]:

- Direct zone 1 extensor tendon repair and/or DIP skin imbrication
- Central slip tenotomy for extensor mechanism rebalancing by the retracting central tendon that pulls on the terminal tendon through the lateral bands
  - Indicated for an extensor lag less than 35° to 40° at the DIP where the extensor tendon is attenuated but remains in-continuity
- Spiral ORL creation using a free tendon graft
  - Indicated for extensor lags over 45° at the DIP or when there is no tendon continuity between the extensor tendon and the distal phalanx
- Salvage procedures
  - Arthrodesis at the DIP

### Tenodermodesis

A K wire is placed to maintain the DIP in full extension for 6 weeks. An elliptical resection of skin and scarred extensor tendon is excised over the DIP. The skin and extensor tendon are sutured together.

### Central Slip Tenotomy

If the extensor tendon is intact, but is attenuated and elongated over the DIP, release of the central slip at its insertion onto the dorsal base of the middle phalanx will permit the extensor tendon mechanism to move proximally, thereby tightening the extensor mechanism distally and improving extension through the DIP. A midlateral approach is typically used. The lateral bands are protected as the central slip is released from its deep surface. The triangular ligament is preserved to prevent a boutonniere deformity.

Postoperatively, the DIP is splinted in extension and the PIP is splinted in a dorsal blocking splint in

**A  PIP flexion**

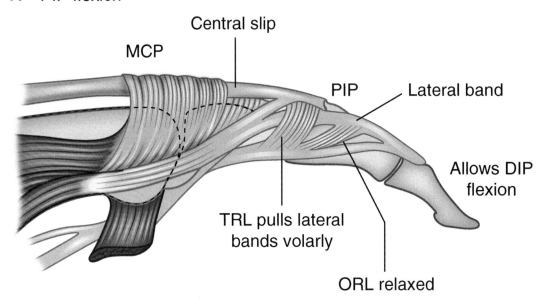

**B  PIP extension**

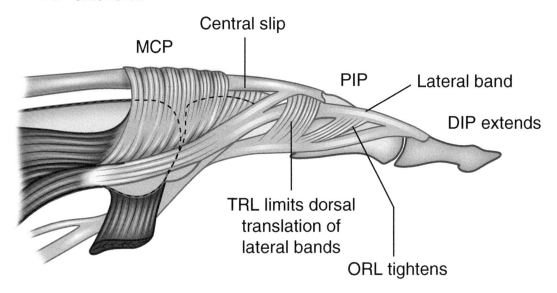

**Fig. 2.** When the PIP flexes, the transverse retinacular ligament (TRL) pulls the lateral bands volarly (aiding PIP flexion) and the oblique retinacular ligament (ORL) relaxes (permitting coordinated DIP flexion) (A). With PIP extension, the TRL limits the dorsal translation of the lateral bands (preventing PIP hyperextension) and the ORL tightens (permitting coordinated DIP extension) (B).

20° of flexion to maximize the tension on the extensor mechanism at the DIP. The dorsal blocking splint is worn for 2 weeks. PIP hyperextension should be avoided. The DIP extension splint is worn for 4 weeks. It is removed several times during the day so the patient can perform active range of motion exercises. From weeks 4 to 8 postoperatively, the DIP extension splint is worn at night.

On average, 36° (range 30°–46°) of extensor tendon lag at the DIP can be corrected with this technique.[5] An improvement in the PIP hyperextension seen in a swan neck deformity also occurs when the insertion the central slip is divided.

## Spiral Oblique Retinacular Ligament Creation

Creation of an ORL restores flexion across the PIP and extension across the DIP. A lateral band[6] or a tendon graft is used. Palmaris or plantaris tendons are most commonly used. The new "ligament" is positioned volar to the PIP and dorsal to the DIP. The tendon graft is fixed distally to the distal phalanx with a suture anchor or a pull-out button, then placed between the flexor tendon sheath and the neurovascular bundle volar to the PIP and secured to the proximal phalanx with a suture anchor or pull-out button (**Fig. 3**). K wires or splints are used to hold the PIP in 10° to 15° of flexion and the DIP in extension. Active motion exercises are started within 3 to 7 days of the reconstruction.

The ORL creates a dynamic tenodesis. When the PIP is actively extended, the DIP will also extend. Equivalent outcomes have been reported for both lateral band and tendon graft reconstructions.[7] Pull-out sutures and bone anchors were also equivalent. On average, the DIP extensor lag improved by 30° for those

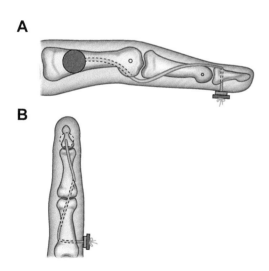

**A**

**B**

**Fig. 3.** In a spiral oblique retinacular ligament reconstruction, a free tendon graft is passed volar to the axis of rotation of the PIP and dorsal to the axis of rotation of the DIP joint (*A-B*). This corrects the PIP hyperextension and the DIP flexion of a swan neck deformity.

treated after a soft tissue injury.[7] There was minimal improvement in the extensor lag, however, for those with distal phalanx fractures.

## Arthrodesis

For a painful DIP with arthritic changes visible on radiographs, DIP arthrodesis is recommended. Splints can be applied to help determine the optimal angle of fusion for each individual patient, typically in neutral to slight flexion. Headless compression screws, K wires, tension band constructs, interosseous wiring, plates and screws, and staples can be used. Clinical union takes 8 weeks on average.[8]

Proximal interphalangeal joint pathology can lead to a swan neck deformity. In rheumatoid arthritis, stretching of the volar plate commonly occurs as a result of inflammation of the synovial pannus, which leads to PIP hyperextension. The lateral bands move dorsally, leading to slack in the extensor mechanism and DIP flexion. When the PIP remains flexible in all positions of the MCP, treatment options for the PIP include splinting, volar plate advancement, dermadesis, flexor digitorum superficialis tenodesis, and ORL reconstruction. If there is additional intrinsic muscle tightness, an intrinsic release is added to the treatment plan. If the dorsal PIP skin is tight, a Z-plasty or full-thickness skin graft can performed. Lateral band mobilization and dorsal capsule release of the PIP can help correct the PIP hyperextension (**Fig. 4**). If the central slip has shortened, a step-cut lengthening can be beneficial (**Fig. 5**).

## BOUTONNIERE RECONSTRUCTION

Boutonniere deformities arise from pathology at the PIP. Central slip injuries and attenuation of the triangular ligament result in a boutonniere deformity. The conjoint lateral bands migrate volarly over the radial and ulnar aspects of the digit, volar to the axis of the PIP. With force through the extensor mechanism, the PIP is subject to a pathologic flexion force. Over time, the conjoint lateral bands contract and create an extension force across the DIP. Proximal interphalangeal joint flexion and DIP hyperextension result. Gradually, the ORL and the transverse retinacular ligament also contract, worsening the DIP hyperextension.

For acute, flexible boutonniere deformities, the PIP is splinted continuously in extension for 6 weeks, with the DIP free to flex to stretch out the contracted lateral bands. Active DIP range of motion exercises are performed hourly to permit distal gliding of the lateral

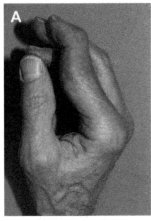
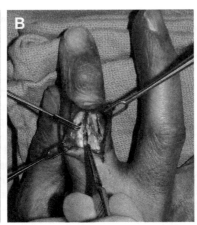
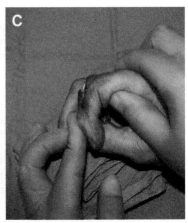

**Fig. 4.** PIP joint hyperextension (*A*) (preoperative image) can be improved by release of the lateral bands over the PIP (*B*) (intraoperative image, dorsal approach), allowing them to move volarly to the axis of the joint. The tight dorsal capsule of the PIP joint can be released to improve passive (*C*) (intraoperative image) and active PIP flexion.

bands and central slip, movement of the lateral bands back into their correct dorsal alignment, stretching of the tight transverse retinacular ligaments, and tightening of the triangular ligament. The splint is then weaned during the day and PIP active flexion exercises begin. The splint is worn at night for an additional 6 weeks.

For patients with chronic supple, passively corrected boutonniere deformities, splinting is the mainstay of treatment, surgery is rarely indicated. Orthoses are used to achieve full PIP extension. Dynamic or serial splinting or casting can be

used. The full extension is maintained for 6 to 12 weeks with splints. Distal interphalangeal joint active and passive flexion exercises are performed throughout. If PIP extension cannot be achieved with therapy alone, operative release of contracted collateral ligaments and/or volar plate can be performed (**Fig. 6**).

For boutonniere deformities unresponsive to splinting, surgical correction focuses on decreasing the extensor tone at the DIP and increasing the extensor force at the PIP. Full passive motion must be present before surgery. Joint releases, in particular volar plate release, must be

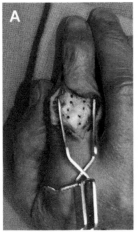
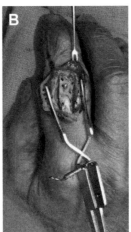
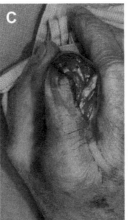
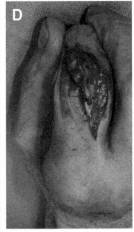

**Fig. 5.** PIP joint hyperextension can be corrected using a dorsal approach to the PIP joint. The lateral bands and central slip are identified and marked (*A*). The radial and ulnar lateral bands are mobilized away from the central slip (*B*), allowing them to move volarly. The central slip can be lengthened (*C*) to further correct the PIP hyperextension and sutured over the dorsal PIP joint in an elongated position (*D*).

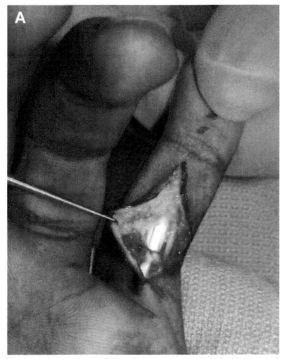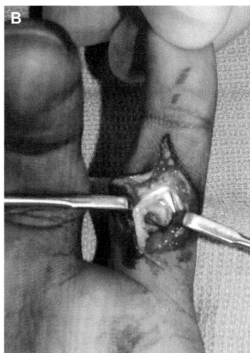

**Fig. 6.** A swan neck deformity can result from a tight volar plate. A volar approach to the PIP joint allows identification of the flexor tendons (*A*), their retraction, and then release of the underlying volar plate (*B*) and improved PIP extension.

performed before any tendon reconstruction. Surgical options include:

- Terminal tendon tenotomy
- Staged Curtis procedure

Boutonniere deformities do not typically limit function. The risks and benefits of surgical intervention must be thoroughly discussed with the patient. Despite surgical correction of a boutonniere deformity, 20° of persistent extensor lag is common at the PIP. Performing surgery for PIP extensor lags less than 30° may not result in marked improvement postoperatively. There is a risk of worsening PIP flexion by attempting to correct the extension of the PIP.

## Terminal Tendon Tenotomy

The extensor tendon is divided over the distal middle phalanx, proximal to the triangular ligament, which in essence preserves the ORLs by avoiding a chronic mallet finger. This corrects the hyperextension deformity at the DIP, but does not result in a mallet finger deformity, also likely owing to the chronically tight collateral ligaments and DIP capsule. A DIP extension splint is worn for 6 to 8 weeks between active range of motion exercises. The extensor mechanism migrates proximally,

increasing the extensor tension at the PIP, thus correcting the flexion deformity of the PIP.

## Staged Curtis Procedure

A staged Curtis reconstruction can be performed for stepwise correction of a boutonniere deformity (**Table 1**).

Local anesthesia is used, permitting the patient to actively test their range of motion during

| Table 1 | |
|---|---|
| **Curtis staged technique for the repair of the traumatic boutonniere deformity** | |
| **Stage** | **Procedure** |
| I | Tenolysis of the extensor tendon and freeing of the transverse retinacular ligament |
| II | Sectioning of the transverse retinacular ligament |
| III | Tendon lengthening of the lateral bands over the middle phalanx |
| IV | Repair of the central extensor tendon |

*Data from* Curtis RM, Reid RL, Provost JM. A staged technique for the repair of the traumatic boutonniere deformity. J Hand Surg Am 1983;8(2):167–71.

the surgery. A dorsal curvilinear incision is used over the PIP. In the first stage, the transverse retinacular ligament is freed and an extensor tendon tenolysis performed. Extension is reassessed, if incomplete, stage II is performed, in which the transverse retinacular ligament is divided and the lateral bands move dorsally (**Fig. 7**). If full extension is still not achieved, stage III or IV is performed depending on the extensor lag. For an extensor lag of 20° or less, a Fowler tenotomy is performed for stage III. The extensor mechanism is divided distal to the triangular ligament (**Fig. 8**). For an extensor lag over 20°, stage IV is performed. The central slip tendon is transected and advanced distally for 4 to 6 mm. It is secured to the dorsal base of the middle phalanx with a suture anchor. The slack lateral bands are loosely sutured to the central slip tendon (**Fig. 9**).

Curtis reported a persistent 10° PIP extensor lag at 1 year follow-up, with an average of 31°

**A** Prior to the TRL division

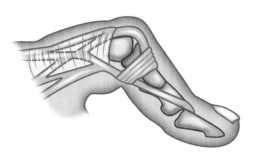

**B** After the TRL division

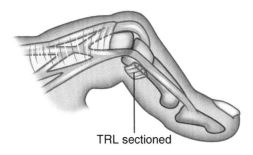

TRL sectioned

**Fig. 7.** During a staged Curtis procedure, tenolysis of the extensor tendon and transverse retinacular ligament is performed as stage I (*A*). The procedure proceeds to stage II if the boutonniere deformity persists after stage I. In stage II, the transverse retinacular ligament is released to allow dorsal movement of the lateral bands (*B*). TRL, transverse retinacular ligament.

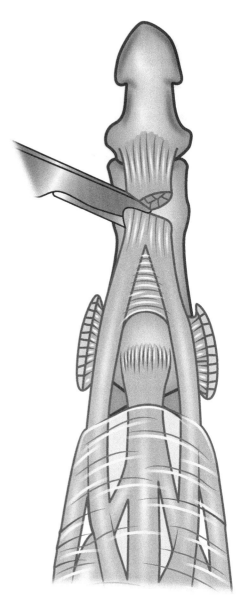

**Fig. 8.** A Fowler tenotomy is performed by releasing the extensor tendon distal to the triangular ligament over the distal middle phalanx. This procedure corrects extensor lags up to 20° at the DIP.

of improvement.[9] A staged approach minimizes the risk of a loss of flexion postoperatively at the PIP.

## Arthroplasty or Arthrodesis

For patients with PIP arthritis, arthroplasty or arthrodesis are recommended to relieve pain. Distal interphalangeal joint arthritis can be surgically treated with arthrodesis.

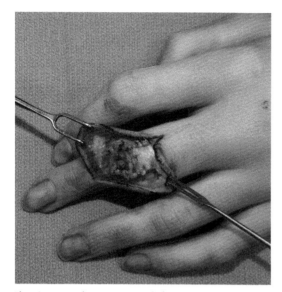

**Fig. 9.** For a boutonniere deformity with a loss of extension through the PIP, the central slip can be advanced and resecured to the dorsal base of the middle phalanx distally using a bone anchor. The lateral bands can be sutured to the radial and ulnar edges of the central slip with nonabsorbable sutures to improve their position over the dorsal PIP joint and thus their ability to extend this joint.

## SUMMARY

Early recognition and treatment of extensor tendon injuries is best to prevent extensor tendon imbalances and resultant swan neck and boutonniere deformities. Once established, these deformities can require prolonged courses of splinting and, less commonly, surgery for correction.

## REFERENCES

1. Shrewsbury MM, Johnson RK. A systematic study of the oblique retinacular ligament of the human finger: its structure and function. J Hand Surg Am 1977; 2(3):194–9.
2. Wehbé MA. Anatomy of the extensor mechanism of the hand and wrist. Hand Clin 1995;11(3):361–6.
3. Lutz K, Pipicelli J, Grewal R. Management of complications of extensor tendon injuries. Hand Clin 2015; 31(2):301–10.
4. Strauch R. Extensor tendon injury. In: Wolfe S, Hotchkiss R, Pederson W, et al, editors. Green's operative hand surgery, vol. 1, 6th edition. Philadelphia: Elsevier; 2011. p. 159–88.
5. Chao JD, Sarwahi V, Da Silva YS, et al. Central slip tenotomy for the treatment of chronic mallet finger: an anatomic study. J Hand Surg Am 2004;29(2):216–9.
6. Chung K. Operative techniques: hand and wrist surgery. 3rd edition. Philadelphia: Elsevier; 2017.
7. Oh JY, Kim JS, Lee DC, et al. Comparative study of spiral oblique retinacular ligament reconstruction techniques using either a lateral band or a tendon graft. Arch Plast Surg 2013;40(6):773–8.
8. Ruchelsman DE, Hazel A, Mudgal CS. Treatment of symptomatic distal interphalangeal joint arthritis with percutaneous arthrodesis: a novel technique in select patients. Hand (N Y) 2010;5(4):434–9.
9. Curtis RM, Reid RL, Provost JM. A staged technique for the repair of the traumatic boutonniere deformity. J Hand Surg Am 1983;8(2):167–71.

# The Pathogenesis and Treatment of the Stiff Finger

Eric D. Wang, MD, Paymon Rahgozar, MD*

## KEYWORDS

- Stiff finger • Contracture • Metacarpophalangeal joint • Proximal interphalangeal joint
- Capsulotomy • Tenolysis • Progressive splinting • Dynamic splinting

## KEY POINTS

- Evaluation and treatment of the stiff finger requires understanding of the complex periarticular anatomy surrounding the metacarpophalangeal and proximal interphalangeal joints.
- Finger joint stiffness is best avoided with appropriate splinting, therapy, and minimizing postinjury swelling, edema, and pain. It is much more difficult to treat as a chronic problem.
- Nonoperative therapy is the mainstay of treatment, with targeted operative interventions reserved for motivated patients who have either plateaued or have not responded to aggressive therapy.
- Surgery for contracted joints sequentially releases pathologic structures, including the joint capsule, volar plate, collateral ligaments, and surrounding tendons, to achieve functional mobility.

## INTRODUCTION

The metacarpophalangeal (MCP) joint, proximal interphalangeal (PIP) joint, and distal interphalangeal (DIP) joint maintain a complementary relationship; injury at one joint may lead to dysfunction of neighboring joints or digits. Many structures are present within a tight joint space, pronouncing the effect of edema and inflammation from the smallest of injuries.

The initial response to injury is inflammation, causing edema and pain. Within a week, proinflammatory leukocytes and mediators surround the injured digit resulting in a fibroblastic phase, which lasts for approximately 3 weeks. Collagen is deposited in a disorganized manner, causing adhesions. Either inadequate or overzealous immobilization at this juncture can be detrimental. The final stage of the response to injury is remodeling of disorganized collagen. Completion of this phase is marked by the end of meaningful gains in therapy, complete healing with supple skin and soft tissue, and resolution of edema.[1]

Prevention of stiffness is a core tenet of hand surgery and therapy. However, approaching the stiff digit requires a nuanced evaluation of the specific pathologic situation in each case. This review addresses the pathogenesis of the stiff finger and the selection, timing, execution, and expected outcomes of surgical treatment.

## ANATOMY
### The Metacarpophalangeal Joint

The MCP joint is a condylar joint with an arc of motion ranging from slight hyperextension to 90° of flexion (**Fig. 1**). The volar plate is the thick, fibrous portion of the volar joint capsule that originates proximally from the metacarpal head and inserts on the base of the proximal phalanx. It primarily limits hyperextension. The dorsal joint capsule is closely associated with the extensor tendon. The

Disclosure Statement: Neither Dr E.D. Wang nor Dr P. Rahgozar has commercial relationships or conflicts of interest to disclose.
Division of Plastic and Reconstructive Surgery, Department of Surgery, UC San Francisco Medical Center, 505 Parnassus Avenue, Suite M593, San Francisco, CA 94143, USA
* Corresponding author.
*E-mail address:* paymon.rahgozar@ucsf.edu

Clin Plastic Surg 46 (2019) 339–345
https://doi.org/10.1016/j.cps.2019.02.007
0094-1298/19/© 2019 Elsevier Inc. All rights reserved.

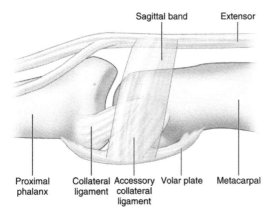

**Fig. 1.** The metacarpophalangeal joint. (*From* Chung KC. Operative techniques: hand and wrist surgery. 3rd edition. Elsevier: Philadelphia; 2018; with permission.)

sagittal bands of the extensor tendon originate from the volar plate, wrap around the joint capsule, and insert on the extensor hood.

Paired proper collateral ligaments originate from the ulnar and radial boundaries of the metacarpal and insert on the base of the proximal phalanx. Accessory collateral ligaments arise volar to the proper collateral ligaments and insert on the volar plate.[2] In extension, the cam-shaped metacarpal head creates redundancy in the collateral ligaments and the dorsal capsule, permitting a limited degree of radial and ulnar deviation. The collateral ligaments are on maximal stretch at 70° of flexion.[3] In the setting of postinjury swelling without appropriate splinting, the MCP joint assumes a position of extension, with laxity of the dorsal capsule and the collateral ligaments. This results in shortening of the collateral ligaments, scarring of the joint capsule, and stiffness of the joint.

## The Proximal Interphalangeal Joint

The PIP joint is a hinge joint, with an arc of motion ranging from slight hyperextension to 110° of flexion. Unlike the MCP joint, it does not permit motion in the coronal plane. This stability arises from the bicondylar geometry of the articular surfaces as well as the thick volar plate and collateral ligaments.[4]

The proper collateral ligaments originate from the lateral portion of the proximal phalanx head and insert on the volar portion of the middle phalanx base and volar plate. Accessory collateral ligaments originate volar to the proper collateral ligaments and insert laterally onto the volar plate.[5] The proximal aspect of the volar plate forms 2 projections known as checkrein ligaments that extend over the transverse digital artery and insert onto the volar aspect of the proximal phalanx (**Fig. 2**A, B). Dorsally, the extensor tendon lies in close association with the joint capsule.

In contrast to the MCP joint, the injured PIP joint adopts a flexed position. Without therapy, fibrosis of the volar plate, shortening of the checkrein ligaments, and contracture of the periarticular soft tissues quickly leads to a flexion deformity.

## EVALUATION AND TREATMENT ALGORITHM

The treatment of a stiff digit requires an educated and motivated patient who is medically and psychologically prepared for treatment and therapy. Persistent hypersensitivity and regional pain syndrome should be controlled, and scars should be matured. Functional goals are tailored to the patient's needs, occupation, and expectations.[6] A hand therapist should be involved to maximize

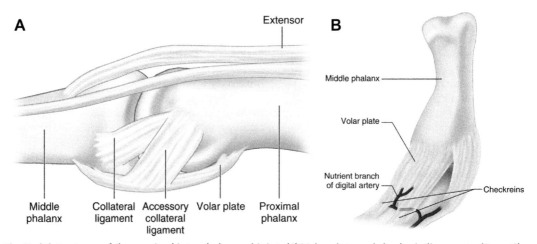

**Fig. 2.** (*A*) Anatomy of the proximal interphalangeal joint. (*B*) Volar plate and checkrein ligaments. (*From* Chung KC. Operative techniques: hand and wrist surgery. 3rd edition. Elsevier: Philadelphia; 2018; with permission.)

passive joint motion and to treat scars, hypersensitivity, and edema.

The goal of the patient examination is to identify the source of the stiffness, which may include pathology of one or more of the following structures:

1. Osseous and articular: metacarpals, phalanges, and joint surface
2. Capsuloligamentous: proper and accessory collateral ligaments, volar plate, and joint capsule
3. Musculotendinous units: extensor mechanism, flexor tendons, intrinsic contributions, and tenosynovium
4. Soft tissue and fascia: skin, subcutaneous tissue, neurovascular structures, and superficial fascia

Radiographs are helpful in identifying a bony block to motion. The stability and compliance of skin, fascial, and neurovascular structures should be assessed. Passive and active motion of each joint is evaluated. Passive motion that exceeds active motion suggests musculotendinous unit disruption, subluxation, or adhesions. However, if active and passive motion are equivalent, the cause of the stiffness is most likely related to intra-articular disorder or capsuloligamentous fibrosis.[6,7]

Decreased passive finger extension with the wrist in maximal extension suggests extrinsic flexor muscle-tendon shortening or adhesions. In cases of extension contracture, the Bunnell test can help determine whether intrinsic muscle tightness is present. The test is positive if there is less PIP joint flexion with MCP joint extension when compared with MCP joint flexion.[8,9]

### Prevention

Secondary dysfunction and deformities can often be prevented if initial care follows the principles of hand surgery. This treatment includes repair or replacement of normal anatomy, elevation to control edema, immobilization in the protective "intrinsic plus" position (30° wrist extension, 90° of MCP joint flexion, and full extension of PIP joint and DIP joint; **Fig. 3**), and early motion protocols when appropriate to prevent fibrosis and adhesions.[6,10]

### NONOPERATIVE INTERVENTION

The initial treatment of the stiff finger consists of a therapy program aimed at softening and stretching scar tissue as well as maximizing passive range of motion (ROM).[11–13] Exercises are supplemented with splinting: dynamic, static-progressive, or serial static splints. All types of splinting apply

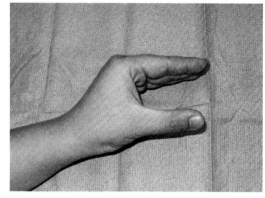

**Fig. 3.** The intrinsic plus "safe" position.

mechanical force to the joint at its end point of motion to encourage stretching of contracted tissues. Static and static-progressive splinting apply inelastic forces to the joint to position it at maximal stretch, but need to be refabricated or adjusted in intervals. Dynamic splints apply a preset force across the joint using springs or elastics to position the joint at maximal stretch. Either type of splinting regimen has been demonstrated to be equally effective.[13]

In a series of 212 stiff joints, therapy alone successfully treated 87% of PIP joint and MCP joint contractures.[14] The groups of Flowers and Glasgow[15–17] demonstrated that passive ROM gains are a function of increasing splint time and force applied. However, the optimal intensity and duration of therapy is not well defined. Excessive external force can cause damage from tearing of soft tissues and ligaments or articular subluxation. Time spent splinting reaches a practical maximum based on the limits of patient tolerance and diminishing returns.[15,17]

Numerous researchers have investigated external devices for mobilizing a PIP joint flexion contracture.[18–21] Placed surgically, these devices apply skeletal traction across the PIP joint in the form of gradual extension or distraction as the device is adjusted. These devices stretch not only the deeper capsuloligamentous tissues and musculotendinous units but also stretch the soft tissue and fascia, as in Dupuytren contracture. Institutional results from these devices have shown promising improvements in PIP joint arc of motion, with a mean of 67° over long-term follow-up.[20]

### SURGICAL INTERVENTIONS

The end point for nonoperative therapy is poorly defined. However, the consensus among most hand surgeons[6,7,22] is to offer operative intervention when nonoperative therapy has failed to produce additional desired gains. The focus of these interventions is the MCP joint and the PIP joint.

## Osseous and Articular Pathology

Bone and joint pathology is addressed first. A fracture malunion, rotational malunion greater than 10°, or presence of exostoses may cause a fixed block to joint motion and is corrected with an osteotomy.[23–26] Joint replacement of the MCP and PIP joints has also been described as a potential treatment. However, multiple reviews have not demonstrated significant improvement in ROM.[20,27–32] Therefore, joint replacement may be more applicable for treatment of pain rather than stiffness.

## Skin and Fascia

A stable, compliant soft-tissue covering is necessary for surgical recovery and early rehabilitation. Contracted scar and prior skin grafts may require excision and reconstruction with vascularized tissue in the form of local or distant flaps. Restricted passive motion caused by skin or fascial contracture is treated with release, fasciotomy, and/or resurfacing.

## Tendon Tenolysis/Reconstruction

Fingers with normal passive extension but limited active extension may have disruption or incompetence of the extensor mechanism, which can be corrected with an extensor tenolysis, rebalancing, or reconstruction. When active flexion is diminished, flexor tendon adhesions can be treated with tenolysis, but flexor incompetence may require a staged tendon reconstruction. These procedures can be performed in combination with capsuloligamentous releases.[33]

## Sequencing of Procedures

Operations are performed in a stepwise sequence designed to facilitate joint mobility during recovery and minimize the need for protective immobilization.[34–36] Motion is reassessed after each step until functional goals are achieved. Performing the procedure with local anesthetic, minimal sedation, and no tourniquet permits immediate intraoperative assessment of improvements in active ROM.[37] A counter-incision at the wrist may be used to simulate active tendon excursion if the patient is under general anesthesia.

In cases of both extension and flexion contracture, a staged approach is recommended, with immediate postoperative therapy after the first stage to maximize passive ROM. Simultaneous surgery on dorsal and volar structures compromises effective therapy because of excessive postoperative pain and edema.[6,7]

## Proximal Interphalangeal Joint Flexion Contracture Release

PIP joint flexion contractures are treated through either a volar or midlateral approach.[36] The authors prefer a midlateral incision dorsal to the neurovascular bundle (**Fig. 4**). The transverse retinacular ligament and A3 pulley are divided. The flexor tendon is retracted in a volar direction, providing exposure to the proper collateral, accessory collateral, and checkrein ligaments. The volar plate is dissected subperiosteally and the checkrein ligaments are incised, taking care to avoid the transverse digital artery. The volar accessory collateral ligaments are then partially incised. The proper collateral ligaments are also released if necessary. Tenolysis is performed if flexor tendon adhesions are further limiting passive extension. The patient should begin aggressive ROM exercises within 48 to 72 hours after surgery.

Brüser and colleagues[38] compared the midlateral with the palmar approach and found that at a minimum of 1.5 years of follow-up, the midlateral technique had a greater improvement in the arc of motion. These investigators concluded that quicker healing with this approach facilitated earlier therapy and superior outcomes.

Overall, reported outcomes in surgical PIP joint flexion contracture release are mixed among series. In contrast to the 30° to 50° gain in extension reported by Brüser and colleagues[38] and the 25° to 30° gain reported by Hogan and Nunley,[39] Ghidella and coworkers[40] found that improvements were modest at 2-year follow-up, with an average of only 5.8° improvement in extension and a 31% reoperation rate. Older patients experienced the worst outcomes in the Ghidella series, emphasizing the importance of surgical patient selection.

## Proximal Interphalangeal Joint Extension Contracture Release

PIP joint extension contracture release is performed through a dorsal curvilinear incision. Once the extensor apparatus is exposed, an incision is made on either side of the extensor tendon to separate it from the lateral bands. A tenolysis is performed, ensuring that the central slip insertion is not violated. A dorsal capsulotomy or capsulectomy is performed. If full passive flexion is not obtained, the proper and accessory collateral ligament fibers are sequentially released from their origin on the proximal phalanx beginning dorsally (**Fig. 5**C). Active flexion of the PIP joint

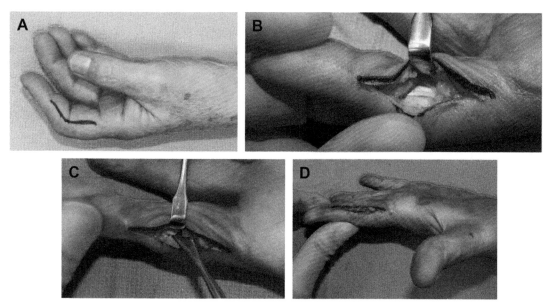

**Fig. 4.** (A) Preferred midlateral approach for index finger PIP joint flexion contracture capsuloligamentous release. (B) Exposure of the flexor tendons after retraction of the neurovascular bundles, division of transverse retinacular fibers, and division of A3 pulley. (C) Volar retraction of the flexor tendon provides exposure to incise proper and accessory collateral ligaments at their origin. Photo shows subperiosteal dissection of the volar plate and release of checkrein ligaments. (D) Immediate correction of PIP flexion contracture. Bilateral incisions can be used to improve exposure. (*Courtesy of* Kevin C. Chung, MD, Ann Arbor, MI.)

is then tested. If incomplete, a flexor tenolysis is performed.[41] Alternatively, adhesions between the central extensor tendon, lateral bands, and dorsal capsule are divided and the finger flexed under anesthesia with placement of a dorsal blocking Kirschner wire.[42]

If the cause of PIP joint extension contracture is intrinsic tightness, the intrinsic contributions to the extensor aponeurosis (lateral band and oblique

fibers) are divided in a distal intrinsic release.[9,43] If the MCP joints are also affected with a flexion deformity caused by interosseous fibrosis, the intrinsic tendons are divided proximally.[9]

Mansat and Delprat[44] described results of PIP joint contracture release in a multicenter study. Among their cohort of extension contractures, a 28° improvement in arc of motion was maintained over long-term follow-up.

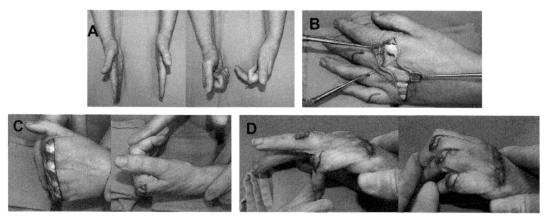

**Fig. 5.** (A) Preoperative extension contracture of left hand PIP joint and MCP joint. (B) Dorsal skin incisions for approach to MCP joint and PIP joint extension contracture release, and release of sagittal bands for exposure to dorsal MCP joint capsule and collateral ligaments. (C) Intraoperative MCP joint flexion following tenolysis, dorsal capsulotomy, and sequential release of collateral ligaments. (D) Intraoperative PIP joint flexion following extensor tenolysis, dorsal capsulotomy, and release of proper and accessory collateral ligaments. (*Courtesy of* Kevin C. Chung, MD, Ann Arbor, MI.)

## Metacarpophalangeal Joint Extension Contracture Release

The MCP joint is approached dorsally by splitting the extensor tendon or by incising the sagittal band.[3,45] An extensor tenolysis may be performed first for exposure, followed by a dorsal capsulotomy or capsulectomy. The most dorsal fibers of the collateral ligament are divided until the MCP joint can be flexed to 60°. If necessary the collateral ligaments can be divided, beginning with the ulnar collateral ligament. If adequate flexion is still not obtained after these maneuvers, capsular adhesions to the volar plate are then released using an elevator (**Fig. 5**A, B). The extensor tenolysis is extended proximally and distally until full extension is achieved. Early therapy is a mainstay of recovery from this operation. Outcomes have demonstrated long-term gains of 29° of passive flexion and 21° of active flexion.[3,45]

Alternatively, Weeks and colleagues[46] advocated for a volar approach to MCP joint contractures. In a study comparing 25 joints treated with a dorsal approach with 31 treated with a volar approach, a higher percentage of joints treated with the volar approach gained greater than 50° of passive ROM (76% versus 29%) and active ROM (44% versus 16%). However, the dorsal approach is still more commonly used because of direct exposure of the joint capsule, ability to perform simultaneous extensor tenolysis, and less risk of injury to tendons and neurovascular structures.[3,6,45,46]

## POSTOPERATIVE CARE

Early postoperative therapy with dynamic splinting and early mobilization protocols are essential for successful treatment of the stiff finger.[39] Following release of joint contractures, a bulky dressing is placed with splinting in the maximum degree of corrected flexion or extension obtained intraoperatively. Strict elevation and edema control is implemented within the first 24 to 48 hours, and therapy is initiated as early as possible. Specific therapy and splinting protocols are tailored to the procedures performed in each case. If protective immobilization is not required, serial static splints are instituted only at night to maximize active motion during the day but still maintain correction of the contracture at night.[6,7,45,46]

## SUMMARY

The specialized anatomy of the MCP joint and PIP joint predisposes the injured finger to stiffness. When evaluating the stiff finger, it is important to identify the pathologic structures. Treatment is based on restoration of normal bony anatomy and articular alignment, release of soft-tissue contractures, and therapy to achieve passive mobilization. Additional surgical interventions are designed to release contracted capsuloligamentous structures and reconstruct dysfunctional muscle-tendon units.

## REFERENCES

1. Brand PW. Mechanical factors in joint stiffness and tissue growth. J Hand Ther 1995;8:91–6.
2. Minami A, An KN, Cooney WP, et al. Ligamentous structures of the metacarpophalangeal joint: a quantitative anatomic study. J Orthop Res 1984;1(4):361–8.
3. Buch VI. Clinical and functional assessment of the hand after metacarpophalangeal capsulotomy. Plast Reconstr Surg 1974;53:452–7.
4. Kuczynski K. The proximal interphalangeal joint. Anatomy and causes of stiffness in the fingers. J Bone Joint Surg Br 1968;50(3):656–63.
5. Lee SWJ, Ng ZY, Fogg QA. Three-dimensional analysis of the palmar plate and collateral ligaments at the proximal interphalangeal joint. J Hand Surg Eur Vol 2014;39(4):391–7.
6. Jupiter JB, Goldfarb CA, Nagy L, et al. Posttraumatic reconstruction in the hand. J Bone Joint Surg Am 2007;89A:428–35.
7. Kaplan FTD. The stiff finger. Hand Clin 2010;26(2): 191–204.
8. Smith RJ. Balance and kinetics of the fingers under normal and pathological conditions. Clin Orthop Relat Res 1974;104:92–111.
9. Smith RJ. Non-Ischemic contractures of the intrinsic muscles of the hand. J Bone Joint Surg Am 1971;53: 1313–31.
10. Glasgow C, Fleming J, Tooth LR, et al. The long-term relationship between duration of treatment and contracture resolution using dynamic orthotic devices for the stiff proximal interphalangeal joint: a prospective cohort study. J Hand Ther 2012;25(1): 38–46.
11. Young VL, Wray RC, Weeks PM. The surgical management of stiff joints in the hand. Plast Reconstr Surg 1978;62:835–41.
12. Houshian S, Jing SS, Chikkamuniyappa C, et al. Management of posttraumatic proximal interphalangeal joint contracture. J Hand Surg Am 2015;40: 2081–4.
13. Michlovitz SL, Harris BA, Watkins MP. Therapy interventions for improving joint range of motion: a systematic review. J Hand Ther 2004;17(2):118–31.
14. Weeks PM, Wray RC, Kuxhaus M. The results of nonoperative management of stiff joints in the hand. PRS 1978;71:58–63.
15. Glasgow C, Wilton J, Tooth L. Optimal daily total end range time for contracture: resolution in hand splinting. J Hand Ther 2003;16(3):207–18.

16. Flowers KR, LaStayo P. Effect of total end range time on improving passive range of motion. J Hand Ther 1994;7(3):150–7.

17. Flowers KR. A proposed decision hierarchy for splinting the stiff joint, with an emphasis on force application parameters. J Hand Ther 2002;15(2):158–62.

18. Agee JM, Goss BC. Use of skeletal extension torque in reversing Dupuytren contractures of the proximal interphalangeal joint. J Hand Surg 2012;37:1467–74.

19. Houshian S, Chikkamuniyappa C, Schroeder H. Gradual joint distraction of post-traumatic flexion contracture of the proximal interphalangeal joint by a mini-external fixator. J Bone Joint Surg Br 2007; 89(2):206–9.

20. Houshian S, Jing SS, Kazemian GH, et al. Distraction for proximal interphalangeal joint contractures: long-term results. J Hand Surg Am 2013;38:1951–6.

21. Houshian S, Chikkamuniyappa C. Distraction correction of chronic flexion contractures of PIP joint: comparison between two distraction rates. J Hand Surg 2007;32(5):651–6.

22. Yang G, McGlinn EP, Chung KC. Management of the stiff finger: evidence and outcomes. Clin Plast Surg 2014;41(3):501–12.

23. Buchler U, Gupta A, Ruf S. Corrective osteotomy for post-traumatic malunion of the phalanges in the hand. J Hand Surg Br 1996;21(1):33–42.

24. Green DP. Complications of phalangeal and metacarpal fractures. Hand Clin 1986;2(2):307–28.

25. Duncan KH, Jupiter JB. Intraarticular osteotomy for malunion of metacarpal head fractures. J Hand Surg 1989;14(5):888–93.

26. Royle SG. Rotational deformity following metacarpal fracture. J Hand Surg Br 1990;15(1):124–5.

27. Field J. Two to five year follow-up of the LPM ceramic coated proximal interphalangeal joint arthroplasty. J Hand Surg Eur Vol 2008;33(1):38–44.

28. Yamamoto M, Malay S, Fujihara Y, et al. A systematic review of different implants and approaches for proximal interphalangeal joint arthroplasty. Plast Reconstr Surg 2017;139(5):1139e–51e.

29. Stoecklein HH, Garg R, Wolfe SW. Surface replacement arthroplasty of the proximal interphalangeal joint using a volar approach: case series. J Hand Surg Am 2011;36(6):1015–21.

30. Jennings CD, Livingstone DP. Surface replacement arthroplasty of the proximal interphalangeal joint using the PIP-SRA implant: results, complications, revisions. J Hand Surg 2008;33:1565.e1-11.

31. Murray PM, Linscheid RL, Cooney WP III, et al. Long Term Outcomes of PIPJ surface replacement arthroplasty. J Bone Joint Surg Am 2012;94A:1120–8.

32. Tarabadkar N, Iorio ML, Huang JI. Proximal interphalangeal joint arthroplasty. JBJS Rev 2015;3:e1–10.

33. Azari KK, Meals RA. Flexor tenolysis. Hand Clin 2005;21(2):211–7.

34. Watson HK, Light TR, Johnson TR. Checkrein resection for flexion contracture of the middle joint. J Hand Surg 1979;4(1):67–71.

35. Schneider LH. Tenolysis and capsulectomy after hand fractures. Clin Orthop Relat Res 1996;327:72–8.

36. Curtis RM. Capsulectomy of the interphalangeal joints of the fingers. J Bone Joint Surg Am 1954; 36:1219–32.

37. Lalonde D, Bell M, Benoit P, et al. A multicenter prospective study of 3,110 consecutive cases of elective epinephrine use in the fingers and hand: the Dalhousie Project clinical phase. J Hand Surg 2005;30(5):1061–7.

38. Brüser P, Poss T, Larkin G. Results of proximal interphalangeal joint release for flexion contractures: midlateral versus palmar incision. J Hand Surg 1999;24(2):288–94.

39. Hogan CJ, Nunley JA. Posttraumatic proximal interphalangeal joint flexion contractures. J Am Acad Orthop Surg 2006;14(9):524–33.

40. Ghidella SD, Segalman KA, Murphey MS. Long-term results of surgical management of proximal interphalangeal joint contracture. J Hand Surg 2002; 27(5):799–805.

41. Diao E, Eaton RG. Total collateral ligament excision for contractures of the PIPJ. J Hand Surg 1993; 18A:395–402.

42. Inoue G. Lateral band release for post-traumatic extension contracture of the proximal interphalangeal joint. Arch Orthop Trauma Surg 1991;110(6): 298–300.

43. Harris C, Riordan DC. Intrinsic contracture in the hand and its surgical treatment. J Bone Joint Surg Am 1954;36-A(1):10–20.

44. Mansat M, Delprat J. Contractures of the proximal interphalangeal joint. Hand Clin 1992;8(4):777–86.

45. Gould JS, Nicholson BG. Capsulectomy of the metacarpophalangeal and proximal interphalangeal joints. J Hand Surg 1979;4(5):482–6.

46. Weeks PM, Young VL, Wray RC. Operative mobilization of stiff metacarpophalangeal joints: dorsal versus volar approach. Ann Plast Surg 1980;5(3):178–85.

# Nerve Tumors of the Upper Extremity

Sophia A. Strike, MD[a],*, Mark E. Puhaindran, MBBS, MMED (Surg)[b]

## KEYWORDS

- Schwannoma • Neurilemmoma • Neurofibroma • Malignant peripheral nerve sheath tumor
- Neurofibromatosis

## KEY POINTS

- Benign peripheral nerve sheath tumors are far more common than malignant peripheral nerve sheath tumors.
- Malignant transformation is more common when tumors are associated with neurofibromatosis.
- A rapid increase in size of a tumor or pain is suggestive of malignant transformation.
- Imaging characteristics suggestive of malignant nerve sheath tumors include larger size, perilesional edema, heterogeneous enhancement, and perilesional enhancement on MRI as well as a standardized uptake value greater than 4.0 on PET with fludeoxyglucose F 18.
- Surgical excision is the treatment of choice. Schwannomas are well encapsulated and typically can be separated from the underlying nerve with microscopic intrafascicular dissection whereas neurofibromas may require nerve excision due to their tendency to intertwine with nerve fascicles.

## INTRODUCTION

Nerve tumors of the upper extremity include benign peripheral nerve sheath tumors (BPNSTs) and malignant peripheral nerve sheath tumors (MPNSTs). The most common peripheral nerve sheath tumors (PNSTs) of the hand and upper extremity are schwannomas, which are benign tumors of Schwann cell origin[1–4] (**Fig. 1**). Multiple schwannomas may occur in schwannomatosis. Neurofibromas, also benign, are classically associated with neurofibromatosis (NF) but can occur as solitary lesions. These tumors also may be associated with gigantism of the underlying anatomy.[1] BPNSTs can be observed or surgically excised with careful microscopic intrafascicular dissection.[4] BPNSTs can transform to MPNSTs, which require more aggressive surgical treatment by a multidisciplinary team. Clinical and radiological factors for identifying malignant tumors and differentiating these from their benign counterparts are discussed. The most current recommended surgical techniques for tumor excision also are reviewed.

## CONTENT
### Clinical Presentation

Classic symptoms of malignant degeneration of an MPNST include rapid growth, pain at night, size greater than 5 cm, previously soft consistency that becomes firm, and any associated constitutional symptoms.[5] Malignant transformation is rare for schwannomas.[1] Neurofibromas associated with NF are more likely to undergo malignant transformation than solitary lesions.[1,2] MPNSTs may occur in 2% to 13% of patients with NF1 compared with 0.001% of the general population[5,6]; 50% of MPNSTs are in patients with NF1 but can occur postradiation or sporadically.[7,8] Rapid growth of a plexiform neurofibroma in NF1 may not necessarily represent malignant transformation. This is a

Disclosure Statement: The authors have nothing to disclose.
[a] Department of Orthopaedic Surgery, Johns Hopkins University School of Medicine, Johns Hopkins Outpatient Center, 601 North Caroline Street, Suite 5252, Baltimore, MD 21287, USA; [b] Department of Hand and Reconstructive Microsurgery, National University Hospital, Level 11, NUHS Tower Block, 1E Kent Ridge Road, Singapore 11928, Singapore
* Corresponding author.
E-mail address: Sstrike1@jhmi.edu

Clin Plastic Surg 46 (2019) 347–350
https://doi.org/10.1016/j.cps.2019.02.008
0094-1298/19/© 2019 The Authors. Published by Elsevier Inc. This is an open access article under the CC BY-NC-ND license (http://creativecommons.org/licenses/by-nc-nd/4.0/).

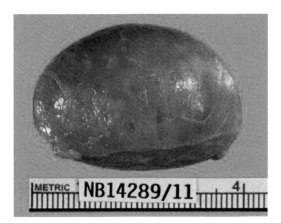

**Fig. 1.** Gross appearance of a schwannoma.

clinical finding that is still being actively studied.[5] A recent study on the impact of family history suggests that a positive family history of MPNST is a risk factor for MPNST development at an earlier age in patients with NF1.[9]

The typical clinical presentation of benign tumors is a firm, slow-growing mass that is either asymptomatic or causes radiating pain or paresthesia along the course of the nerve.[1,2] On physical examination, a positive Tinel sign may be present over the mass.[1]

## Investigations

Evaluation should begin with plain radiographs, which are likely to be normal in cases of most PNSTs.[3] In general, a soft tissue mass of unknown character in the upper extremity that is concerning for a PNST requires further work-up with MRI because this is the most useful imaging modality for these tumors.[3,10,11] Nerve sheath tumors classically are homogeneously hypointense centrally with a peripheral hyperintensity, known as the target sign, although this is not specific to nerve sheath tumors.[11,12] Nilsson and colleagues[10] reported MRI to be diagnostic in 75% of their series of nerve tumors of the upper extremity. In a study by Hung and colleagues,[11] the diagnostic accuracy of ultrasound and of MRI in the evaluation of nerve tumors of the upper extremity was reported as 77% and 100%, respectively. MPNSTs are more likely to be larger and have perilesional edema, heterogeneous enhancement, and perilesional enhancement.[12] The target sign is more specifically associated with BPNSTs.[12] Diffusion-weighted imaging and apparent diffusion coefficient mapping can be used to help differentiate between benign and MPNSTs.[12]

The role of PET with fludeoxyglucose F 18 ([18]F FDG)-PET/CT in identifying PNSTs that have undergone malignant transformation is still being developed.[5] A standardized uptake value (SUV) of 4.0 has been suggested as a cutoff to help distinguish between benign and MPNSTs. In a study of pediatric patients with NF1, sensitivity and specificity of 1.0 and 0.94, respectively, were reported when using this SUV.[13] PET-CT in conjunction with high-resolution MRI has been studied with potential objective features unique to MPNSTs. These technical imaging features may be more useful for radiologists in assisting surgeons with diagnosis. Serial [18]F FDG-PET/CT scans have been used for monitoring lesions in patients with NF1 for malignant transformation.[14]

When clinical and radiological findings are not clearly consistent with a benign nerve sheath tumor, a core needle biopsy should be performed, although it can be painful.[11] For a lesion without suspicious malignant characteristics and clinical and radiological findings of a benign nerve sheath tumor, a marginal excision can be performed.

## Management

BPNSTs can be observed if they remain stable in size and asymptomatic. Surgical management of BPNSTs is with marginal excision. Due to their encapsulated nature, schwannomas are more amenable to intraneural dissection than neurofibromas, allowing preservation of the associated nerve.[1–4] Intracapsular dissection and meticulous tumor removal under magnification preserve nerve structures and are recommended for schwannomas of the hand and wrist[4,15] (**Fig. 2**). In a series of 14 patients treated with intracapsular dissection, no recurrences were reported at a mean follow-up of 12.6 years.[15] Neurofibromas classically intertwine with the underlying nerve, and thus intraneural dissection and fascicular preservation may not be possible.[1,2] If there is significant morbidity with resection of the associated nerve, it is reasonable to perform a biopsy to ensure the tumor is not malignant and then observe. If the affected nerve is not of functional importance, then tumor excision with primary nerve repair versus nerve grafting is the recommended treatment.[1–3] Cutaneous nerves can be easily excised with sacrifice of the nerve.[3] Intraneural dissection with microscopic magnification may be possible for neurofibromas associated with large nerves, which allows preservation of function.[1,3] We prospectively studied patients with schwanommas and neurofibromas who underwent marginal excision using microscopic intrafascicular dissection and found, on histological analysis, that nerve fascicles may even run through the main tumor and may require sacrifice if a marginal excision is performed (**Fig. 3**). Plexiform neurofibromas, which

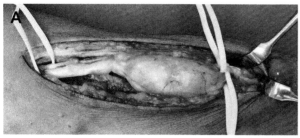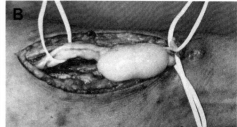

**Fig. 2.** Neurofibroma in a patient with NF1, before (*A*) and after (*B*) microscopic intraneutral intrafascicular dissection.

are almost exclusively associated with NF1, typically are difficult to separate from the surrounding nerve.[16] In a recent review of a large series of 62 patients with NF1 and plexiform neurofibromas of the upper extremity and hand, a majority of patients underwent 3 or fewer surgical procedures for these tumors and 74% of the procedures had no complications, with only 0.6% of procedures resulting in a temporary sensibility disorder.[16] Postoperative neurologic disorder usually is temporary but has been reported to occur in up to 50% of patients and patients should be counseled accordingly.[11]

MPNSTs require wide excision. Nerve reconstruction may not be helpful, and amputation should be considered for large or recurrent tumors.[5,7] Radiotherapy for MPNSTs may provide local control but has not been shown to prolong survival.[5,7] Chemotherapy generally is reserved for metastatic disease, although its role in MPNST management has not been fully elucidated.[5,7] Tyrosine kinase inhibitors and anti-RAS pathway drugs may show some promise in management of MPSNTs.[5]

Percutaneous radiofrequency ablation has been described with reasonable success in the treatment of benign and MPNSTs in patients who are poor surgical candidates.[17] This treatment modality has not been studied in the upper extremity. The anatomy of the upper extremity is more amenable to local surgical excision than the retroperitoneal PNSTs for which this technique has primarily been used.[17]

Recurrence after excision of a schwannoma is relatively rare.[1,12] MPNSTs have a poorer prognosis, with 50% of patients presenting with metastases and 5-year survival rates ranging from 15% to 50%.[7]

## SUMMARY

BPNSTs and MPNSTs in the upper extremity can occur as solitary or as syndrome-related lesions. Classically, Tinel sign is positive over the tumor. Clinical features of rapid growth, new neuro- logic symptoms, and increased pain are suggestive of but not specific for malignant transformation. Radiological evaluation with MRI can provide diagnostic information in 75% of cases and [18]F FDG-PET/CT may be used to help differentiate benign from malignant lesions, with an SUV greater than 4.0 suggestive of malignant lesions. Treatment in the upper extremity is with surgical excision. Intraneural dissection is recommended for all schwannomas and many neurofibromas, although some degree of fascicular sacrifice may be necessary and the degree of excision should be tailored to the nerve involved. MPNSTs have a poor prognosis and require multidisciplinary care and a wide surgical excision, which may lead to amputation.

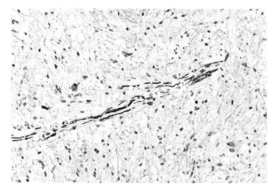

**Fig. 3.** Neurofilament stain demonstrating nerve fiber running through lesion near periphery (immunohistochemistry, ×250).

## REFERENCES

1. Hsu CS, Hentz VR, Yao J. Tumours of the hand. Lancet Oncol 2007;8:157–66.
2. Longhurst W, Khachemoune A. An unknown mass: the differential diagnosis of digit tumors. Int J Dermatol 2015;54:1214–25.
3. Payne WT, Merrell G. Benign bony and soft tissue tumors of the hand. J Hand Surg 2010;35A:1901–10.

4. Lai CS, Chen IC, Lan HC, et al. Management of extremity neurilemmomas: clinical series and literature review. Ann Plast Surg 2013;71(Suppl 1):S37–42.

5. Ferner RE1, Gutmann DH. International consensus statement on malignant peripheral nerve sheath tumors in neurofibromatosis. Cancer Res 2002;62(5): 1573–7.

6. Ducatman BS, Scheithauer BW, Piepgras DG, et al. Malignant peripheral nerve sheath tumors. A clinicopathologic study of 120 cases. Cancer 1986;57(10): 2006–21.

7. Farid M, Demicco EG, Garcia R, et al. Malignant peripheral nerve sheath tumors. Oncologist 2014; 19(2):193–201.

8. Longo JF, Weber SM, Turner-Ivey BP, et al. Recent advances in the diagnosis and pathogenesis of neurofibromatosis type 1 (NF1)-associated peripheral nervous system neoplasms. Adv Anat Pathol 2018;25(5):353–68.

9. Malbari F, Spira M, Knight PB, et al. Malignant peripheral nerve sheath tumors in neurofibromatosis: impact of family history. J Pediatr Hematol Oncol 2018;40(6):e359–63.

10. Nilsson J, Sandberg K, Søe Nielsen N, et al. Magnetic resonance imaging of peripheral nerve tumours in the upper extremity. Scand J Plast Reconstr Surg Hand Surg 2009;43(3):153–9.

11. Hung YW, Tse WL, Cheng HS, et al. Surgical excision for challenging upper limb nerve sheath tumours: a single centre retrospective review of

treatment results. Hong Kong Med J 2010;16: 287Y291.

12. Ahlawat S, Fayad LM. Imaging cellularity in benign and malignant peripheral nerve sheath tumors: utility of the "target sign" by diffusion weighted imaging. Eur J Radiol 2018;102:195–201.

13. Tsai LL, Drubach L, Fahey F, et al. [18F]-Fluorodeoxyglucose positron emission tomography in children with neurofibromatosis type 1 and plexiform neurofibromas: correlation with malignant transformation. J Neurooncol 2012;108(3):469–75.

14. Ren J, Yang G, Zhou J, et al. The value of 18F-FDG PET/CT in patient with neurofibromatosis type 1: a case report and literature review. Medicine 2018; 97:20.

15. Ozdemir O, Ozsoy MH, Kurt C, et al. Schwannomas of the hand and wrist: long-term results and review of the literature. J Orthop Surg (Hong Kong) 2005; 13(3):267–72.

16. Friedrich RE, Diekmeier C. Peripheral nerve sheath tumors of the upper extremity and hand in patients with neurofibromatosis type 1: topography of tumors and evaluation of surgical treatment in 62 patients. GMS Interdiscip Plast Reconstr Surg DGPW 2017; 6:Doc15.

17. Mrowczynski O, Mau C, Nguyen DT, et al. Percutaneous radiofrequency ablation for the treatment of peripheral nerve sheath tumors: a case report and review of the literature. Cureus 2018;10(4): e2534.

# Managing Mutilating Hand Injuries

Amitabha Lahiri, MBBS, MS, MCh (Plast), FRCS (Edin), FAMS (Hand Surgery), MRes (tissue engineering)

## KEYWORDS

• Hand • Trauma • Reconstruction • Microsurgery • Rehabilitation

## KEY POINTS

- Management of mutilating injuries is complex and should be based on clear understanding of principles of wound management, fracture fixation, and soft-tissue reconstruction.
- The surgeon must be able to anticipate the effects of the trauma and set clear goals of reconstruction directly from the first surgery.
- Debridement, bony stabilization, revascularization, and soft-tissue cover should be achieved in the primary surgery. Nerve and tendon reconstruction can be performed as delayed procedures.

## INTRODUCTION

The hand is a complex organ that is unique in several ways. It has a mechanical component consisting of bones, joints, tendons, and muscles, and a sensory component comprising the skin and the sensory nerves. The components work seamlessly to give rise to the function of the hand, which is referred to as prehension.

Prehension includes the integration of 2 components: feeling, which is transfer of information from the environment to the brain, and response, the manipulation of objects.

Both the components are of equal importance. Loss or damage to any component in the system results in suboptimal function. An insensate hand in leprosy is as dysfunctional as a sensate but paralyzed hand in poliomyelitis.

"Mutilating hand injuries" is a group of injuries that is difficult to define. The English dictionary defines mutilate as "to damage something severely, especially by violently removing a part."

Mutilation of the hand may be taken to include injuries that result in significant damage to several tissues at once.

The patterns of these injuries are so variable because of the nearly unlimited permutations and combinations of the severity, extent, and the number of tissues involved that the treatment can never be standardized; however, clear principles for surgical management can be established.

The surgeon managing such injuries must have a clear understanding of the principles that would influence decisions and hence the outcomes. A clear treatment plan based on precise goals leads to rapid functional and psychological recovery. However, repeated surgeries and failures often may lead to opposite outcomes.

The ability to restore function in the injured hand nowadays is the result of the culmination of developments in several fields.

- Principles of debridement
- Antibiotic therapy and infection
- Principles and techniques of skeletal stabilization
- Principles and techniques of tendon repair
- Microvascular surgery
- Peripheral nerve surgery
- Tissue transfer
- Rehabilitation

*Thus, a surgeon or a team dealing with mutilating hand injuries must be conversant with these principles in order to provide the optimal management.*

For the purpose of the present discussion, pure amputation injuries are excluded; however,

The author has nothing to disclose.
Department of Hand and Reconstructive Microsurgery, National University Hospital, Level 11, NUHS Tower block, 1E Kent Ridge Road, Singapore 119228, Singapore
*E-mail address:* amitabha27r@gmail.com

Clin Plastic Surg 46 (2019) 351–357
https://doi.org/10.1016/j.cps.2019.02.009

amputation in the context of a mutilating injury is discussed.

## THE INJURY

In the current day and age, such an injury usually results from heavy machinery or automobile accidents. It may also arise from explosives in war zones or from the hand being trapped under heavy rubble in natural disasters.

The common characteristics of mutilating injuries can be summarized as follows.

- Loss of skin and soft-tissue cover
- Multiple tendon injuries with loss of tendon substance
- Wide zone of injury to the vessels with devascularization of parts
- Nerve injuries with loss
- Fractures and dislocations
- Contamination of tissues with foreign material

## DEFINING THE GOALS OF SURGICAL MANAGEMENT

The final functional outcome of each injury is unique and varies with the severity of structural damage and contamination, as well as the surgery and rehabilitative care; however, some generalization can be established.

The overall goal of reconstruction is summarized as:

- Restoration of maximal function
- In shortest possible time
- Through minimum number of procedures
- If multiple procedures are planned, each procedure should be performed with clear goals

and should set the stage for the next procedure

## DEFINING THE FUNCTIONAL HAND

As already mentioned, the function of the hand is summarized by the word "prehension" and is a composite function of dynamic interaction between the motor and sensory loops that connect the hand and the nervous system.

The motor function relies on the integrity of the motor nerves, muscles, tendons, bones, and joints. Sensory function relies on the integrity of skin cover, receptors, and the sensory nerves.

In 1979 Midgley and Entin[1] summarized the 6 basic requirements in a functioning hand:

- Strength
- Position
- Length
- Stability
- Mobility
- Sensibility

## FUNCTIONAL ASPECTS OF THE HAND

Essentially the functional hand depends on an opposable thumb and one or more mobile digits.[2]

The opposable thumb provides a post against which the digits grip objects.

A pinch can be achieved with the thumb and a single mobile digit.

A tripod pinch requires the thumb and 2 digits (**Figs. 1** and **2**).

The power grip requires 3 to 4 digits and the thumb.

Span requires ulnar digits.

*The ability of the hand to adapt.* The surgeon must remember that the hand shows extraordinary

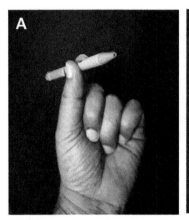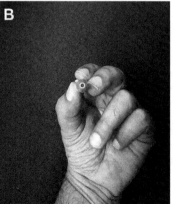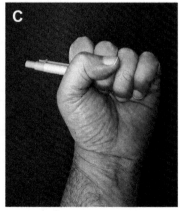

**Fig. 1.** (*A*) Pinch can be achieved using one finger and the thumb; however, it lacks strength and the ability to stabilize the object being held. (*B*) A tripod pinch requires 2 fingers and the thumb. It has precision strength and control, but large objects cannot be held using this grip. (*C*) Power grip using all the fingers and the thumb demonstrates strength and stability.

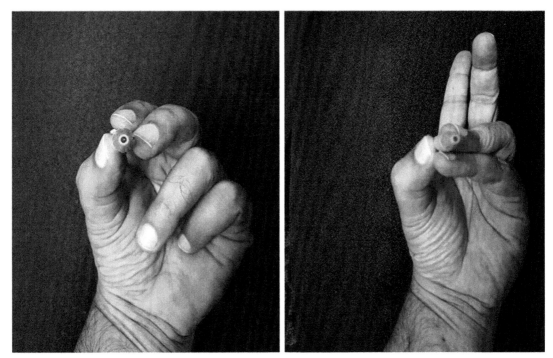

**Fig. 2.** The ability for the hand to adapt and compensate for the loss of digits. A tripod pinch can be achieved with the radial or ulnar digits against an opposable thumb.

plasticity. In situations of significant structural loss, the remaining functional elements can adapt to compensate for the lost function.

In general the functions involving precision are performed by the radial 2 digits and the thumb, whereas the functions for holding large objects are performed by the entire hand and needs the ulnar digits and the thumb. The thumb plays the crucial part in both forms, although the digits can adapt to the function.

The implication of this concept is that fewer but functional digits, whether radial or ulnar, may provide equal or better outcomes than a greater number of stiff or nonfunctional digits.

## APPROACH TO A PATIENT WITH A MUTILATING INJURY OF THE HAND

The management starts with a precise clinical assessment of the patient followed by the creation of a surgical plan.

*Clinical assessment.* The most essential part of clinical assessment of a patient with major hand trauma is the assessment of the patient as a whole, and exclusion of severe life-threatening trauma and exsanguination (**Fig. 3**).

It is also essential to examine the whole upper limb including the axilla, shoulder, and clavicular region in such cases.

Once the patient is stabilized, attention is focused on the hand.

A history of comorbidities and possible drug allergies that may compromise the safety of major surgery is extremely important.

Three essential questions need to be asked regarding the trauma to the hand.

1. When: the time at which injury took place
2. How: the mechanism
3. Where: the environment in which the injury occurred (possible contaminants)

Most of the time the patient is in severe pain and in a state of psychological shock, at which point a conventional examination may not be feasible; however, a detailed knowledge of the structural damage is essential in formulating the surgical strategy.

Careful observation and synthesis of information is gained from:

- Knowledge of surface anatomy
- A visual "feel" for the depth of trauma
- Understanding the mechanism of injury
- Plain radiographs

These factors provide an extraordinary amount of information without the need to touch the patient.

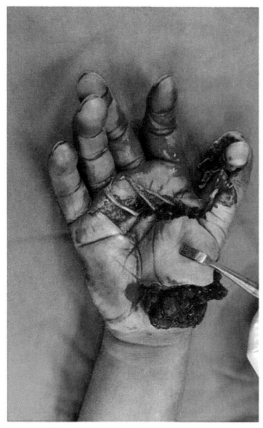

**Fig. 3.** A hand crushed by heavy machinery. Conventional examination is practically impossible in the awake patient; however, a thorough visual examination can provide a great amount of information that is necessary for planning. On visual assessment, the thumb shows separation of soft tissue from bone and the distal soft tissue is rotated, indicating likely devascularization of distal phalanx. The thenar muscles are crushed and seen protruding and are likely to be unsalvageable, while the thenar skin is likely to be devascularized because of separation from muscles. Avulsed digital nerves are seen, indicating a high possibility of neurovascular trauma even though the color of the digits is pink. The middle finger is rotated, indicating a possible fracture.

The wound may be irrigated with saline in the emergency department and photographs taken so that repeated examinations by different specialists are avoided.

## PLANNING

**Table 1** and a sketch can enhance preoperative planning.

*Surgical preparation.* It is useful to refer to the plan for surgical preparation. Anticipation of potential donor sites must be included in the patient's preparation on the table. Failure to anticipate may require interruption of surgery to prepare additional sites for donor tissues.

Common examples are:

Skin graft: thighs
Pedicled flaps: abdominal flap/groin flap
Free/flow-through flaps: anterolateral thigh flap, dorsalis pedis, radial artery forearm flap, and lateral arm flap from the opposite limb
Vein graft: leg (saphenous vein)
Nerve graft: leg (sural nerve)

*Spare parts.* Considering spare parts is one of the essential components of surgery, which reduces the burden on healthy donor sites in the body.[3]

Tissues that are not crushed or contaminated but are being sacrificed can be used as spare parts.

For example, a digit with double-level injury that is not being replanted can be a source of nerve graft, artery, and skin.

Free flaps can be fashioned from amputated parts that are not being replanted.

Degloved or sheared skin can be used as a skin graft after removal of fat.

## STEPS OF SURGERY

*Debridement.* Debridement is the first and essential component of surgery, and is performed in a methodical fashion to include skin, subcutaneous tissue, muscle, and bone while preserving nerves and intact vessels and tendons.

The debridement should create unquestionably healthy surgical margins for each tissue. A temptation to preserve devitalized tissue should be avoided.

A good debridement sets the stage for clear reconstruction goals and prevents postoperative complications such as ongoing tissue necrosis and infection that require repeated debridement.

*Intraoperative "triaging" and the sequence of salvage and prioritization (thumb).* In mangling injuries the different structures suffer different degrees of damage. The surgeon must make decisions on the spot regarding the order in which the structures are to be addressed to achieve the best outcomes.[4]

Fatigue from spending several frustrating hours on salvaging a severely damaged digit may compromise the reconstruction of the better preserved digits and worsen the surgical outcome in comparison with successfully salvaging the less severely damaged digits and sacrificing an unsalvageable digit.

However, the decision to sacrifice a digit is not simple. A digit may be deemed unsalvageable if

**Table 1**
**Summary of procedures and potential donor sites as an aid to planning surgical reconstruction in mutilating hand injuries**

| Structures | Extent of Injury | Plan | Donor |
|---|---|---|---|
| Immediate priority for repair/reconstruction | | | |
| Dorsal and palmar skin | Area of loss | Flap/graft | Thigh/groin flap |
| Palmar arch and digital arteries | What level/possible segmental loss | Vein graft | Foot/leg/forearm/ flow-through flap |
| Fractures | Level/bone loss/ comminution | Plating/bridge plating external fixation/bone graft? | Donor? |
| Possible secondary reconstruction | | | |
| Median/ulnar and digital nerves | Level of trauma/possible segmental loss | Primary repair/graft | Forearm/sural |
| Flexor and extensor tendons | Which level and digit Possible segmental loss | Primary repair/delayed grafting | |

the anticipated outcome is a short or a nonfunctional digit.

1. The skin and neurovascular bundles are crushed or avulsed over a significant length
2. Large segments or multiple phalanges have bone loss or loss of multiple joints
3. Severe contamination of tissues

Priority is given to salvaging the thumb. However, if the thumb is not salvageable, reconstruction must set the stage for further reconstruction.

Midgley and Entin's[1] parameters of strength, position, length, stability, mobility, and sensibility can be used here to anticipate the functional outcome of the digits.

In summary, following adequate debridement,

1. Reconstruction should begin with salvage of best-preserved digits (author's opinion)
2. High priority must be given to salvage the thumb
3. If the thumb or several digits are not salvageable, using another amputated digit may be considered to reconstruct the thumb if possible (transposition). If transposition is not thought to be suitable, flap cover for secondary reconstruction of the thumb (osteoplastic reconstruction), or a toe transfer, may be incorporated in the procedure. Essentially the end point of the first procedure should prepare the stage for a secondary reconstruction.

## Essential Components of Primary Surgery

The primary surgery has three essential components.

*Skeletal stabilization.* Skeletal stability forms the foundation for soft-tissue reconstruction.

The aim is to maintain length and alignment of the skeletal elements. In many cases shortening of bones can provide a platform for primary co-optation of neurovascular structures and assist in achieving soft-tissue cover. However, excessive shortening of skeletal elements may deform the hand and compromise function.

The options include internal fixation with plates and screws or Kirschner wires.

In situations of bone loss, external fixators or bridging plates are used.

When using external fixators, it must be kept in mind that positioning of the hand for microvascular procedures may become extremely difficult and, similarly, application of groin or abdominal flaps may be impossible.

The choice of fixation is also dictated by the contamination and the anticipated risk of infection during and following the debridement. The assessment is entirely subjective; however, in situations of biological contamination (e.g., barnyard injuries, contamination with meat or fish), external fixation may be preferred because of the higher risk of deep infection, which may necessitate removal of implants.

*Revascularization.* Following skeletal stabilization, the immediate concern is to establish blood flow to the ischemic structures. One or several digits may be devascularized, and crush injuries resulting in mutilation commonly result in loss of large segments of blood vessels, meaning that vein grafts are necessary.

Vein grafts can be harvested from the same limb if the proximal forearm is not injured. Saphenous vein may also be used.

Although vein grafts are possible for veins they have a higher propensity to fail, and in this situation the veins should not be reversed. Once revascularization has been performed, nerves and tendons can be repaired at the same sitting or planned for a secondary reconstruction (**Fig. 4**).

*Soft-tissue cover.*[5] The next crucial component of primary reconstructive surgery is soft-tissue cover. Bones, implants, or vessels cannot be left exposed. If these structures are covered, the remaining soft-tissue defect can be reconstructed as an early secondary reconstruction within 48 to 72 hours.

Pedicled groin and abdominal flaps alone or in combination provide a versatile solution for emergency flap coverage of the hand. These flaps can be raised rapidly to cover a variety of defects and may be combined to provide coverage for large areas.[6]

Anterolateral thigh flaps can provide reliable soft-tissue cover for the injured hand. They can also be used as flow-through flaps to provide simultaneous revascularization.[7]

Free flaps also provide an opportunity for single-stage reconstruction of composite soft-tissue defects of the hand. A dorsalis pedis flap can be harvested with extensor tendons[8] to reconstruct dorsal defects with loss of tendons. Similarly, radial forearm flaps and lateral arm flap can be harvested with vascularized bone to treat bone and soft-tissue defects (**Fig. 5**).

### Late Secondary Procedures

The primary procedure should set the stage for necessary secondary procedures.[9]

Secondary procedures should be carried out when the wounds have healed and the scars have stabilized. Such procedures include bone grafts to bridge bone defects, tendon grafts, tendon transfers, nerve grafts, and toe transfer.

## HINDRANCES TO IDEAL OUTCOME AND THE ROLE OF REHABILITATION

Beyond soft-tissue cover and survival of digits, there are several barriers to establishment of function.

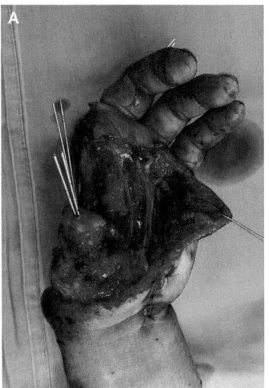
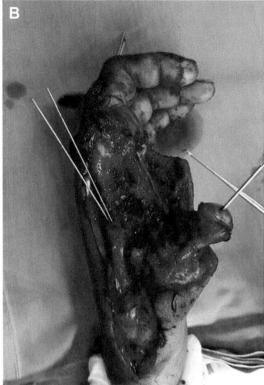

**Fig. 4.** Complete debridement of crushed tissues. Following revascularization of digits using vein grafts, the index finger could not be perfused. Exploration showed thrombosis of both digital arteries up to the distal phalanx. The decision was made to amputate. (*A*) The thumb metacarpal, completely devoid of soft-tissue cover, was preserved. (*B*) Skeletal stabilization of the thumb metacarpal to the trapezium in the position of function, and stabilization of the third carpometacarpal joint.

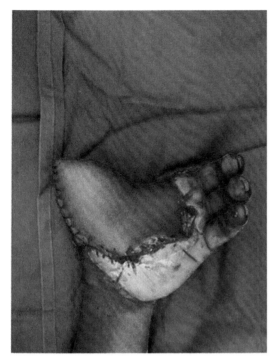

**Fig. 5.** Combined groin and abdominal flap transfer was performed during the primary surgery to reconstruct the palm, the thumb, and the dorsum. The soft-tissue cover over the thumb metacarpal was planned for secondary debulking, and also provided a platform for a possible great toe transfer.

Mutilating injuries involve multiple tissue planes that heal by fibrosis. Adhesions and loss of gliding planes through scarring impair tendon function and joint motion. Nerve repairs in general have partial recovery, which is caused by axonal entrapment at the site of repair and loss of axons caused by fascicular mismatch.

The surgeon must anticipate individual problems and initiate rehabilitative measures as early as possible.

The rehabilitation in such cases is complex, and set protocols cannot be applied. Each patient requires an individualized protocol. For example, combined flexor and extensor injuries in different digits and at different anatomic zones along with fractures would produce unique scenarios for each patient. There has to be clear communication between the surgeon and the occupational therapist in formulating a plan that is safe to ensure maximal functional recovery.

## THE FUTURE: BIONIC PROSTHESES

At present the prosthetics designed for the upper limb are still in the stage of infancy. Hence a good reconstruction, even with a partial hand, is superior to a prosthetic hand.

Although great progress has been made in terms of design and control systems, all the current prostheses are myoelectric. Each movement relies on one voluntary muscle contraction, resulting in a slow stepwise motion as opposed to the fluid composite movement of the natural limb. A second issue is that the prostheses are insensate.

Considerable research is under way around the world to establish a neural interface between the nerve and prostheses.[10] In the near future bionic replacements will become commonplace and part of the armamentarium for upper limb reconstruction.

## SUMMARY

The successful treatment of mutilating injuries of the hand depends on correct assessment and execution of the surgical plan.

## REFERENCES

1. Midgley RD, Entin MA. Management of mutilating injuries of the hand. Clin Plast Surg 1976;3(1):99–109.
2. Moran SL, Berger RA. Biomechanics and hand trauma: what you need. Hand Clin 2003;19(1): 17–31.
3. Peng YP, Lahiri A. Spare-part surgery. Semin Plast Surg 2013;27(4):190–7.
4. Soucacos PN. Indications and selection for digital amputation and replantation. J Hand Surg Br 2001; 26(6):572–81.
5. Buchler U. Traumatic soft-tissue defects of the extremities. Implications and treatment guidelines. Arch Orthop Trauma Surg 1990;109(6):321–9.
6. Sabapathy SR, Bajantri B. Indications, selection, and use of distant pedicled flap for upper limb reconstruction. Hand Clin 2014;30(2):185–99, vi.
7. Qing L, Wu P, Liang J, et al. Use of flow-through anterolateral thigh perforator flaps in reconstruction of complex extremity defects. J Reconstr Microsurg 2015;31(8):571–8.
8. Caroli A, Adani R, Castagnetti C, et al. Dorsalis pedis flap with vascularized extensor tendons for dorsal hand reconstruction. Plast Reconstr Surg 1993; 92(7):1326–30.
9. Katsaros J. Indications for free soft-tissue flap transfer to the upper limb and the role of alternative procedures. Hand Clin 1992;8(3):479–507.
10. Lahiri A, Delgado IM, Sheshadri S, et al. Self-organization of "fibro-axonal" composite tissue around unmodified metallic micro-electrodes can form a functioning interface with a peripheral nerve: a new direction for creating long-term neural interfaces. Muscle Nerve 2016;53(5):789–96.

# Efficiency in Digital and Hand Replantation

Shimpei Ono, MD, PhD[a],*, Kevin C. Chung, MD, MS[b]

## KEYWORDS

• Digit • Finger • Hand • Replantation • Amputation

## KEY POINTS

- Multiple factors should be considered before conducting replantation: patient's age, occupation, hand dominance, severity and level of injury, warm ischemia time, general condition, motivation, economic factors.
- Strong indications to replantation include thumb, multiple digits, transmetacarpal and proximal, and any pediatric amputations whatever the level.
- For successful replantation, the usefulness of a 2-team approach, bone shortening, tension-free anastomosis, and vein graft is emphasized. Early recognition of postoperative vascular compromise is also important.
- Recent studies have shown high survival rates after fingertip replantation by providing excellent functional and aesthetic outcomes. Artery-only fingertip replantation requires several methods to restore venous outflow: removal of the nail bed, use of medical leeches, and heparin-soaked gauze dressing.

## INTRODUCTION

Digital and hand replantation has progressed since the first replantation of a completely amputated digit by Japanese orthopedic surgeons, Tamai and Komatsu, in 1965, which was reported in 1968.[1] With the advancement of microsurgery techniques and instrumentation, replantation is effective in treating digital and hand amputations. Successful digital and hand replantation can provide excellent aesthetic outcomes by maintaining the number and length of the digits. However, replantation should not be done routinely without considering postoperative functional outcomes. For example, a severely injured digit involving multiple tissue, usually more than 3 injured categories of 5 tissues in digital and hand components (bone or joint, tendon, vessels, nerves, and skin), may be considered a contraindication for replantation given presumed poor functional outcomes. Achieving best outcomes after replantation is not solely related to the success of microvascular anastomosis but also to the adequacy of bone fixation, tendon and nerve repair, and soft-tissue coverage. The aim of this article is to review the literature relating to surgical technique and recent evidence in microsurgical digital and hand replantation and describe our surgical pearls for overcoming various pitfalls.

## INDICATIONS AND CONTRAINDICATIONS FOR REPLANTATION

There is much controversy regarding the indications and contraindications for digital and hand replantation. Because there are multiple factors to consider (eg, patient's age, occupation, dominant hand, severity and level of injury, warm ischemia time, general condition, motivation, economic factors), the final decision regarding replantation depends on the surgeon and the patient. Moreover, the suitability of this procedure is usually done under the

Funding sources: Supported in part by grants from a Midcareer Investigator Award in Patient-Oriented Research (2 K24-AR053120-06).
[a] Department of Plastic, Reconstructive and Aesthetic Surgery, Nippon Medical School, 1-1-5 Sendagi, Bunkyo-ku, Tokyo 113-8603, Japan; [b] Section of Plastic Surgery, Department of Surgery, The University of Michigan Health System, 1500 E. Medical Center Drive, Ann Arbor, MI 48109, USA
* Corresponding author.
*E-mail address:* s-ono@nms.ac.jp

plasticsurgery.theclinics.com

microscope in the operating theater after inspecting the amputated digit and proximal stump. Although it is difficult to definitively specify the indications for replantation, there are several rules that help the decision. First, replantation is only considered in a stable patient. In the case of associated life-threatening injuries, replantation should be avoided. Second, amputated levels, number of digits, and patient background are important. Thumb, multiple digit, or transmetacarpal amputations are considered strong indications for replantation.[2] There is no age limitation for replantation. However, patients with diabetes mellitus or obliterative vascular diseases, or smokers have a higher failure rate.[3,4] Patients with active psychiatric illness or self-amputation should be contraindications. On the other hand, any pediatric amputation is considered for replantation, because children have good potential for recovery and regeneration, resulting in better functional outcomes than adults.[5] Our indications for digital and hand replantation based on injury and patient factors are summarized in **Table 1**. Third, the factors affecting the severity of injury that can achieve good outcomes after replantation include (1) guillotine: clean and sharp amputation (eg, knife); (2) crush amputation (eg, saw), with minimal local tissue damage, and (3) avulsion amputation (eg, machine press or door) with minimal vascular injury. Guillotine injuries are favorable for replantation, on the other hand, crush or avulsion injuries are less likely to be salvageable. Predictive signs of severe vascular injury of amputated digits, red line sign (small hematomas seen in the skin along the course of the neurovascular bundle) (**Fig. 1**) and ribbon sign (a corkscrew appearance of the arteries), are considered contraindications for replantation because of extensive zone of injury.

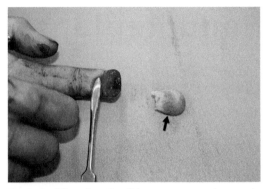

**Fig. 1.** Red line sign. Small hematomas can be seen in the skin along the course of the neurovascular bundle (*black arrow*).

Fourth, replantation should be undertaken emergently to minimize ischemia time and maximize clinical outcomes. Warm ischemia time for a successful digit (no muscle) replantation should be up to 12 hours and cold ischemia to 24 hours.[6] However, with a hand amputation, ischemia time is shorter because of muscle necrosis, leading to myoglobinuria, acidosis, and hyperkalemia after reperfusion. Thus, minimizing warm ischemia and total ischemia time is crucial for successful replantation.

## CLASSIFICATIONS BASED ON THE LEVEL OF AMPUTATION

Amputations can be classified based on the anatomic level of amputation. Upper extremity amputations can be classified into 2 groups: major amputation (amputations proximal to the radiocarpal joint) and minor amputation (amputations distal to the radiocarpal joint). With regard to digital amputation, Tamai's classification[7] is the most frequently used system. He classified digital amputation into 5 zones (**Fig. 2**). Each zone has anatomic characteristics that influence the technique and outcome of replantation. Fingertip amputation has been classified by many authors (**Fig. 3**).[7–9] Tamai's classification of zone 1 (from the fingertip to the base of the nail) and zone 2 (from the base of the nail to the distal interphalangeal joint) is also used for amputation classification of the fingertip.

## A STEP-BY-STEP OPERATIVE APPROACH
### *Step 1: Emergency Management and Care of the Amputated Digit*

On arrival to the emergency care unit, a complete trauma assessment is essential; life-threatening conditions must be investigated and controlled. Most patients with digital and hand amputations are cared for initially by nonspecialists, before referral to hand surgery centers or microsurgical

| Table 1 |
|---|
| **Indications for replantation** |

| Strong Indications | |
|---|---|
| Patient factors | Any pediatric amputation |
| Injury factors | Thumb amputation<br>Multiple digit amputation<br>Transmetacarpal amputation |
| **Relative Indications** | |
| Patient factors | Special needs (eg, musician, craftworker's dominant hand, young lady, small finger replantation in Japan) |
| Injury factors | Single digit zone I amputation<br>Ring finger avulsion injury |

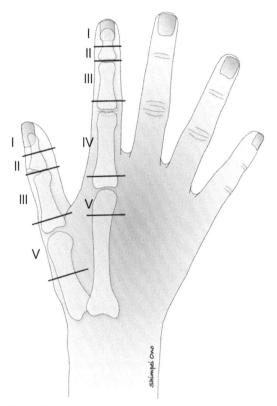

**Fig. 2.** Tamai's classification of fingertip amputation.

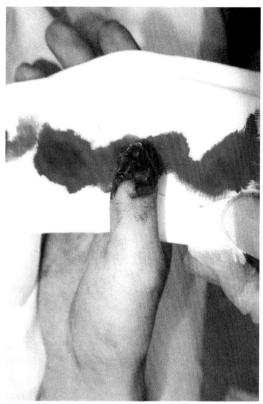

**Fig. 4.** Bleeding vessels at the stump should be controlled with external gauze pressure to avoid additional damage to vessels.

units. Appropriate initial management is a key factor of good outcomes. Actively bleeding vessels at the stump should never be clamped and should be controlled with hand elevation and external gauze pressure to avoid additional damage to vessels (**Fig. 4**).[10] The amputated digit and hand should

be immediately wrapped in saline-moistened gauze (**Fig. 5**), placed in a plastic bag (**Fig. 6**), in a container with ice and water (approximately 4°C). Cooling below 4°C and ice in direct contact

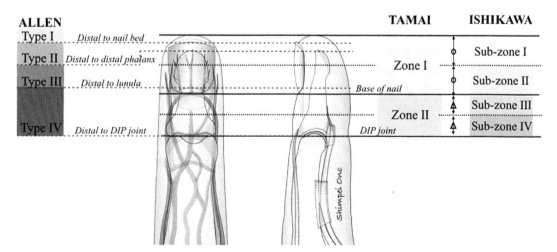

**Fig. 3.** Classifications of distal digital amputations. DIP, distal interphalangeal. Ishikawa and colleagues subdivided Tamai's classification into 4 subzones: subzone I, the distal to the midpoint of the nail; subzone II, from the nail base to the midpoint of the nail; subzone III from midway of the nail base and DIP joint to the nail base; subzone IV, from the DIP joint to the midway point.

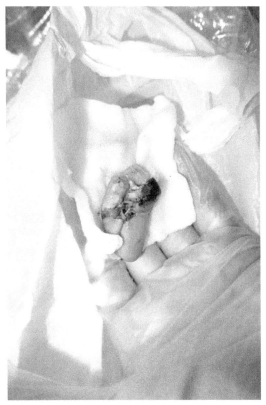

**Fig. 5.** Amputated digit should be immediately wrapped in saline-moistened gauze.

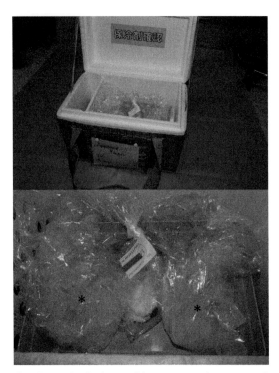

**Fig. 7.** A plastic bag with amputated segment is placed in a container. Particular care must be taken so that the amputated segment does not come in direct contact with the ice (*asterisk*).

with the tissue cause frostbite damage.[11] Thus care must be taken that the amputated segment does not come in direct contact with the ice (**Fig. 7**). Radiographic examination of the hand and the amputated segment should be performed to evaluate the extent of the bone injury (**Fig. 8**).

A 2-team approach is ideal; while one team evaluates and prepares the patient, the other assesses the amputated segment. Ideally, the amputated segment is taken immediately to the operating room to be examined under a microscope or loupe magnification (**Fig. 9**). The amputated segment is then dissected to expose important structures

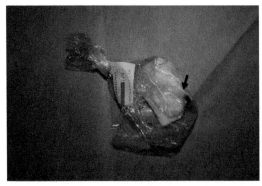

**Fig. 6.** Amputated digit in saline-moistened gauze (*black arrow*) placed in a plastic bag.

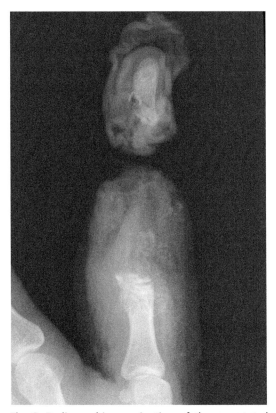

**Fig. 8.** Radiographic examination of the amputated segment should be performed to evaluate the extent of the bone injury.

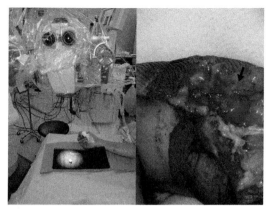

**Fig. 9.** The amputated segment is taken to the operating room to be examined under a microscope and dissected to allow exposure of important structures such as the digital artery (*black arrow*).

(arteries, veins, and nerves), and they are tagged with sutures of 9-0 or 10-0 nylon.

## Step 2: Anesthesia

Replantation surgery is usually performed under regional anesthesia, axillary nerve block, alone or in combination with general anesthesia. Regional anesthesia provides the benefit of sympathetic blockade, which optimizes vasodilatation and facilitates vascular anastomosis.[12] Moreover, the regional anesthesia can be maintained in the postoperative period.

## Step 3: Preparation of the Proximal Stump

A tourniquet is used during the dissection in the proximal stump. Midlateral incisions (**Fig. 10**) provide rapid and excellent exposure for the dorsal veins located just above the extensor tendons and volar neurovascular bundle. The flexor tendons are retracted proximally; they are retrieved and held out to length by transfixing them with 23G needles. The artery is located dorsal to the nerve in the digit, whereas the common digital artery is volar to the common digital nerve in the palm. Each end is identified and tagged before skeletal fixation.

## Step 4: Order of Repair

After all vital structures have been identified, repair is begun. Two methods are available when multiple digits are replanted. One is digit by digit, wherein each digit is replanted one after the other. The other method is structure by structure[13]; skeletal fixation of all digits is done first, and the extensors, flexors, palmar arteries and nerves, and dorsal veins are then repaired in this order. The author prefers the structure-by-structure method to reduce operating time and avoid accidental

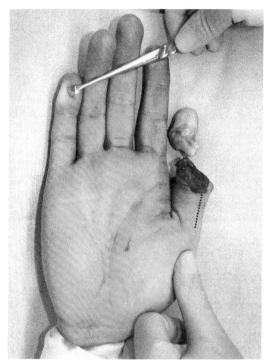

**Fig. 10.** Midlateral incisions are used for exposure to raise volar and dorsal skin flaps.

damage to repaired adjacent neurovascular structures. The logical sequence of replantation is to progress from deeper structures to superficial structures: (a) bone stabilization, (b) repair extensor tendons, (c) repair flexor tendons, (d) repair arteries, (e) repair nerves, (f) repair veins, and (g) close or cover wound. In the case of excess tension at the anastomosis site, vein grafts should be harvested from the volar aspect of the wrist to provide tension-free anastomoses (**Fig. 11**).

## Step 5: Bone Stabilization

Digital and hand replantation requires bone stabilization first. Various bony stabilization methods

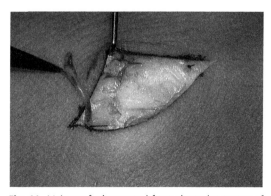

**Fig. 11.** Vein grafts harvested from the volar aspect of the wrist.

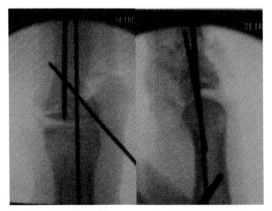

**Fig. 12.** Crossed K wires were used to obtain skeletal fixation.

are available: Kirschner (K) wire, intraosseous wiring, screw, peg, and small plate. Digital amputations at the distal or middle phalanx are most often secured with single or crossed K wires (**Fig. 12**) and at the proximal phalanx with crossed K wires or intraosseous wiring. Care must be taken to avoid twisting the neurovascular bundle or tethering the tendons by the K wires. On the other hand, transmetacarpal amputations often require mini-plate fixation (**Fig. 13**) for rigid fixation strong enough to withstand the rigors of hand therapy after replantation surgery. Wires and plates should be placed to allow joint motion, if possible. Care should be taken to achieve anatomic alignment and correct rotation of the replanted segments. Bone shortening is 1 method to make replantation easier and permits tension-free vascular anastomosis and nerve repairs. The amount of bone shortening depends on the extent of tissue involved. Less than 0.5 to 1.0 cm in the digits and 2 to 4 cm in the hand is

safer to prevent postoperative functional impairment.

### Steps 6 and 7: Tendon Repair

After rigid bony stabilization is performed, extensor and flexor tendon repair is performed. Extensor tendons are repaired with a figure-of-eight, horizontal mattress, or (locked) running suture of 5-0 or 4-0 nylon. Repair of the intrinsic tendons, lateral bands, is important for extension of distal interphalangeal joints.

After repair of the extensor mechanism, flexor tendons are then repaired (**Fig. 14**). As for the flexor tendons, primary repair is the rule. However, secondary repair, usually with the 2-stage silicone rod method, is required in some cases. Four-strand core sutures are now used for primary flexor tendon repair. We prefer to use 4-stand modified Kessler of 4-0 double-loop sutures for making core sutures. In zone II level amputation, only the profundus tendon is repaired to avoid adhesions between the superficialis and profundus tendon. Some surgeons prefer to repair not only the profundus but also a half-slip of the superficialis to improve postoperative motion compared with single profundus fingers. Subsequent tenolysis may be required 6 months after replantation.

### Step 8: Vessel and Nerve Repair

Once tendons are repaired, arteries are anastomosed (**Fig. 15**). Some surgeons recommend repairing all the arteries that can be restored; however, 1 digital artery repair for 1 digit is enough for replantation and can save total operating time. If only 1 digital artery is repaired, the dominant artery should be repaired if selectable. In the thumb, index, long, and ring fingers, the ulnar digital artery is dominant, whereas in the small finger the radial artery is dominant. If possible, multiple venous

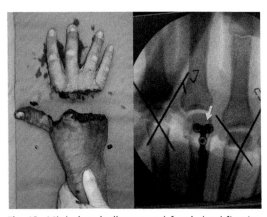

**Fig. 13.** Mini-plate (*yellow arrow*) for skeletal fixation in a transmetacarpal amputation.

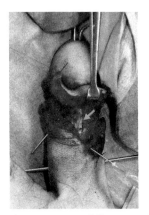
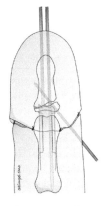

**Fig. 14.** Repaired flexor tendon (*green arrow*).

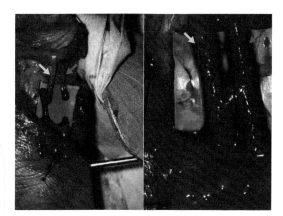 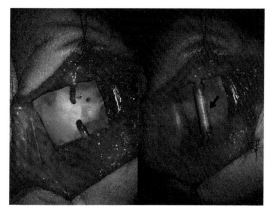

**Fig. 15.** Tension-free arterial anastomosis using a vein graft (*red arrow*) and nerve repair (*yellow arrow*).

**Fig. 16.** Artificial nerve conduit (*black arrow*) repair for a nerve defect.

anastomoses are recommended to improve outflow and increase the chances of survival. Although bone shortening is useful for tension-free vessels anastomosis, vein grafts are often required for bypassing vasospastic or damaged segments of vessels at the amputation site. Vein grafts are usually harvested from the volar wrist or dorsal foot, which are similar in caliber to digital vessels, whereas saphenous veins are suitable for hand vessels. The damaged artery has separation of the endothelial layer and must be resected until normal intima is visualized. Insufficient resection and arterial tension repair without vein grafts decrease the survival rate. Moreover, arterial anastomosis should not be done until spurting and pulsating arterial flow from proximal arteries have been identified. If vasospasm of proximal arteries is identified, useful methods for vasodilatation include (a) relief of arterial tension or compression, (b) warming of the room, patient, and proximal artery, (c) gentle intraluminal flushing with papaverine (1:20 dilution), (d) continuous intravenous prostaglandin E1 (PGE1), and (e) waiting.

The digital nerves are then repaired (see **Fig. 15**) because they are located in the same surgical field. After bone shortening, nerve repair is easy because there is no tension at the suture site. In digital nerve repair, 2 or 3 epineural sutures with 9-0 to 10-0 nylon are necessary. If a nerve defect occurs, autologous nerve grafting is usually performed. The medial antebrachial cutaneous nerve or posterior interosseous nerve is ideal as a donor for digital nerve grafting, whereas the sural nerve best matches the common digital nerve. However, the use of autologous nerve grafts carries the risk of donor-site morbidity, including sensory loss, neuroma, and scar. Recently, artificial nerve conduit repair can be chosen for replantation treatment of the nerve defect when direct tension-free coaptation is not possible (**Fig. 16**).

Further studies are required to estimate its role in nerve reconstruction for digital and hand replantation.[14]

After the arteries and nerves are repaired, dorsal veins are anastomosed finally (**Fig. 17**). It is difficult to find the dorsal veins because they are usually collapsed. Thus, by releasing the arterial clamps, the veins will enlarge and be easier to find. Before releasing the arterial clamps, a bolus of 3000 U of heparin is injected intravenously. If the dorsal veins are not available for repair, the thin, smaller volar veins can be used. Ideally, 2 vein repairs are necessary for 1 arterial repair.

### Step 9: Skin Closure

The skin is closed loosely with a few interrupted nylon sutures (**Fig. 18**). Small defects, less than 1 cm in a diameter, can be covered with artificial dermis (**Fig. 19**). If skin defects are large, a local flap or split-thickness skin grafts may be

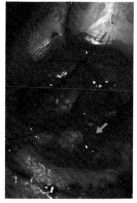 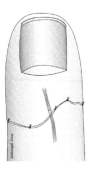

**Fig. 17.** Venous anastomosis on the dorsal side. Blue arrow: anastomosed vein.

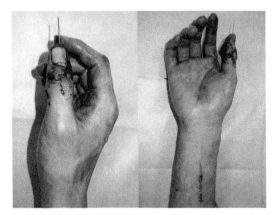

**Fig. 18.** Skin closure with a few interrupted nylon sutures.

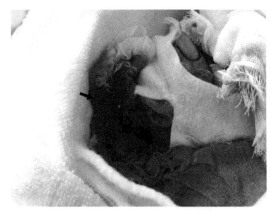

**Fig. 20.** A small area of skin is left exposed for evaluation of the circulation. Black arrow indicates heparin-soaked gauze.

required. A large volar defect with an arterial defect can be reconstructed by a venous flap harvested from the volar wrist as a flow-through flap.[15]

### Step 10: Postoperative Care

A bulky and noncompressive dressing and dorsal plaster splint are applied for postoperative

protection and comfort. The affected hand is kept elevated above the heart or slightly higher to increase circulation. The fingertips and a small area of skin are left exposed for evaluation of the circulation (**Fig. 20**). Postoperative management is important to improve the success rate of replantation. Skin color, temperature, turgor, and capillary refilling time should be monitored closely and frequently; every 1 to 3 hours for the first 24 hours, then every 6 to 8 hours until the fifth postoperative day (**Table 2**). More objective and quantitative evaluation can be measured with transcutaneous oxygen measurements, an easy and reliable method to predict the viability of the tissue (**Fig. 21**). The patient is kept warm and well hydrated. Pain and anxiety are controlled to avoid an adrenergic response and vasoconstriction. Smoking and caffeinated drinks are prohibited. The use of anticoagulants is

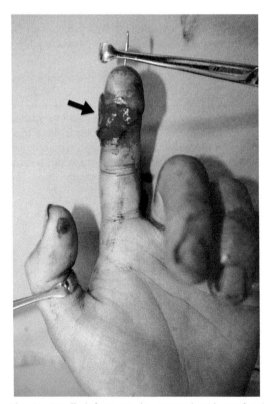

**Fig. 19.** Small defects can be covered with artificial dermis (*black arrow*).

| Table 2 |
|---|
| **Indicators for arterial and venous crisis** |

| Indicators for Vascular Crisis | Arterial Crisis (Arterial Vasospasm or Thrombosis) | Venous Crisis (Venous Thrombosis) |
|---|---|---|
| Skin color | White, pale | Dark purple |
| Skin temperature | Decreased | First high then low |
| Skin turgor | Decreased tension | Increased tension |
| Capillary refilling time | Prolonged (>2 s) | Shorten (<1 s) |
| Pin-prick test | Slow and decreased bleeding | Fast and excessive bleeding |

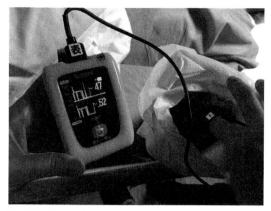

**Fig. 21.** Transcutaneous oxygen measurements are an easy and reliable method to predict the viability of the tissue.

controversial. The authors do not use postoperative anticoagulation routinely because there are no prospective randomized data to support a standard regimen of any of these medications. One exception is crush or avulsion injury, for which intravenous heparin, 1000 U per hour, is used for 5 to 7 days.

If there is suspicion of a vascular crisis (arterial or venous insufficiency), the patient is immediately transferred to the operating room for exploration of the vascular anastomosis. Early recognition of vascular crisis is essential for improving outcomes of replantation surgery. In patients with arterial obstruction, there is usually a thrombosis of an anastomosis that invariably requires re-anastomosis or vein grafting. In patients with venous obstruction, the solutions are a fish-mouth incision, dermal de-epthelization, periodic puncture of the fingertip, continuous nail bed bleeding by removing a portion of the nail bed, use of medical leeches, and a heparin-soaked gauze dressing to the wound. These methods are more useful in distal replants. A postoperative view at 2 months is shown in **Fig. 22**.

## OUTCOMES

Functional outcomes depend on the level of amputation. In general, the more distal the amputation, the better the functional result of replantation. A recent systematic review by Sebastin and Chung[16] revealed the following outcomes for distal digital replantation: mean survival rate, 86%; mean 2-point discrimination (2-PD), 7 mm; 98% returned to work; complications include pulp atrophy in 14% and nail deformity in 23%. For more proximal digital amputations, the outcomes are similar, with reported survival rates

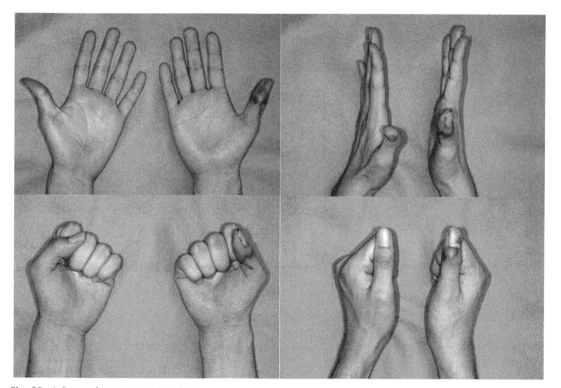

**Fig. 22.** A 2-month postoperative view.

between 80% and 90%[17–19] and an average 2-PD of 8 to 15 mm.[20] Range of motion is also related to amputation level. Active proximal interphalangeal (PIP) joint motion in replantation proximal to flexor digitorum superficialis (FDS) insertion is 35°, and 82° distal to FDS insertion.[21] For transmetacarpal amputations, the survival rate is relatively high (86%–90%), however, the functional outcomes are poorer. Sensory recovery is poor (78% achieved 2-PD; among those the mean 2-PD was 14.7 mm), less than 50% return to previous work, and the mean total active motion is 109 to 154°. Despite these poorer outcomes, patient satisfaction with the replantation surgery is high.[22,23]

## FINGERTIP REPLANTATION

Fingertip is defined as distal to the flexor and extensor tendon insertion site on the distal phalanx. Fingertip amputation was traditionally considered to be a contraindication for replantation. However, after the first report by Yamano,[24] recent studies have shown high survival rates (>80%–90%)[16] and excellent functional and aesthetic outcomes, providing a high degree of patient satisfaction. Nowadays, it is recognized that successful fingertip replantation is superior to any other reconstructive choice.[25] Fingertip replantation is more demanding than proximal digital replantation because veins are small and sometimes difficult to find. If a suitable vein cannot

be found, artery-only fingertip replantation is a good treatment option (**Fig. 23**); however, venous congestion is an inevitable phenomenon. Venous congestion of the replanted segment can be managed by pin-prick every 3 to 6 hours for 5 to 7 days, but the surviving fingertip often becomes painful with atrophy (**Fig. 24**). Several methods have been described to prevent venous congestion until internal circulation is established: removal of the nail bed,[26] use of medical leeches,[27] and a heparin-soaked gauze dressing. Koshima and colleagues[28] has devised 2 useful methods: arteriovenous anastomosis to eliminate venous drainage and delayed venous repair[29] (arterial anastomosis first and veins become engorged after 24 hours). Some surgeons mentioned that obligatory external bleeding to restore venous outflow is not always necessary, and venous outflow could be managed by the bleeding that occurred from the wound edge and bone marrow reflux.[30,31]

Another useful choice for fingertip replantation is the cap technique[32] and pocket plasty,[33] nonmicrosurgical reattachment. These techniques strive to increase venous outflow. The cap technique enhances composite graft survival by increasing the contact surface between the distal amputated fingertip and the stump. Pocket plasty involves de-epithelializing the pulp and choosing a suitable site on the palm and suturing them together. The pulp and palm are separated 2 to 3 weeks later after the initial operation.

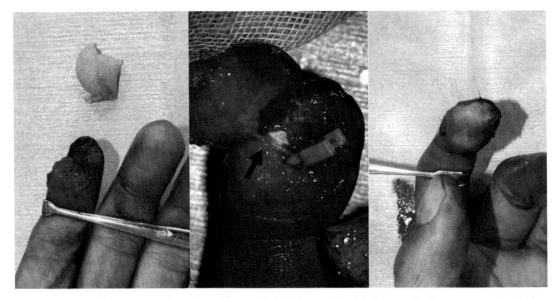

**Fig. 23.** Artery-only fingertip replantation of zone I digital amputation. Black arrow indicates a reconstructed artery with a vein graft.

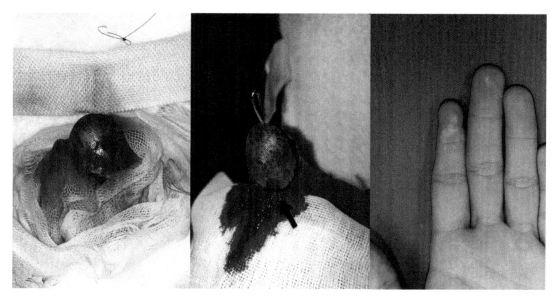

**Fig. 24.** Artery-only fingertip replantation of zone II digital amputation. Venous congestion of the replanted segment can be managed by pin-prick venous drainage, but the surviving fingertip often becomes painful with atrophy. Black arrow indicates venous drainage by pin-prick at the edge of the wound.

## SUMMARY

Surgical technique and recent evidence in microsurgical digital and hand replantation are comprehensively reviewed. Best outcomes after replantation are not solely related to the success of microvascular anastomosis but also to functional and aesthetic outcomes. More prospective studies are necessary to evaluate the quality of life, patient satisfaction, and cost-effectiveness of replantation compared with revision amputation.

## REFERENCES

1. Komatsu S, Tamai S. Successful replantation of a completely cut-off thumb: case report. Plast Reconstr Surg 1968;42:374–7.
2. Chung K, Alderman A. Replantation of the upper extremity: indications and outcomes. J Am Soc Surg Hand 2002;2:78–94.
3. Kleinert HE, Juhala CA, Tsai TM, et al. Digital replantation-selection, technique, and results. Orthop Clin North Am 1977;8:309–18.
4. Dec W. A meta-analysis of success rates for digit replantation. Tech Hand Up Extrem Surg 2006;10: 124–9.
5. Cheng GL, Pan DD, Zhang NP, et al. Digital replantation in children: a long-term follow-up study. J Hand Surg Am 1998;23:635–46.
6. Van Beek AL, Kutz JE, Zook EG. Importance of the ribbon sign, indicating unsuitability of the vessel, in replanting a finger. Plast Reconstr Surg 1978;61: 32–5.
7. Tamai S. Twenty years' experience of limb replantation–review of 293 upper extremity replants. J Hand Surg 1982;7A:549–56.
8. Allen MJ. Conservative management of fingertip injuries in adults. Hand 1980;12:257–65.
9. Ishikawa K, Ogawa Y, Soeda H, et al. A new classification of the amputation level for the distal part of the fingers. J Jpn Soc Microsurg 1990;3:54–62.
10. Wilhelmi BJ, Lee WP, Pagenstert GI, et al. Replantation in the mutilated hand. Hand Clin 2003;19: 89–120.
11. Sapega AA, Heppenstall RB, Sokolow DP, et al. The bioenergetics of preservation of limbs before replantation. The rationale for intermediate hypothermia. J Bone Joint Surg Am 1988;70:1500–13.
12. Maricevich M, Carlsen B, Mardini S, et al. Upper extremity and digital replantation. Hand 2011;6:356–63.
13. Camacho FJ, Wood MB. Polydigit replantation. Hand Clin 1992;8:409–12.
14. Paprottka FJ, Wolf P, Harder Y, et al. Sensory recovery outcome after digital nerve repair in relation to different reconstructive techniques: meta-analysis and systematic review. Plast Surg Int 2013;2013: 704589.
15. Pederson WC. Upper extremity microsurgery. Plast Reconstr Surg 2001;107:1524–37.
16. Sebastin SJ, Chung KC. A systematic review of the outcomes of replantation of distal digital amputation. Plast Reconstr Surg 2011;128:723–37.
17. Yoshizu T, Katsumi M, Tajima T. Replantation of untidily amputated finger, hand, and arm: experience of 99 replantations in 66 cases. J Trauma 1978;18: 194–200.

18. Cheng GL, Pan DD, Qu ZY, et al. Digital replantation. A ten-year retrospective study. Chin Med J 1991; 104:96–102.

19. Waikakul S, Sakkarnkosol S, Vanadurongwan V, et al. Results of 1018 digital replantations in 552 patients. Injury 2000;31:33–40.

20. Glickman LT, Mackinnon SE. Sensory recovery following digital replantation. Microsurgery 1990; 11:236–42.

21. Urbaniak JR, Roth JH, Nunley JA, et al. The results of replantation after amputation of a single finger. J Bone Joint Surg Am 1985;67A:611–9.

22. Weinzweig N, Sharzer LA, Starker I. Replantation and revascularization at the transmetacarpal level: long-term functional results. J Hand Surg Am 1996; 21:877–83.

23. Paavilainen P, Nietosvaara Y, Tikkinen KA, et al. Long-term results of transmetacarpal replantation. J Plast Reconstr Aesthet Surg 2007;60:704–9.

24. Yamano Y. Replantation of the amputated distal part of the fingers. J Hand Surg Am 1985;10: 211–8.

25. Yabe T, Tsuda T, Hirose S, et al. Treatment of fingertip amputation: comparison of results between microsurgical replantation and pocket principle. J Reconstr Microsurg 2012;28:221–6.

26. Yabe T, Muraoka M, Motomura H, et al. Fingertip replantation using a single volar arteriovenous anastomosis and drainage with a transverse tip incision. J Hand Surg Am 2001;26:1120–4.

27. Han SK, Chung HS, Kim WK. The timing of neovascularization in fingertip replantation by external bleeding. Plast Reconstr Surg 2002;110:1042–6.

28. Koshima I, Soeda S, Moriguchi T, et al. The use of arteriovenous anastomosis for replantation of the distal phalanx of the fingers. Plast Reconstr Surg 1992;89:710–4.

29. Koshima I, Yamashita S, Sugiyama N, et al. Successful delayed venous drainage in 16 consecutive distal phalangeal replantations. Plast Reconstr Surg 2005;115:149–54.

30. Tanaka K, Kobayashi K, Murakami R, et al. Venous drainage through bone marrow after replantation: an experimental study. Br J Plast Surg 1998;51: 629–32.

31. Peterson SL, Peterson EL, Wheatley MJ. Management of fingertip amputations. J Hand Surg Am 2014;39:2093–101.

32. Rose EH, Norris MS, Kowalski TA, et al. The "cap" technique: nonmicrosurgical reattachment of fingertip amputations. J Hand Surg Am 1989;14: 513–8.

33. Brent B. Replantation of amputated distal phalangeal parts of fingers without vascular anastomoses, using subcutaneous pockets. Plast Reconstr Surg 1979;63:1–8.

# Hand Infections

Wendy Z.W. Teo, BA (Cantab), BM BCh (Oxon), LLM[a],*, Kevin C. Chung, MD, MS[b]

## KEYWORDS

- Hand • Infections • Superficial • Deep • Bites

## KEY POINTS

- Hand infections can lead to devastating impact on functional outcomes and should be treated promptly and properly.
- Detailed history and examination, and occasionally radiological imaging, are necessary to guide a physician to the correct diagnosis.
- Antimicrobial treatment and/or surgical drainage are mainstays of treatment of hand infections.

## INTRODUCTION

Hand infections can lead to debilitating and permanent disability, particularly if they are not treated promptly or properly treated.[1] The unique anatomy of the hand, with its numerous enclosed and confined spaces, warrants special considerations. For instance, infections in deep spaces of the hand may require surgical drainage despite an appropriate course of antimicrobial treatment. A majority of hand infections are found in young, active, and healthy adults who defer treatment of seemingly minor trauma.[2] Progression of infection depends on the immune status of patients, virulence of the offending organisms, and anatomic location of tissue.[3]

## HISTORICAL BACKGROUND ON MANAGEMENT

In 1912, Allen B. Kanavel penned *Infections of the Hand: A Guide to the Surgical Treatment of Acute and Chronic Suppurative Processes in the Fingers, Hand and Forearm*,[4] which proved a seminal work on the management of hand infections. His understanding and recommendations on management of hand infections were firmly grounded on a detailed study on anatomy of the hand. The general principles on diagnosis

and conservative management espoused in his work are still largely relevant today. A few decades later, Sterling Bunnell, who is widely acknowledged as the founding father of hand surgery in the United States, made extraordinary steps toward advancing hand surgery as an independent specialty; he believed a combination of plastic, orthopedic, and neurosurgery skills is a prerequisite to master the specialty. His work, *Surgery of the Hand*, distills the vast developments in hand surgery during and after World War II. The book outlined the devastating and permanent deformities, with its attendant functional debilitation, that can arise from hand infections.[5,6] As Adrian E. Flatt, an eminent hand surgeon who was the former chief of the Department of Orthopaedic Surgery at Baylor University Medical Centre in Dallas wrote, "Hand surgery is an area specialty, not a tissue specialty."[7] Likewise, optimal management of hand infections warrants unique considerations in addition to issues dealt with in the management of general infections. The advent of antibiotics marks another revolutionary leap forward in managing hand infections; it decreased the morbidity of hand surgery considerably and reduced the mortality rate to almost zero.[8] Development of new classes of antibiotics over the past 50 years, however, has slowed down drastically and new strains of

Disclosure Statement: There are no conflicts of interest or financial interests to disclose.
a Department of Hand and Reconstructive Microsurgery, National University Health System, 1E Kent Ridge Road, Level 11, Singapore 119228, Singapore; b The University of Michigan Health System, 1500 East Medical Center Drive, 2130 Taubman Center, SPC 5340, Ann Arbor, MI 48109-5340, USA
* Corresponding author.
*E-mail address:* wendy_zw_teo@nuhs.edu.sg

antibiotic-resistant bacteria are continuing to emerge, which may pose a problem in the treatment of hand infections in the coming decades.[9,10]

## PATHOPHYSIOLOGY

Inoculation induces a reaction characterized by inflammation and an immune response, otherwise known as the inflammatory phase.[11] The immune response mounted results in the release of enzymes and toxins against the offending pathogen but also induces edema and swelling, leading to an increase in tissue pressure. Tissue necrosis may be an inadvertent consequence caused by the purulent phase. Although lymphangitis and lymphadenopathy can be seen in some cases, the bacterial load in hand infections often is of low volume, and systemic symptoms are rare. Consequently, signs, such as fever and elevated levels of C-reactive protein, are not present in approximately three-fourths of hand infections.[12]

## GENERAL PRINCIPLES OF MANAGEMENT
### History

It is crucial to obtain a focused and pertinent history because this provides a firm guide for definitive treatment. In addition to information that is obtained in a typical history, such as age and hand dominance, it is recommended that the following information are elicited:

- Occupation: a patient's occupation should be elicited for numerous reasons—to explore possible risks that a patient's occupation, such as manual labor, may predispose to hand injuries; to tailor the postoperative rehabilitation program to accommodate a patient's working schedule; and to better understand the extent to which a patient's livelihood depends on the function of the hands.[13] Although knowledge of the extent to which a patient's livelihood depends on his hands does not alter the optimal treatment option, it serves to underscore the gravity of the injury from the patient's perspective and facilitate shared decision making.
- Mode of inoculation: it is helpful to establish the mode of inoculation, because this guides examination and treatment options, especially empiric antibiotic choices, while culture results are pending. The most common mechanism of injury is trauma, such as penetrating injuries or bites.[12] Specific organisms are of relevance to certain occupations—animal handlers may be exposed to Pasteurella

through animal bites, gardeners to Sporothrix, and divers in aquariums to mycobacterium.
- Symptoms: pertinent symptoms must be elicited with all infections, including location and character of pain (excruciating throbbing pain is suggestive of abscess in a confined area), radiation (proximal extension along forearm should alert physician to possible ascending lymphangitis), duration and progression (indolent, acute, or rapidly progressing), fever or chills, spontaneous discharge and character of discharge (puslike or clear), worsening or improvement of symptoms over time, aggravating factors, (movement, heat, and pressure), and factors that offer relief (elevation and analgesia). Prior recurrent episodes that resolved spontaneously or with anti-inflammatories may point toward a different pathology, such as gout or pseudogout.
- Previous treatment: it is not uncommon for patients to have sought medical attention elsewhere, for example, family physicians prior to presentation. Hence, it is imperative to obtain information on previous treatment methods, including extended courses of antibiotics. A lack of response to conservative management offers valuable clues to the nature and severity of the infections and may prompt physicians to lean toward surgical interventions. Other physicians or patients themselves may have attempted drainage, and it is helpful to note the method of drainage, for example, an unsterile needle as well as the character of discharge if applicable.
- Immune status: it should be established if a patient has any underlying medical conditions that impairs immunologic function and hence predisposes to infections, including diabetes, HIV infection, malignancies, or previous organ transplant necessitating immunosuppressive medications. An immunocompromised patient is more susceptible to rapid clinical progression, increased complication rates, and poorer outcomes.[12] Immunosuppressive patients may not mount an inflammatory response marked by erythema or pus collection. Therefore, the clinical findings may mask an indolent infection, which requires more aggressive open drainage to ascertain the extent and the severity of the infection. If a patient has other comorbidities, skillful coordination of care between different specialties during a single episode of care can improve overall clinical outcomes and the patient's sense of well-being.

## Examination

As with any suspected cases of infection, findings, such as erythema, swelling, and fluctuance, can help localize the infection and assist in assessment of severity. Early demarcation of the extent of visible erythema with a marker helps monitor progression of infection. Specific examination findings also may provide clues on the nature of infection—central skin necrosis with surrounding erythema is associated with methicillin-resistant *Staphylococcus aureus*; crepitus can be caused by gas-forming organisms, including *Clostridium*, anaerobic streptococcus, and some coliforms; and Kanavel cardinal signs. Although Kanavel highlighted only 3 signs deemed cardinal (tenderness over the course of sheath, finger held in a partially flexed posture, and pain on passive extension), he did discuss a fourth sign in the same initial work published in 1912 ("the whole of the finger is uniformly swollen"),[14] which later became the fourth cardinal sign ("fusiform swelling of entire digit").[4] Proximal extension of erythema and epitrochlear or axillary lymphadenopathy are indicative of lymphangitic spread. A detailed neurovascular examination also is crucial because complications may arise due to compressive effect, with immunocompromised patients especially susceptible. Maneuvers also can be done to localize the infection—tenderness is elicited if the volume of an infected compartment is reduced.

## Investigations

1. Blood tests—white blood cell count, erythrocyte sedimentation rate, and C-reactive protein can be measured at baseline to assess for severity and subsequent response to treatment.
2. Radiological imaging—radiographs are helpful for identifying radio-opaque foreign bodies that act as nidus for infections as well as possible osteomyelitis and accompanying fractures. MRI can be used to assess accompanying soft tissue and bony abnormalities whereas ultrasound can assist with localization of deep abscesses or fluid collection along tendon sheaths.[15–17]
3. Cultures—fluid and tissue cultures (both aerobic and anaerobic) as well as Gram stain, if possible, should be obtained prior to embarking on antibiotic therapy.

## Treatment

1. Conservative treatment: antibiotic therapy is vital in the treatment of hand infections, and empiric antibiotics should be administered in the early stages before culture results are obtained. Empiric antibiotics, such as first-generation cephalosporins, cover skin flora, such as *S aureus* and β-hemolytic streptococcus. The lack of clinical response to antibiotic treatment after 12 hours to 24 hours of initiating treatment can mean either that the choice of antibiotic was inappropriate or that antibiotic treatment alone is inadequate, and surgical intervention should be undertaken.
2. Surgical intervention: in cases of severe infection or infection that does not respond to antibiotic treatment, surgical incision and drainage as well as débridement of necrotic or nonviable tissue are necessary and may need to be repeated at regular intervals until tissue cultures are negative or the wound is deemed cleared of infection. The placement of incisions must be given careful consideration—although accessibility and extensibility of incision are crucial factors, the incision should not expose critical structures, for example, nerves, arteries, and vessels; exposing critical structures risks desiccation because the wound often is left open to allow drainage. The incision also should be designed to minimize functional limitations from possible scar contracture. Local anesthetic agents may not be effective in view of the acidic nature of infections and may inadvertently spread infection along tissue planes.
3. Postoperative: dressings must be kept clean and dry at all times, and regular dressing changes must be done under aseptic technique. Splinting can minimize pain, reduce flexion contracture and stiffness, and speed up functional rehabilitation. Elevation of hand reduces edema by improving venous and lymphatic drainage whereas early rehabilitation of the hand can speed up functional recovery. Heat can increase a patient's comfort and causes vasodilatation, hence allowing antibiotics to reach tissues faster.[18]

## Miscellaneous

- Tetanus: the tetanus immunization status of the patient should be reviewed and tetanus immune globulin or toxoid should be administered if necessary.
- Management of expectations: the optimal treatment of hand infections often requires a prolonged duration of recovery and may necessitate repeated surgical interventions. It is sensible to counsel patients about the possible recovery process at initial presentation so as to tailor expectations and allow patients to make plans accordingly.

## INFECTIONS
### Superficial

1. Onychomycosis: onychomycosis is a fungal infection of the nail apparatus and typically is chronic in nature. Patients may reveal a history of prolonged or repeated exposure of digits to water; Trichophyton rubrum and Candida species are the most common organisms involved. Topical antifungals can be used for distal onychomycosis whereas oral antifungals can be used to treat proximal cases. Systemic treatment, however, may not be sufficient and nail removal may be required.

2. Cellulitis: cellulitis is a diffuse superficial infection involving the subcutaneous tissues and presents with warmth, erythema, and edema, which all can progress over time. The treatment of cellulitis in the hand is similar to treatment of cellulitis elsewhere—rest, elevation, warm soaks, antibiotics, and monitoring for progress. Compared with any area of the body, however, patients with cellulitis in the hand have a higher likelihood of requiring hospital admission for intravenous antibiotics to treat the infection adequately.[19] Initial delineation of the boundaries can assist in monitoring of progress of cellulitis. The lack of response to conservative management points toward the possibility of a deeper infection.

3. Lymphangitis: lymphangitis presents with erythematous streaks that spread proximally up the arm and may be associated with palpable epitrochlear or axillary lymphadenopathy. It can be managed conservatively and, like cellulitis, a deep hand infection should be considered if there is a lack of response.

4. Paronychia: acute paronychia is a bacterial infection of the lateral nail fold that is less than 6 weeks in duration and presents with erythema, swelling, tenderness, and occasionally spontaneous discharge of purulent material. It may progress to involve the proximal nail fold (acute eponychia) and opposite lateral nail fold (runaround abscess); in extreme cases, it can extend to the pulp space.[20] S aureus is the most common infecting organism, with Streptococcus pyogenes and oral anaerobes present in patients who bite their nails.[21] In early stages of acute paronychia, it may be treated conservatively with warm soaks and oral antibiotics, but if an abscess is present, surgical drainage is necessary, with a skin incision to be made on the eponychium or a portion of the nail plate to be removed.[22] Chronic paronychia is characterized by symptoms of at least 6 weeks in duration and is common in patients whose hands are constantly exposed to water or chemical irritants, like dishwashers, florists, swimmers, and medical professionals.[9,23] Antifungal treatment, both topical and oral, are of marginal benefit and surgical intervention is often necessary. Eponychial marsupialization often is carried out, but a different school of thought is that chronic paronychia is due to exposure dermatitis (and not infection), and topical corticosteroids have been able to achieve satisfactory results.[24,25]

5. Felon: a felon is a severe infection of the pulp space that generally arises from direct inoculation. It accounts for 15% to 20% of all hand infections, with the thumb and index fingers most commonly affected.[26] Patients with felon present with pain, cellulitis, and a tender fluctuant swelling; occasionally, a focal area of skin blanching can be seen. The pain often is characterized as severe and throbbing and has an adverse impact on the quality of sleep.[27] Because the pulp is divided into multiple compartments by fibrous septae, swelling in a restricted compartment can increase pressure and lead to ischemic necrosis of surrounding tissue. It also can spread the infection and cause osteomyelitis, flexor tenosynovitis, and septic arthritis of the distal interphalangeal joint.[28] A radiograph is valuable in excluding retained foreign bodies of involvement of the distal phalanx. Although conservative management with rest, elevation, warm soaks, and oral antibiotics can be considered in early presentations, most patients require surgical drainage. Purulent materials should be cultured before starting antibiotics. Some investigators believe antibiotics are not necessary after surgical intervention for uncomplicated cases.[29,30]

6. Herpetic whitlow: herpetic whitlow is an infection of the finger caused by herpes simplex virus-1 (HSV-1) in children (who put their hands in their mouth) and by HSV-1 or HSV-2 in nurses, dental workers, and sexually active adults.[31] The lesions in herpetic whitlow often present as a single vesicle or a cluster of vesicles that are initially clear but become yellow with an erythematous base and may coalesce to form large blisters. The vesicles eventually evolve into shallow ulcers that form crusts, and the process often takes place over 14 days, during which the patients are infectious.[32] Pain often is out of proportion to the clinical presentation and often precedes the appearance of vesicles. If the vesicles are found on multiple digits, an alternative diagnosis, such as coxsackievirus, should be considered. Although a diagnosis of herpetic

whitlow often is made based on clinical findings, diagnostic tests, including Tzanck smear, lesion-specific antigen detection tests, viral culture, and serum antibody cultures, are helpful.[32] The treatment of herpetic whitlow is conservative, with rest, elevation, and anti-inflammatory agents, and does not require antibiotics unless a secondary bacterial infection is suspected, for example, blistering dactylitis in children with herpetic whitlow. The use of oral acyclovir can be used in immunocompetent patients with recurrent disease or primary disease at multiple sites whereas topical acyclovir therapy may be of benefit for those with primary herpetic whitlow.[33] The recurrence rate is 20%.[33]

## Deep Infections

1. Synovial space infections: there are a few synovial spaces in the hand—flexor tendon sheaths, radial and ulnar bursa, and space of Parona. Synovial spaces are in communication and provide optimum conditions for bacterial growth because they are poorly vascularized and rich in synovial fluid.[1,34,35] The flexor tendons in the hand are enclosed in a double-layered synovial sheath. An infection within this enclosed sheath is called pyogenic flexor tenosynovitis. Bacterial proliferation within the sheath can severely impair the tendon's gliding mechanism, whereas the increased pressure within the enclosed sheath can impair vascular supply and cause tendon necrosis and tendon rupture.[36] Flexor tenosynovitis of a digit may result from direct inoculation or a spread from a contiguous deep space infection. The 4 cardinal signs of flexor tenosynovitis (Kanavel signs) are, in descending order of frequency, fusiform swelling of the entire finger, pain with passive extension, a partially flexed resting posture of the finger, and volar tenderness along the length of the finger and into the palm[4,37] (**Fig. 1**). Not all 4 signs need to be present, however, to diagnose pyogenic flexor tenosynovitis.[38] The tendon sheath of the flexor pollicis longus continues proximally as radial bursa whereas the tendon sheaths of the fingers (ulnar digits) continue proximally as the ulnar bursa. Both bursae communicate with each other via the space of Parona, which is a potential space between the profundus tendons and pronator quadratus.[1] Infection of the radial or ulnar bursa hence can track proximally and spread to the other, forming a horseshoe abscess. Patients with such infections often present with a flexed attitude of the wrist, swelling, and tenderness along the thenar, hypothenar, and distal wrist crease because of an associated thumb or small finger flexor tenosynovitis. Surgical drainage often is warranted: a systematic review of 28 case series articles by Giladi and colleagues in 2015[35] concluded that closed sheath catheter irrigation achieved improved range of motion compared with open washout. Factors associated with a

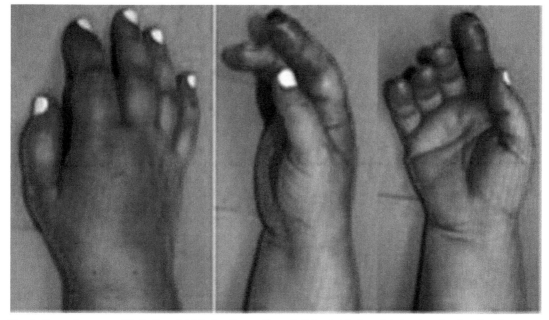

**Fig. 1.** Flexor tenosynovitis in the right index finger (from left to right: dorsal, lateral and volar views).

poorer outcome include comorbidities like diabetes, renal failure, peripheral vascular disease, subcutaneous purulence, and ischemic changes on presentation.[38]

2. Hand space infections

- Deep fascial space infections: deep fascial space infections are emergencies and warrant immediate surgical intervention. There are 3 potential closed spaces in the palm with well-defined anatomic boundaries that are susceptible to infections: thenar, midpalmar, and hypothenar spaces.[39] These spaces are located deep to the flexor tendons but are superficial to the interosseous muscles and infections in these compartments remain confined. Ultrasound imaging can help differentiate a deep hand space infection from pyogenic flexor tenosynovitis or hematogenous spread from a distant site.

    a. Thenar space abscess presents with a widely abducted thumb and swelling on the dorsum of the first webspace, with severe pain on abduction or opposition of the thumb. Drainage can be achieved through a volar incision or a combined volar and dorsal approach, taking care to avoid the neurovascular bundle to the thumb.

    b. Midpalmar space infection leads to loss of the normal palmar concavity with the long and ring fingers by assuming a partially flexed posture and pain on passive extension of these fingers. This space may communicate with Parona space anterior to pronator quadratus and drainage can be achieved through a palmar incision.

    c. Hypothenar space infections have less swelling and do not involve the digits or flexor tendons. Drainage can be achieved via a volar longitudinal incision.

- Webspace infections: webspace infections may exist on both volar and dorsal sides of webspaces (collar button abscess), although this rarely has been seen since the advent of antibiotics. The adjacent fingers typically are held in an abducted position, and a combined palmar and dorsal surgical approach is necessary to achieve adequate drainage and débridement.

- Dorsal subaponeurotic space lies deep to extensor tendons on the dorsal surface of hand. Drainage can be achieved through 2 longitudinal incision or 2 longitudinal incisions with a wide skin bridge. Extensor tendons should not be left exposed or allowed to desiccate.

3. Septic arthritis: patients with septic arthritis present with an erythematous, swollen, warm, and tender joint that elicits pain on passive motion. Septic arthritis is uncommon in the hand and wrist, however, so mimickers of infection, such as gout, pseudogout, arthritis, and Lyme disease, should be given serious consideration. Finger joint infections often occur after direct inoculation, whereas wrist infections can be sequelae of bacteremia. Fluid that is aspirated should be sent for culture, cell count, peripheral blood white cell counts, and erythrocyte sedimentation rate. S aureus commonly is found, although gonococcal infections should be suspected in young, sexually active individuals.[9] Likewise, polymicrobials should be suspected in immunocompromised individuals or infections resulting from human bites. The presence of a white, pasty substance and absence of pus are highly suggestive of gout, although gout and septic arthritis can coexist. Radiographs should be taken to exclude osteomyelitis and can also be helpful in differentiating from pseudogout—calcification of the triangular fibrocartilage complex is indicative of pseudogout. Appropriate antibiotic treatment is indispensable and should be adjusted after close monitoring and culture results. A study of 97 patients by Meier and colleagues[40] in 2017 found that the median antimicrobial treatment duration was 14 days. Surgical drainage should be done with care to avoid contamination of surrounding structures or injury to nearby structures, and patients should be advised that some degree of joint stiffness often is inevitable, especially in patients who presented after a few days of infection or whose proximal interphalangeal joints are affected.[41]

4. Necrotizing fasciitis: necrotizing fasciitis is a rapidly progressive, potentially lethal soft tissue infection with widespread fascial necrosis.[42,43] Initial presentation in early stages may be similar to that of cellulitis but the presence of the following symptoms point toward necrotizing fasciitis: severe pain that is out of proportion to clinical appearance, rapid spread and progress of symptoms, bullae, skin numbness, subcutaneous crepitus, systemic toxicity, patient sense of impending doom, and a lack of response to appropriate antibiotics. Group A hemolytic streptococcus is the most common offending organism for necrotizing fasciitis of the upper limbs, although S aureus and other microorganisms can be involved.[44] Necrotizing fasciitis requires urgent surgical intervention, with initial treatment involving resuscitation, stabilization of the patient, and empirical

broad-spectrum intravenous antimicrobial therapy, after which repeated surgical débridement should be carried out as soon as possible. Skin, subcutaneous tissue, fascia, and any necrotic muscle should be excised, if necessary, and fascia radically débrided well beyond the zone of obvious infection. The prognosis is poor, with approximately half of patients with extremity necrotizing fasciitis requiring amputation, and approximately one-third die, including young healthy patients who have undergone aggressive treatment.[45,46] Negative wound pressure dressing has not proved to improve morbidity or mortality in the treatment of necrotizing fasciitis in the extremities.[47]

5. Osteomyelitis: osteomyelitis is uncommon in the hand and wrist, and route of inoculation usually is from direct trauma or contiguous spread from adjacent areas that are infected. The distal phalanx is most commonly infected and radiographs are useful, although it may take up to 2 weeks to 3 weeks to reflect osteolysis.[48] Surgical débridement of infected and necrotic bone is required, and a prolonged course of antibiotics should be administered (minimum 4–6 weeks) until all signs and symptoms have resolved.[49]

## Postsurgery Infection

1. Infection after elective surgeries of the hand is rare. A study of 2337 elective hand and upper extremity surgeries done by Kleinert and colleagues[50] in 1997 revealed an overall infection rate of 1.4%, with a deep infection rate of 0.3%. Likewise, Hansen and colleagues assessed 3620 cases of elective carpal tunnel release and found an overall infection rate of less than 1%.[51] Both retrospective and prospective studies have revealed that operations that last longer than 2 hours are at a higher risk of postoperative infection.[52–54]

Consequently, elective procedures that may take longer than 2 hours may benefit from prophylactic antibiotics.[55]

## Bites

### Animal bites

The most common animal bites are dog and cat bites. Dog bites account for 80% to 90% of all animal bite injuries whereas cat bites are responsible for an overwhelming majority of bites that go on develop infections (76%).[56–59] The reason underlying this phenomenon is that cats have sharp, long teeth that can inoculate bacteria deep in soft tissue, and patients often present late when infection has already set in, in view of the seemingly innocuous puncture wounds and in part for fear of punitive action toward their pets. Dog bites usually consist of abrasions and lacerations (**Fig. 2**). The immunization status of the animals (including rabies) should be established. All animal bite wounds should be opened and irrigated as soon as possible, either in an emergency department under local anesthesia, if presented early, or in an operating room. The bites are often polymicrobial, and the most commonly isolated organisms from dog and cat bite infections are *Pasteurella multocida*, viridans streptococci, *S aureus*, and anaerobes.[28,57] Both aerobic and anaerobic cultures of bite wounds hence should be obtained. Prophylactic antibiotics have not been shown of much benefit in uncomplicated cat and dog bites.[60]

### Human bites

Human bites are are the products of physical confrontations. Patients hence are often reluctant to offer an accurate history, and the innocuous outward appearance of such wounds means that patients often present late. Patients may be more willing to divulge crucial information if they are reassured of complete confidentiality. Human

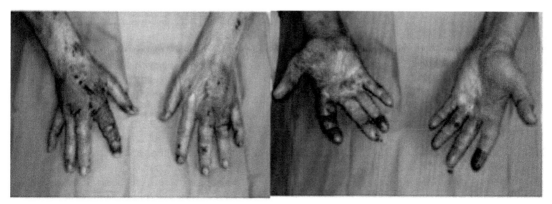

**Fig. 2.** Bilateral hand wounds sustained from dog bites (from left to right: dorsal and volar views).

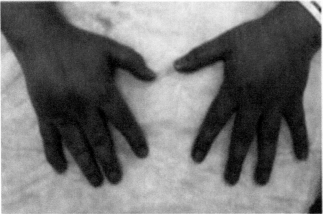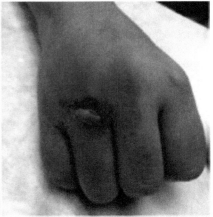

**Fig. 3.** Wound sustained from a human bite (from left to right: dorsal view of bilateral hands, close up of wound).

bites must be considered when a young male patient presents with a laceration over the metacarpophangeal joints, especially if on the dominant hand (**Fig. 3**). Any open wound that results from a human bite should be considered contaminated regardless of absence of signs of infection.

It is crucial to note that the bite is often sustained with the fist held in a clenched position, therefore unlikely that the skin laceration corresponds to the site of underlying injuries to bone, cartilage, or joint when the hand is held in extended position. Tenosynovitis, septic arthritis, osteomyelitis, and residual stiffness are common serious complications.[61] Patients who present more than 8 days after sustaining bite injury have a 18% chance of undergoing amputation.[62] A radiograph (Brewerton view) can reveal fracture of the metacarpal head, retained foreign body (tooth fragment), or osteomyelitis. A depression of metacarpal head seen on radiograph, however minute, suggests an impaction by a tooth, and, subsequently, intra-articular penetration. Although *Eikenella* is characteristic of human bite wounds, the wounds commonly have polymicrobial bacterial infections with a mixture of both anaerobic and aerobic organisms.[57] The human oral flora is highly virulent and hence human bites often require hospital admission, repeated débridement and irrigation, antibiotics, and delayed closure. Tissue cultures are indispensable; intravenous antibiotics should be used and tailored postoperatively to reduce risk of infection.

## Uncommon Infections

1. *Sporothrix schenckii*: infections with *sporothrix schenckii* arise from rose thorn inoculation and present with granuloma at inoculation site with proximal lymphadenopathy.

2. *Mycobacterium marinum*: infections with *mycobacterium marinum* are associated with water exposure or fish handling with the upper extremity being the most common site of infection.

3. *Vibrio vulnificus*: inoculation usually is from a puncture by a fish spine, and infection typically is rapidly progressive, causing extensive skin and soft tissue necrosis. It can lead to necrotizing fasciitis, and urgent surgical débridement often is necessary.

## DIFFERENTIALS/MIMICKERS

There are a few inflammatory conditions that may present with signs and symptoms similar to those of hand infections, making it clinically difficult to between among them. A physician should make every possible effort to reach a unifying diagnosis because the treatment can be vastly different, with potentially deleterious impact on the patient.

1. Gout and pseudogout: gout is a disorder of urate metabolism that leads to high levels of uric acid and formation of urate crystals that can be deposited under the skin and joints and within tendon sheaths as gouty tophi (**Fig. 4**). Pseudogout is caused by the deposition of calcium pyrophosphate crystals. Both conditions easily can be confused with a felon, subcutaneous abscess; pyogenic flexor tenosynovitis; or septic arthritis, which can lead to unnecessary or even damaging treatment options. The keys to differentiating between hand infections and gout or pseudogout are a comprehensive history, exploring the possibility of preexisting gout or previous similar flare-ups, and clinical presentation. Serum uric acid values and radiographs can be useful in differentiating gout. If still in doubt, a trial of colchicine may be of

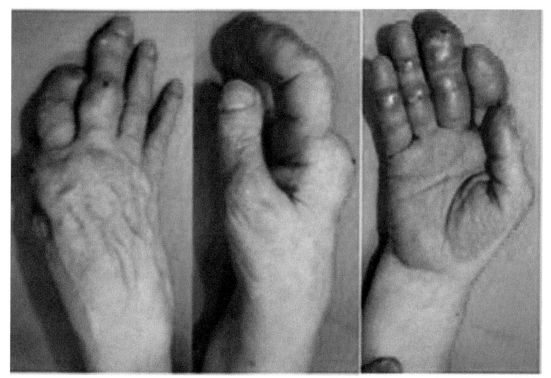

**Fig. 4.** Gouty tophi in digits (from left to right: dorsal, lateral and volar views).

value. For definitive confirmation, aspiration of the involved joint and examining the synovial fluid under a polarizing microscope may reveal negatively birefringent needle-shaped intracellular monosodium urate crystals (gout) or positively birefringent rhomboid-shaped calcium pyrophosphate crystals (pseudogout).

2. Acute calcific tendinitis: deposition of calcium salts around tendons and ligaments can result in acute calcific tendonitis in which patients present with pain, swelling, erythema, and tenderness overlying tendons or ligaments. Other telltale signs of infection, including fever and abnormal laboratory values, often are absent and radiographs can reveal characteristic homogenous calcific densities in the area of tenderness. The treatment of acute calcific tendinitis is conservative, with analgesics, rest, and splintage; differentiation from infection hence is crucial to prevent unnecessary antibiotic treatment or surgical intervention.

3. Retained foreign bodies: foreign bodies, such as splinters and thorns, can cause an inflammatory response, which has a presentation similar to that of infection. A detailed history is crucial in helping the physician distinguish between the 2, and often the removal of the foreign body is necessary for definitive treatment.

4. Iatrogenic injury: extravasation of irritants (such as vesicant chemotherapeutic agents) or injection of illicit drugs at sites of intravascular access can mimic infection, with signs, such as erythema and swelling.[63]

5. Pyoderma gangrenosum: pyoderma gangrenosum is an inflammatory skin disease that is associated with systemic disorders, such as inflammatory bowel disease, arthritis, and lymphoproliferative disorders. In the early stages, it appears as small papules on extremities (and trunk as well) but it rapidly progresses to central necrosis that results in a central ulcer and a raised border and ultimately forms cribriform scars. A diagnosis of pyoderma gangrenosum often is a diagnosis of exclusion, that is, after all infectious etiologies are ruled out.

6. Metastatic tumor: metastatic or primary tumors in the hand are rare. Primary lesions often are dermatologic in nature, for example, squamous cell carcinoma, basal cell carcinoma, melanoma, and keratoacanthoma. Metastatic tumors can be mistaken for chronic infections, with more than 50% involving the distal phalanx. Lung tumors most commonly are the source of metastatic tumors, but other primary tumors, such as breast, kidney, colon, thyroid, and prostrate, should be considered.[64–66] If in

doubt, the adage to "biopsy what you culture, and culture what you biopsy" can be of help.[67]

## REFERENCES

1. Patel DB, Emmanuel NB, Stevanovic MV, et al. Hand infections: anatomy, types and spread of infection, imaging findings, and treatment options. Radiographics 2014;34(7):1968–86.
2. Tosti R, Ilyas AM. Empiric antibiotics for acute infections of the hand. J Hand Surg Am 2010;35(1):125–8.
3. Ong Y, Levin LS. Hand infections. Plast Reconstr Surg 2009;124(4):225–33.
4. Kanavel A. Infections of the hand: a guide to the surgical treatment of acute and chronic suppurative processes in the fingers, hand and forearm. Philadelphia: Lea & Febiger; 1925.
5. Bunnell S. Surgery of the Hand. Philadelphia, PA: JB. Lippincott; 1944.
6. Contractures of the hand from infections and injuries. In: Bunnell S, editor. Surgery in World war II, hand surgery. Washington, DC: Office of the Surgeon General, Department of the Army; 1995.
7. Flatt AE. Surgery in World War II: Hand Surgery. AMA Arch Intern Med 1958;101(5):1009–10.
8. Finland M. Emergence of antibiotic-resistance bacteria. N Engl J Med 1956;253:909–22.
9. Osterman M, Draeger R, Stern P. Acute hand infections. J Hand Surg Am 2014;39(8):1628–35.
10. Kistler JM, Thoder JJ, Ilyas AM. MRSA incidence and antibiotic trends in urban hand infections: a 10-year longitudinal study. Hand (N Y) 2018. 1558944717750921. [Epub ahead of print].
11. Michon J, Bour C. Les infections de la main. Ann Med Nancy 1989;231–8.
12. Houshian S, Seyedipour S, Wedderkopp N. Epidemiology of bacterial hand infections. Int J Infect Dis 2006;10:315–9.
13. Wong KY, Maw J, Gillespie P. Assessment of hand injuries. Br J Hosp Med (Lond) 2016;77(3):C41–4.
14. Kanavel AB. The symptoms, signs, and diagnosis of tenosynovitis and major fascial-space abscesses. In: Kanavel AB, editor. Infections of the Hand. 6th edition. Philadelphia, PA: Lea & Febiger; 1933. p. 364–95.
15. McDonald LS, Bavaro MF, Hofmeister EP, et al. Hand infections. J Hand Surg Am 2011;36:1403–12.
16. Gottlieb J, Mailhot T, Chilstrom M. Point-of-Care ultrasound diagnosis of deep space hand infection. J Emerg Med 2016;50(3):458–61.
17. Marvel BA, Budhram GR. Bedside ultrasound in the diagnosis of complex hand infections: a case series. J Emerg Med 2015;48(1):63–8.
18. Leaper D. Effects of local and systemic warming on postoperative infections. Surg Infect (Larchmt) 2006;7(Suppl 2):S101.
19. Volz KA, Canham L, Kaplan E, et al. Identifying patients with cellulitis who are likely to requiring inpatient admission after a stay in an ED observation unit. Am J Emerg Med 2013;31(2):360–4.
20. Shafritz AB, Coppage JM. Acute and chronic paronychia of the hand. J Am Acad Orthop Surg 2014;22:165–74.
21. Rockwell PG. Acute and chronic paronychia. Am Fam Physician 2001;63(6):1113–6.
22. Ritting AW, O'Malley MP, Rodner CM. Acute paronychia. J Hand Surg Am 2012;37:1068–70.
23. Leggit JC. Acute and chronic paronychia. Am Fam Physician 2017;96(1):44–51.
24. Bednar MS, Lane LB. Eponychial marsupialization and nail removal for surgical treatment of chronic paronychia. J Hand Surg Am 1991;16(2):314–7.
25. Tosti A, Piraccini BM, Ghetti E, et al. Topical steroids versus systemic antifungals in the treatment of chronic paronychia: an open, randomized double-blind and double dummy study. J Am Acad Dermatol 2002;47:73–6.
26. Stern PJ. Selected acute infections. Instr Course Lect 1990;39:539.
27. Nardi NM, Schaefer TJ. Felon. StatPearls [Internet]. Treasure Island (FL): StatPearls Publishing; 2019.
28. Franko OI, Abrams RA. Hand infections. Orthop Clin North Am 2013;44:625–34.
29. Tannan S, Deal DN. Diagnosis and management of the acute felon: evidence-based review. J Hand Surg Am 2012;37(12):2603–4.
30. Pierrart J, Delgrande D, Mamane W, et al. Acute felon and paronychia: antibiotics not necessary after surgical treatment. Prospective study of 46 patients. Hand Surg Rehabil 2016;35(1):40–3.
31. Wu I, Schwartz R. Herpetic whitlow. Cutis 2007;79(3):193–6.
32. Rubright JH, Shafritz AB. The herpetic whitlow. J Hand Surg Am 2011;36(2):340–2.
33. Patel R, Kumar H, More B, et al. Paediatric recurrent herpetic whitlow. BMJ Case Rep 2013;2013 [pii: bcr2013010207].
34. Hyatt BT, Bagg MR. Flexor tenosynovitis. Orthop Clin North Am 2017;48:217–27.
35. Giladi AM, Malay S, Chung KC. A systematic review of the management of acute pyogenic flexor tenosynovitis. J Hand Surg Eur Vol 2015;40:720–8.
36. Schnall SB, Vu-Rose T, Holtom PD, et al. Tissue pressures in pyogenic flexor tenosynovitis of the finger: compartment syndrome and its management. J Bone Joint Surg Br 1996;78(5):792–5.
37. Pang HN, Teoh LC, Yam AK, et al. Factors affecting the prognosis of pyogenic flexor tenosynovitis. J Bone Joint Surg Am 2007;89(8):1742–8.
38. Dailiana ZH, Rigopoulos N, Varitimidis S, et al. Purulent flexor tenosynovitis: factors influencing the functional outcome. J Hand Surg Eur Vol 2008;33(3):280–5.

39. Crosswell S, Vanat Q, Jose R. The anatomy of deep hand space infections: the deep thenar space. J Hand Surg Am 2014;39:2550.

40. Meier R, Wirth T, Hahn F, et al. Pyogenic arthritis of the fingers and the wrist: can we shorten antimicrobial treatment duration? Open Forum Infect Dis 2017;4:ofx058.

41. Boustred AM, Singer M, Hudson DA, et al. Septic Arthritis of the metacarpophalangela and interphalangeal joints of the hand. Ann Plast Surg 1999;42:623-9.

42. Chauhan A, Wigton MD, Palmer BA. Necrotizing fasciitis. J Hand Surg Am 2014;39:1598-601.

43. Wong CH, Chang HC, Pasupathy S, et al. Necrotizing fasciitis: clinical presentation, microbiology, and determinants of mortality. J Bone Joint Surg Am 2003;85-A:1454-60.

44. Gonzalez M. Necrotizing fasciitis and gangrene of the upper extremity. Hand Clin 1998;14(4):635-45.

45. Tang WM, Ho PL, Fung KK, et al. Necrotizing fasciitis of a limb. J Bone Joint Surg 2001;83B:709-14.

46. Gonzalez MH, Kay T, Weinzweig N, et al. Necrotizing fasciitis of the upper extremity. J Hand Surg 1996;21A:689-92.

47. Corona PS, Erimeiku F, Reverté-Vinaixa MM, et al. Necrotising fasciitis of the extremities: implementation of new management technologies. Injury 2016;47(Suppl 3):S66-71.

48. Reilly K, Linz J, Stern P, et al. Osteomyelitis of the tubular bones of the hand. J Hand Surg Am 1997;22(4):644-9.

49. Honda H, McDonald J. Current recommendations in the management of osteomyelitis of the hand and wrist. J Hand Surg Am 2009;34(6):1135-6.

50. Kleinert JM, Hoffmann J, Miller Crain G, et al. Postoperative infection in a double-occupancy operating room. A prospective study of two thousand four hundred and fifty-eight procedures on the extremities. J Bone Joint Surg Am 1997;79(4):503-13.

51. Hanssen AD, Amadio PC, DeSilva SP, et al. Deep postoperative wound infection after carpal tunnel release. J Hand Surg Am 1989;14(5):869-73.

52. Haley RW, Culver DH, Morgan WM, et al. Identifying patients at high risk of surgical wound infection. A simple multivariate index of patient susceptibility and wound contamination. Am J Epidemiol 1985;121(2):206-15.

53. Classen DC, Evans RS, Pestotnik SL, et al. The timing of prophylactic administration of antibiotics and the risk of surgical-wound infection. N Engl J Med 1992;326(5):281-6.

54. Henley MB, Jones RE, Wyatt RW, et al. Prophylaxis with cefamandole nafate in elective orthopedic surgery. Clin Orthop Relat Res 1986;209:249-54.

55. Eberlin KR, Ring D. Infection after hand surgery. Hand Clin 2015;31(2):355-60.

56. Lee R, Lee HY, Kim JH, et al. Acute osteomyelitis in the hand due to dog bite injury: a report of 3 cases. Arch Plast Surg 2017;44(5):444-8.

57. Stevens D, Bisno A, Chambers H, et al. Practice guidelines for the diagnosis and management of skin and soft-tissue infections. Clin Infect Dis 2005;41(10):1373-406.

58. Aghababian R, Conte JE. Mammalian bite wounds. Ann Emerg Med 1980;9(2):79-83.

59. Kennedy SA, Stoll LE, Lauder AS. Human and other mammalian bite injuries of the hand: evaluation and management. J Am Acad Orthop Surg 2015;23:47-57.

60. Medeiros I, Sacaonato H. Antibiotic Prophylaxis for mammalian bites. Cochrane Database Syst Rev 2001;(2):CD001738.

61. Smith HR, Hartman H, Loveridge J, et al. Predicting serious complications and high cost of treatment of tooth-knuckle injuries: a systematic literature review. Eur J Trauma Emerg Surg 2016;42:701-10.

62. Shoji K, Cavanaugh Z, Rodner C. Acute fight bite. J Hand Surg Am 2013;18(8):1612-4.

63. Foster SD, Lyons MS, Runyan CM, et al. A mimic of soft tissue infection: intra-arterial injection drug use producing hand swelling and digital ischemia. World J Emerg Med 2015;6(3):233-6.

64. Afshar A, Farhadnia P, Khalkhali H. Metastases to the hand and wrist: an analysis of 221 cases. J Hand Surg Am 2014;39(5):923-32.

65. Amadio P, Lombardi R. Metastatic tumors of the hand. J Hand Surg 1987;12A(2):311-6.

66. Chaput B, Nouaille de Gorce H, Courtaide-Saidi M, et al. The role of a systematic second look at 48-72 hours in high pressure injection injuries to the hand: a retrospective study. Chir Main 2012;31(5):250-5.

67. Rauh MA, Duquin TR, McGrath BE, et al. Spread of squamous cell carcinoma from the thumb to the small finger via the flexor tendon sheaths. J Hand Surg 2009;34A(9):1709-13.

# Management of Acute Extensor Tendon Injuries

Alfred P. Yoon, MD[a], Kevin C. Chung, MD, MS[b],*

## KEYWORDS

- Extensor tendon injury • Extensor tendon repair • Tendon reconstruction • Swan neck deformity
- Boutonniere deformity • Extensor tendon mechanism

## KEY POINTS

- Extensor tendon injuries are common, and early diagnosis and treatment are essential to optimal outcome.
- If the extensor mechanism is intact, conservative management with splinting in extension is usually appropriate.
- If there is greater than 50% tendon laceration or anomalies in the extensor mechanism, surgical exploration and repair may be warranted.

## INTRODUCTION

More than half of acute tendon traumas consist of extensor tendon injuries, with a reported incidence rate of 14 cases per 100,000 person-years.[1] Extensor tendons are susceptible to damage because of their relatively thin soft tissue coverage. Extensor tendon injuries are differentiated into 9 zones, with odd-numbered zones corresponding to the injuries over the joints and the even-numbered zones referring to the segments between 2 joints (eg, zone 1 distal interphalangeal joint, zone 3 proximal interphalangeal joint, zone 5 metacarpophalangeal joint). The 4 extensor digitorum communis (EDC) tendons share a common muscle belly, while extensor indicis proprius (EIP) and extensor digitorum minimi (EDM) tendons have independent muscle bellies, making EIP and EDM suitable donor tendons in tendon transfers. There are 3 overarching treatment strategies

for extensor tendon injuries: conservative management with splinting, primary repair, or tendon grafts. This article illustrates the intricacies associated with different types of extensor tendon injury and the appropriate treatment strategy for each.

## ZONE 1 EXTENSOR TENDON INJURY

A 19-year-old woman presents with left middle finger injury while playing football. She has tenderness on the distal interphalangeal (DIP) joint and has no open wounds. Radiographs are shown in **Fig. 1**.

### What Is the Relevant Anatomy of This Injury?

Zone 1 extensor tendon injuries are superficial to the DIP joint. The most common mechanism of injury is sudden and forceful flexion of the DIP joint while in extension. Disruption of the terminal

Disclosure Statement: This publication was supported by the National Institute of Arthritis and Musculoskeletal and Skin Diseases of the National Institutes of Health under Award Number 2 K24-AR053120-06. The content is solely the responsibility of the authors and does not necessarily represent the official views of the National Institutes of Health.

[a] Section of Plastic Surgery, Department of Surgery, Michigan Medicine, University of Michigan, 2130 Taubman Center, SPC 5340, 1500 East Medical Center Drive, Ann Arbor, MI 48109-5340, USA; [b] Section of Plastic Surgery, Department of Surgery, Michigan Medicine Comprehensive Hand Center, Michigan Medicine, University of Michigan, 2130 Taubman Center, SPC 5340, 1500 East Medical Center Drive, Ann Arbor, MI 48109-5340, USA
* Corresponding author.
E-mail address: kecchung@umich.edu

Clin Plastic Surg 46 (2019) 383–391
https://doi.org/10.1016/j.cps.2019.03.004

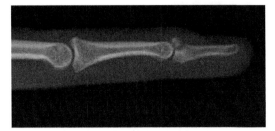

**Fig. 1.** Avulsion fracture at the distal phalanx (mallet fracture).

extensor tendon at the DIP joint is called a mallet deformity. Zone 1 extensor tendon injuries are classified into 4 types based on the severity of anatomic derangement and structures affected (**Table 1**).

### How Should One Manage Zone 1 Extensor Tendon Injuries?

Chronic zone 1 extensor tendon injuries may lead to swan-neck deformity; therefore, correct management is imperative. Closed injuries with or without fracture (type 1) can be managed with 6 to 8 weeks of DIP joint extension splinting followed by gentle active flexion range of motion (**Fig. 2**). Type 2 injuries can be repaired with figure-of-eight suture through the tendon or dermatotenodesis and subsequent DIP joint extension splinting. Type 3 injuries generally require immediate soft tissue coverage and primary grafting versus free tendon graft secondarily. Type 4A and 4B injuries are managed with closed reduction and splinting, while 4C injuries require k-wire fixation and splinting (**Table 2**).[2–5]

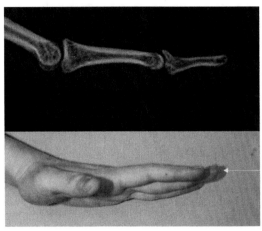

**Fig. 2.** 3-month postoperative result after splinting without surgical intervention for type 1 zone 1 extensor tendon injury.

**Table 1**
**Classification of zone 1 extensor tendon injuries**

| Classification | Definitions |
|---|---|
| Type 1 | Closed with or without avulsion fracture |
| Type 2 | Loss of tendon continuity with skin laceration |
| Type 3 | Loss of skin, subcutaneous tissue, and tendon substance |
| Type 4 | A: Transepiphyseal plate fracture in children<br>B: Hyperflexion injury with <50% fracture of articular surface<br>C: Hyperextension injury with >50% fracture of articular surface with palmar subluxation of distal phalanx |

**Table 2**
**Management of zone 1 extensor tendon injuries**

| Classification | Management |
|---|---|
| Type 1 | Continuous splinting with DIP in extension for 6–8 weeks, followed by up to 3 months of night splinting<br>Week 6: gentle active flexion ROM to 30°<br>Week 8: active flexion to 60°–90°<br>Week 10: resistive exercises |
| Type 2 | Figure-of-eight suture through tendon or dermatotenodesis (suture through skin and tendon)[2] - using a K-wire in addition to suture and splint may have higher incidence of extensor lag[3]<br>Splint protocol as type 1 |
| Type 3 | Immediate soft tissue coverage, primary grafting or late reconstruction using free tendon graft |
| Type 4 | A: Closed reduction, splinting with DIP extension for 3–4 weeks<br>B: Splinting with DIP extended for 6 weeks, subsequent 2 weeks of night splinting<br>C: K-wire fixation, 6 weeks of splinting with DIP extension<br>• Use of hook plate reported[4]<br>• Nonsurgical treatment with splinting only reported[5] |

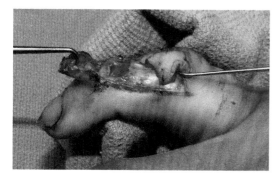

**Fig. 3.** 80% extensor tendon laceration in zone 2.

## ZONE 2 EXTENSOR TENDON INJURY

A 23-year-old male car mechanic sustained a right dorsal small finger middle phalanx trauma from a work-related crush injury. The patient has an extensor lag with 80% extensor tendon laceration (**Fig. 3**).

### What Is the Relevant Anatomy in Zone 2 Extensor Tendon Injuries?

Zone 2 injuries occur in the segment between the DIP and PIP joints in the fingers and between the IP and metacarpophalangeal (MCP) joints in the thumb. The conjoined lateral bands and the triangular ligament are frequently affected. The most common mechanism of injury is direct laceration or crush.

### What Is the Treatment Algorithm for Zone 2 Extensor Tendon Injuries?

Conservative management with splinting and active range of motion therapy are recommended for tendon lacerations less than 50%. Primary repair is recommended for tendon lacerations greater than 50% (**Fig. 4, Table 3**).[6]

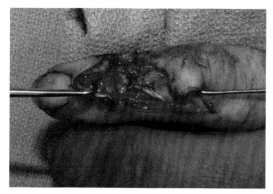

**Fig. 4.** Primary repair with 4-0 Ethibond horizontal mattress sutures.

| Table 3 | |
|---|---|
| **Management of zone 2 extensor tendon injuries** | |
| **Extent of Tendon Laceration** | **Management** |
| <50% | 1–2 weeks of splinting in finger extension, then active motion |
| >50% | Primary repair of extensor tendon - figure-of-eight suture, Silverskiold cross stitch,[6] horizontal mattress<br>6 weeks of splinting with DIP in extension, PIP and MCP free |

## ZONE 3 EXTENSOR TENDON INJURY

A 41-year-old woman presents to the emergency room after sustaining a laceration to her index finger with a kitchen knife over the PIP joint. The patient has loss of extension at the PIP joint.

### What Is the Classic Presentation of Zone 3 Extensor Tendon Injury?

Loss of extension at the PIP joint and hyperextension at the DIP joint, a Boutonniere deformity, is the classic presentation (**Fig. 5**). However, this clinical presentation may only occur 10 to 14 days after the initial injury. **Table 4** illustrates the pathoanatomy of a Boutonniere deformity.

### What Is the Key Physical Examination to Perform in a Suspected Zone 3 Injury?

The Elson test is performed to discern whether a central slip injury is present. While keeping the PIP joint flexed at 90°, the patient is asked to extend the DIP joint. A lax DIP joint despite the patient's effort to extend it is a negative or normal

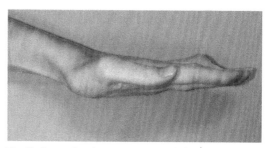

**Fig. 5.** Example of a Boutonniere deformity.

**Table 4**
**Pathoanatomy of boutonniere deformity**

| Anatomic Structure | Pathoanatomy |
| --- | --- |
| Central slip | Rupture of central slip causes loss of extension at the PIP joint because of disruption of EDC |
| Triangular ligament | Attenuation of the triangular ligament causes lumbricals to act as flexor of the PIP joint |
| Lateral bands | Palmar subluxation of lateral bands, unopposed lumbrical pull at the volar base of the distal phalanx causing PIP flexion and DIP extension |

**Table 5**
**Central slip reconstruction for zone 3 injury**

| 1. Snow central slip turndown[7] | Lateral band rerouting from adjacent unaffected finger, then threaded through dorsal cortical perforation, and secured to the lacerated end of injured central slip |
| --- | --- |
| 2. Aiache central lateral band mobilization[8] | Lateral bands of the injured fingers dissected free and split longitudinally for 2 cm and middle segment approximated in the midline over the base of the middle phalanx |
| 3. FDS tendon slip[9] | Free ulnar slip of the FDS tendon of affected finger at A1 level then weave through drilled hole at base of middle phalanx and weave to the proximal extensor tendon |

finding. If the central slip is intact, the loose lateral bands when the PIP is flexed prevent DIP extension. A positive finding is a rigid DIP joint because of increased unopposed pull through the lateral bands.

### How Is a Closed Zone 3 Extensor Tendon Injury Managed?

Splinting with PIP in extension with DIP, MCP, and wrist joints free for 3 to 6 weeks followed by 6 weeks of night time splinting is the recommended treatment for closed injuries. Flexion stretching exercises of the DIP joint while holding the PIP joint in extension promote retraction of the lateral bands dorsally from a volarly subluxed position and tighten the triangular ligament. Surgical indications for closed zone 3 injuries are illustrated in **Box 1**.

### What Is the Surgical Management of Zone 3 Extensor Tendon Injury?

Primary repair of the central tendon and securement of the tendon to the middle phalanx can be considered. Alternative reconstructive options of central slips that are not reparable primarily are described in **Table 5**.[7–9] In patients with

**Box 1**
**Surgical indications of closed zone 3 injuries**

1. Displaced avulsion fracture of middle phalanx base
2. Axial and lateral instability of PIP joint with loss of active or passive extension
3. Failed nonoperative treatment[a]

[a] Even for open injury, tendon ends tend not to retract, recommend attempting splinting first.

Boutonniere deformity or an unstable PIP joint, the PIP joint can be further immobilized with K-wire fixation (**Fig. 6**). If there is a displaced avulsion fracture of the middle phalangeal base, the finger is splinted in extension until bony union. In the setting of isolated tendon injury, some authors propose less immobilization and controlled early active range of motion therapy. Evans[10] advocated for early active short arc motion protocol after observing overall shorter treatment time, less extensor lag, and better flexion in the early motion protocol patients (started 2–11 days postoperatively) compared with immobilized patients. Pratt and colleagues[11] advocated for extension immobilization for 3 weeks then controlled mobilization in Capener coil splints for 3 weeks.

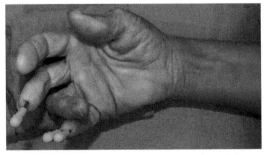

**Fig. 6.** K-wire fixation of right middle and small finger Boutonniere deformity.

## ZONE 4 EXTENSOR TENDON INJURY

A 32-year-old man presented to the emergency room after punching through a glass door now with a 1 cm full-thickness laceration on the right dorsal ring finger proximal phalanx.

### What Is the Appropriate Management in Patients with and Without Extension Deficits in Zone 4 Injuries?

Patients without extension deficits can be splinted with PIP joint in extension for 3 to 4 weeks without

any tendon repair after appropriate soft tissue management. If the patient has extension deficits, surgical exploration and tendon repair are warranted. After repair, the patient should be splinted for 3 weeks. Core suture techniques for proximal tendon zone injuries are depicted in **Fig. 7**.[12–14]

### How Is a Severe Open Injury with Tendon Loss Precluding Primary Repair Treated?

If the tendon defect is less than 1 cm, a local turnover tendon flap using a rectangular flap from the

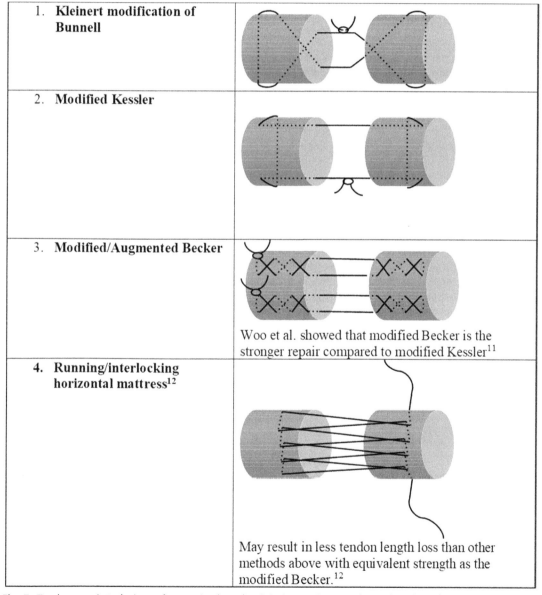

| 1. Kleinert modification of Bunnell | |
| 2. Modified Kessler | |
| 3. Modified/Augmented Becker | Woo et al. showed that modified Becker is the stronger repair compared to modified Kessler[11] |
| 4. Running/interlocking horizontal mattress[12] | May result in less tendon length loss than other methods above with equivalent strength as the modified Becker.[12] |

**Fig. 7.** Tendon repair techniques for proximal tendon injuries. Various mechanical studies of core suture strength have been performed. Woo and colleagues demonstrated that the modified Becker technique is a stronger repair compared with the modified Kessler technique. (*From* Woo SH, Tsai TM, Kleinert HE, et al. A biomechanical comparison of 4 extensor tendon repair techniques in zone IV. *Plast Reconstr Surg* 2005; 115(6):1674–81; with permission.)

proximal portion can be used for reconstruction.[15] A longer gap can be repaired with a distal tendon graft or an L-shaped tendon turnover flap from both the distal and proximal end.[16]

## ZONE 5 EXTENSOR TENDON INJURY

A 22-year-old male presented to the emergency room after being involved in a physical altercation while intoxicated. There is an open wound above the index finger MCP joint.

### What Is the Most Common Cause of Zone 5 Extensor Tendon Injury, and What Is the Classification for Sagittal Band Injuries?

Human bites are the most common source of zone 5 extensor tendon injuries. A thorough washout of the wound before any tendon repair is essential. Also, when exploring the wound to find the tendon end, it will likely be more proximal than the skin edge because the injury usually occurs while the hand is in flexion. The Rayan and Murray system classifies closed sagittal band injuries into 3 types. From type 1 to type 3, the severity of sagittal band subluxation increases (**Table 6**).[17]

### What Is the Management of Zone 5 Injuries?

Zone 5 treatments differ based on presentation: closed, open, or bite injury. Closed injuries are relatively uncommon and often only manifest with sagittal band rupture. These patients can be splinted with the affected MCP joint in extension. Similar to zone 2 injuries, tendons with greater than 50% laceration in zone 5 should be repaired primarily. Sagittal bands must also be repaired to prevent EDC subluxation and MCP extension loss, which can induce quadriga effect if left untreated. The patient should be splinted with wrist in 30° to 45° of extension, MCP joint in 20° to 30° of flexion, and the PIP joint free. Finally, patients with bite injuries should undergo thorough washout of the wound before tendon repair, if greater than half width of the extensor tendon is lacerated (**Table 7**).[18]

| Table 6 |
|---|
| **Rayan and Murray classification** |

| Type I | Sagittal band injury without extensor tendon instability |
|---|---|
| Type II | Sagittal band injury with extensor tendon subluxation but still maintaining contact with the metacarpal heads |
| Type III | Sagittal band injury and dislocation of tendon from metacarpal head |

| Table 7 |
|---|
| **Zone 5 extensor tendon injury management** |

| Closed | MCP extension splinting for 4–6 weeks |
|---|---|
| Open | • Tendon repair if >50% tendon laceration<br>• Sagittal bands must be repaired to prevent EDC subluxation and MCP extension loss - usually reconstructed with distally based slip of extensor tendon, junctura, or lumbrical muscle transfer[18]<br>• Immobilization of wrist in 30°–45° of extension, and MCP joint in 20°–30° of flexion with PIP free. |
| Bite | In addition to management of open injury described previously<br>• Debride wound, thorough washout, and leave wound open or loosely closed; repair extensor tendon if injury >50%<br>• Broad spectrum antibiotics with oral flora coverage (commonly Eikenella corrodens)<br>• If septic arthritis is suspected: arthrotomy |

## ZONE 6 EXTENSOR TENDON INJURY

A 70-year-old man with a history of 4-corner fusion and scaphoid resection for scaphoid nonunion and arthritic wrist presented 16 years after surgery with complaints of left dorsal wrist pain and decreased ability to extend his middle and ring fingers. The patient had a mild extensor lag of the ring finger on examination (**Fig. 8**).

### Why Are Zone 6 Extensor Tendon Injuries Difficult to Diagnose, and What Is the Surgical Indication?

Partial or single tendon injuries in zone 6 may be masked by adjacent junctura tendinum that may

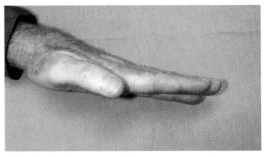

**Fig. 8.** Patient with history of 4-corner fusion 16 years previous presenting with slight extensor lag of the left ring finger.

maintain extension of the injured digit through adjacent intact extensor tendons. Because of this, diagnosing a zone 6 extensor tendon injury may be challenging, and any amount of extension deficit is an indication for surgical exploration and repair.

### What Is the Management of Zone 6 Extensor Tendon Injuries?

If primary repair is possible, techniques illustrated in **Fig. 7** are appropriate for repairing tendon injuries in zone 6 (**Fig. 9**). If primary repair is difficult, tendon reconstruction with tendon grafting or transfers should be performed. After repair, the patient should be splinted with the wrist and MCP joint in 15° to 20° extension for 3 to 4 weeks. A systematic review concluded that early active motion protocols after zone 6 extensor tendon repair result in better total active motion, stronger grip strength, and improved overall outcomes when compared with static splinting.[19] Early dynamic splinting also has been shown to improve outcomes compared with static splinting.[20]

## ZONE 7 EXTENSOR TENDON INJURY

A 14-year-old girl suffered a rotational injury to the left wrist while playing softball 5 months previous and presented with a snapping sensation on the dorsoulnar wrist on supination.

### What Structure Is Subluxing in This Patient, and Why Do Zone 7 Extensor Tendon Injuries Have Poor Outcomes?

The ECU tendon is the likely structure subluxing (snapping ECU). Because of the overlying capsule and retinaculum, tendon adhesion in zone 7 is common. Partial excision of the extensor retinaculum to prevent postoperative adhesion is controversial.

### What Is the Treatment Strategy for Zone 7 Extensor Tendon Injuries?

Primary repair of the tendon using techniques described in **Fig. 7** followed by splinting of the wrist in 40° extension and MCP joint in 20° flexion for 3 to 4 weeks is the preferred management. At least a portion of the extensor retinaculum must be left intact or repaired to prevent bowstringing of the tendons. The ECU tendon subluxation in the presenting case was repaired with a segment of extensor retinaculum wrapped around the ECU tendon to secure it in position (**Fig. 10**).

## ZONE 8 EXTENSOR TENDON INJURY

A 31-year-old man was struck with a knife just proximal to the dorsal surface of the distal radius during an altercation. Subsequently, he was unable to extend his thumb, middle, ring, and small fingers.

### What Is the Challenge and Management Strategy of Zone 8 Extensor Tendon Injuries?

Multiple tendon lacerations prevalent in zone 8 injuries make identifying individual tendons challenging. When repairing zone 8 injuries, restoration of independent thumb and wrist extension is prioritized. Because the injury is proximal, muscle bellies may be lacerated, which are repaired with multiple slow-absorbing figure-of-eight sutures. After repair, the wrist is splinted in 45° extension and the MCP joints in 15° to 20° of flexion for 3 to 4 weeks (**Box 2**).

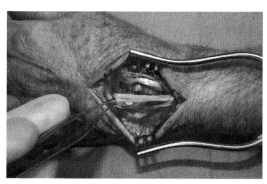

**Fig. 9.** This patient was explored operatively and was found to have ruptured the ring finger EDC tendon. In this case, the EIP tendon was transferred to the EDC tendon for reconstruction.

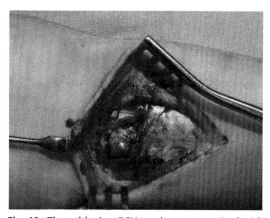

**Fig. 10.** The subluxing ECU tendon was repaired with a segment of extensor tendon retinaculum to wrap around the ECU tendon to secure it in position.

> **Box 2**
> **Management strategies for zone 8 injury**
>
> 1. Prioritize restoration of independent wrist and thumb extension
> 2. Use multiple slow-absorbing figure-of-eight sutures for muscle belly repair; try to place sutures through fibrous raphe in the middle of muscle belly
> 3. Splint wrist in 45° extension and MP joints in 15° to 20° of flexion for 4 to 5 weeks; splinting in elbow flexion may be beneficial

## THUMB EXTENSOR TENDON INJURY

A 35-year-old man punctured his radial wrist with an arrow and felt a popping sensation. Subsequently the patient was unable to extend his thumb at the IP joint (**Fig. 11**).

### What Is the Likely Affected Tendon in This Injury, and What Is the Management of Thumb Extensor Tendon Injuries?

This patient sustained a traumatic rupture of the extensor pollicis longus (EPL) tendon. EPL laceration will cause extension lag of the thumb MCP and IP joints and must be repaired (**Fig. 12**). Isolated extensor pollicis brevis (EPB) laceration is rare, and its repair is optional but recommended. For closed-thumb extensor tendon injuries, splinting for 6 weeks in extension and re-evaluating for surgical repair is appropriate. For open injuries, the tendon should be repaired primarily, the wrist splinted in 40° extension, and the thumb MCP in full extension for 3 to 4 weeks.

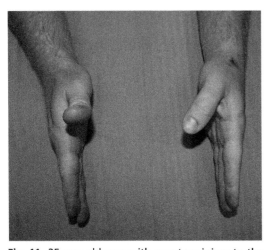

**Fig. 11.** 35-year-old man with puncture injury to the left thumb base with an arrow, unable to extend the thumb.

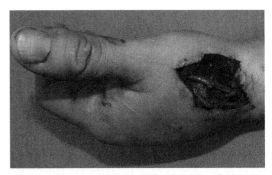

**Fig. 12.** The proximal and distal ends of the EPL tendon were identified, and 6-0 locking Ticron 6-strand suture repair was performed to primarily repair the tendon.

### How Should One Treat Chronic Extensor Pollicis Longus Injuries or Segmental Tendon Loss?

Chronic tendon injuries and segmental tendon loss may not be amenable to primary repair because of retraction or loss of tendon length. Tendon transfer, preferably from the extensor indicis proprius (EIP) tendon to EPL, is recommended (**Fig. 13**). Other donor tendons to consider are palmaris longus, flexor digitorum superficialis (FDS), abductor pollicis longus (APL), or extensor carpi radialis longus (ECRL) partial turn-over tendon if no other tendons are available.[21] The ECRL partial turn-over tendon technique is performed by detaching the ECRL from its insertion on the second metacarpal and turning over the radial half-slip of the tendon to join the distal ruptured EPL tendon.[21]

### What Are the Special Considerations of Abductor Pollicis Longus Laceration Management?

In zones 6 and 7, the APL tendon retracts considerably, and a first dorsal compartment release is likely necessary for successful repair. Postoperatively, immobilize the wrist in radial deviation and

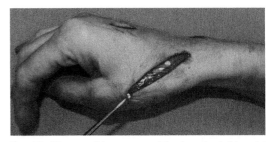

**Fig. 13.** 47-year-old woman with chronic right wrist pain who had increasing pain of her right thumb and wrist with loss of right thumb extension over several months. Atraumatic rupture of EPL tendon was diagnosed, and EIP tendon was suture-weaved into the EPL for tendon transfer.

the thumb in maximal abduction for approximately 4 to 5 weeks.

## SUMMARY

Extensor tendon injuries are classified into 9 zones depending on their location relative to the joints. Extensor tendons are commonly affected in trauma because of thin soft tissue coverage. In some injury patterns, early diagnosis may be difficult but critical to prevent long-term deformities and functional deficits. Understanding of the anatomy and armamentarium of treatment options in extensor tendon injuries is critical to ensure favorable outcomes.

## REFERENCES

1. de Jong JP, Nguyen JT, Sonnema AJM, et al. The incidence of acute traumatic tendon injuries in the hand and wrist: a 10-year population-based study. Clin Orthop Surg 2014;6(2):196–202.
2. Doyle J. Extensor tendons: acute injuries. Green's operative hand surgery. New York: Churchill Livingstone; 1993.
3. Simonian M, Dan M, Graan D, et al. Suture and splint compared with K-wire fixation for open zone 1 extensor tendon injuries. Ann Plast Surg 2018; 81(2):176–7.
4. Teoh LC, Lee JY. Mallet fractures: a novel approach to internal fixation using a hook plate. J Hand Surg Eur Vol 2007;32(1):24–30.
5. Kalainov DM, Hoepfner PE, Hartigan BJ, et al. Nonsurgical treatment of closed mallet finger fractures. J Hand Surg Am 2005;30(3):580–6.
6. Silfverskiöld KL, May EJ. Flexor tendon repair in zone II with a new suture technique and an early mobilization program combining passive and active flexion. J Hand Surg 1994;19(1):53–60.
7. Snow JW. A method for reconstruction of the central slip of the extensor tendon of a finger. Plast Reconstr Surg 1976;57(4):455–9.
8. Aiache A, Barsky AJ, Weiner DL. Prevention of the Boutonniere deformity. Plast Reconstr Surg 1970; 46(2):164–7.
9. Ahmad F, Pickford M. Reconstruction of the extensor central slip using a distally based flexor digitorum superficialis slip. J Hand Surg Am 2009;34(5): 930–2.
10. Evans RB. Rehabilitation techniques for applying immediate active tension to the repaired extensor system. Tech Hand Up Extrem Surg 1999;3(2): 139–50.
11. Pratt AL, Burr N, Grobbelaar AO. A prospective review of open central slip laceration repair and rehabilitation. J Hand Surg Br 2002;27(6):530–4.
12. Howard RF, Ondrovic L, Greenwald DP. Biomechanical analysis of four-strand extensor tendon repair techniques. J Hand Surg Am 1997;22(5): 838–42.
13. Woo SH, Tsai TM, Kleinert HE, et al. A biomechanical comparison of four extensor tendon repair techniques in zone IV. Plast Reconstr Surg 2005; 115(6):1674–81.
14. Lee SK, Dubey A, Kim BH, et al. A biomechanical study of extensor tendon repair methods: introduction to the running-interlocking horizontal mattress extensor tendon repair technique. J Hand Surg Am 2010;35(1):19–23.
15. Kochevar A, Rayan G, Angel M. Extensor tendon reconstruction for zones II and IV using local tendon flap: a cadaver study. J Hand Surg Am 2009;34(7): 1269–75.
16. Cerovac S, Miranda BH. Tendon 'turnover lengthening' technique. J Plast Reconstr Aesthet Surg 2013;66(11):1587–90.
17. Rayan GM, Murray D. Classification and treatment of closed sagittal band injuries. J Hand Surg Am 1994; 19(4):590–4.
18. Segalman KA. Dynamic lumbrical muscle transfer for correction of posttraumatic extensor tendon subluxation. Tech Hand Up Extrem Surg 2006;10(2): 107–13.
19. Wong AL, Wilson M, Girnary S, et al. The optimal orthosis and motion protocol for extensor tendon injury in zones IV-VIII: a systematic review. J Hand Ther 2017;30(4):447–56.
20. Merritt WH, Howell J, Tune R, et al. Achieving immediate active motion by using relative motion splinting after long extensor repair and sagittal band ruptures with tendon subluxation. Operat Tech Plast Reconstr Surg 2000;7(1):31–7.
21. Chetta MD, Ono S, Chung KC. Partial extensor carpi radialis longus turn-over tendon transfer for reconstruction of the extensor pollicis longus tendon in the rheumatoid hand: case report. J Hand Surg Am 2012;37(6):1217–20.

# Considerations in Flap Selection for Soft Tissue Defects of the Hand

Soumen Das De, MBBS (Hons), FRCSEd (Ortho), MPH*,
Sandeep Jacob Sebastin, MBBS, MRCS (UK), FAMS (Hand Surgery)

## KEYWORDS

- Hand defects • Soft tissue reconstruction • Decision making • Flaps

## KEY POINTS

- Soft tissue defects of the hand often involve composite tissue loss.
- Important decision-making parameters include location and size of the defect, associated digital soft tissue loss, and the technical complexity of the planned procedure.
- Aesthetic considerations are important in the choice of flap.

## INTRODUCTION

Soft tissue defects of the hand are commonly encountered in the setting of trauma, infection, or burns and after resection of tumors. Small to moderate-sized defects are amenable to repair or reconstruction using linear closure, skin grafts, and/or local flaps. The usefulness of these procedures is limited, however, in larger defects or if there is a wide zone of injury and the adjacent tissue is of questionable viability. Free tissue transfers have obviated these issues of size and tissue availability but come at the cost of specialized expertise, resources, and risks. Furthermore, the aim of surgical reconstruction has extended from mere coverage of defects to optimizing both functional and aesthetic outcomes.[1] The aim of this article is to discuss the considerations in soft tissue reconstruction of the hand and provide an approach that helps with decision making.

## CONSIDERATIONS IN RECONSTRUCTION OF THE HAND
### Anatomic and Functional Considerations

The hand spans the region between the distal wrist crease and the metacarpophalangeal joints (MPJs). It has dorsal and palmar surfaces that are distinctly different. The dorsal skin is thin, pliable, and designed for mobility. This hair-bearing skin has a certain amount of redundancy, especially over the wrist and MPJs. This allows it to accommodate wrist and finger flexion. The subcutaneous layer is thin and there is an underlying microvacuolar system that permits smooth gliding over the tendons and joints.[2] There are well-defined points at which perforators emerge to nourish the overlying skin, and these form the basis of local perforator flaps. The palmar surface is designed for stability and load bearing. The specialized glabrous skin has a thick stratum corneum and numerous interdigitating dermal folds to withstand shear stresses. The epidermal ridges and the high density of sweat glands increase the surface area and frictional forces for grip. The palmar skin is firmly tethered to the underlying fibrous framework—particularly at the creases—and this confers stability during grasp and pinch. These numerous septations, however, also make palmar skin relatively immobile and limit the availability of local flap options from the palm.

The upper limb has a tapering design, becoming progressively narrower from proximal to distal.[1,3]

Disclosures: No conflicts of interest.
Department of Hand & Reconstructive Microsurgery, National University Health System, 1E Kent Ridge Road, Singapore 119 228, Singapore
* Corresponding author.
E-mail address: das_de_soumen@nuhs.edu.sg

Clin Plastic Surg 46 (2019) 393–406
https://doi.org/10.1016/j.cps.2019.03.010

Thus, there is greater availability of soft tissue proximally. There also is more laxity of skin along the longitudinal axis compared with the transverse axis of the limb. These anatomic concepts form the basis of regional flaps from the forearm to resurface hand defects. These flaps may contain an axial pedicle (eg, radial artery or posterior interosseous artery [PIA]) or perforators from the axial vessels. The maximum length and width of perforator flaps are smaller than axial pedicle flaps.

### Aesthetic Considerations

The aesthetic principles of hand reconstruction deserve special mention. Summers and Siegle described a facial cosmetic unit as "a major structural unit of the face that shares similar skin characteristics of color, texture, thickness, elasticity, pore density and size, hairiness, and sebaceousness."[4] Rehim and colleagues[5] expanded on the cosmetic units of the hand that were originally described by Tubiana. The palmar unit is divided into the thenar, opposition, central triangular, hypothenar, and metacarpal subunits. The dorsal surface of the hand is a single unit. The skin over each phalanx of the fingers and thumb is considered a single subunit. The nail complex and pulp are special subunits because of their unique functional and aesthetic properties (**Fig. 1**).

## PREREQUISITES FOR SOFT TISSUE COVERAGE IN THE HAND

Definitive reconstructive procedures are undertaken only when the wound is free of infection, all nonviable tissue has been removed, and there is a stable skeletal framework. Other considerations in planning soft tissue reconstruction for hand defects include the following.

### Avoid Excessive Granulation and Scar Formation

The use of vacuum-assisted closure devices promotes granulation, even over poorly vascularized tissue, such as tendon and bone. In the hand, excessive granulation obliterates the gliding planes that exist between the joints, tendons, and skin and leads to adhesions and stiffness.[6] Skin grafts that are applied to such surfaces may take, but the period of immobilization required for skin grafts take along with graft contracture lead to more adhesions and further limitation of motion. For this reason, the authors do not recommend prolonged application of negative-pressure dressings unless the defects are small and/or other patient factors preclude more complex reconstructive procedures. A cutaneous flap is preferred because it allows earlier mobilization and restoration of the gliding plane between tendon and skin.

### Use a Thin Flap

The primary goal of soft tissue reconstruction in the hand is to ensure that the fingers regain normal or near-normal motion. This requires thin and pliable skin that allows digital flexion and gliding of the underlying tendons. A bulky flap may impair finger flexion if used for reconstruction of the palm. Although an adipofascial flap with a skin graft provides a thin flap, the authors have had poor outcomes with adipofascial flap reconstructions in the hand. The skin graft contracts significantly, limiting motion, obviating any perceived advantages of the thin flap. In addition, it is easier to elevate a cutaneous flap compared with the adipofascial flap for any secondary surgery.

### Determine if There Are Digital Soft Tissue Defects that Need Coverage

The presence of finger and/or thumb defects that require concomitant soft tissue coverage significantly affects the reconstructive strategy. Propeller flaps based on perforators of the radial and ulnar arteries are not long enough to safely resurface the web space and skin over the proximal phalanx. The pivot points of these flaps are approximately 2 cm to 5 cm proximal to the wrist crease, and the maximum safe dimensions of these flaps are 12 cm by 4 cm.[3] Regional flaps from the forearm based on an axial pedicle (eg, reverse radial forearm flap [RFF] or posterior interosseous artery [PIA] flap) require an extended pedicle design to safely reach the web space and proximal phalanx. Larger hand defects extending beyond the proximal interphalangeal joint require a distant (eg, groin) or free flap and creation of a syndactyly with subsequent division, if multiple digits require resurfacing.

### Maintain the Aesthetics of the Hand

Although aesthetics traditionally were not the primary goal of reconstruction, they do affect a patient's acceptance of a reconstructive procedure. An unsightly outcome may result in a hand that is hidden in a pocket and an anxious and depressed patient. Factors that influence the aesthetic outcome of a reconstruction are color and texture match, donor-recipient tissue interface, hairiness, scar location and propensity for contractures, nail deformities, presence of amputations, and donor site appearance.[5] Every effort should be made to incorporate these factors when deciding on the reconstructive strategy. Skin incisions

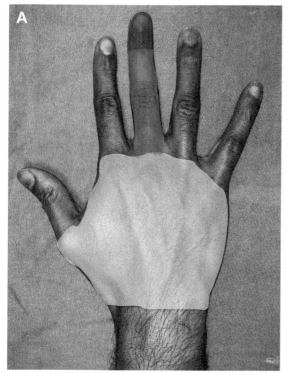
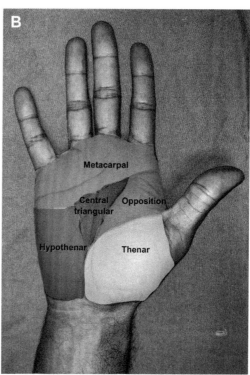

**Fig. 1.** The functional aesthetic units of the hand. (*A*) The dorsum of the hand is a single unit, comprising thin, pliable, hair-bearing skin. The skin over each of the phalanges of the fingers and thumb is a functional subunit. The nail complex is a specialized subunit because of its unique functional and aesthetic properties. (*B*) The palmar unit of the hand is made up of 5 functional subunits—thenar, opposition, central triangular, hypothenar, and metacarpal. As in the dorsum, the skin over each phalanx is a separate subunit and the pulp has unique functional properties. The boundaries of these subunits are demarcated by skin creases and the undulating surfaces reflect light to differing degrees, accounting for the typical light-dark contrasts of the normal hand. Incisions planned in the boundaries of these functional subunits tend to be concealed and are aesthetically pleasing. Scars, skin grafts, or flaps that break up this normal color contrast confer an abnormal 3-D appearance, and the result is a cosmetically unattractive hand.

should be planned in relatively concealed regions (eg, medial forearm) or along boundaries of functional units (eg, the midaxial surface of the hand or digit). Skin grafts used by themselves provide poor volume replacement and are reserved for small defects with a healthy subcutaneous bed. The authors prefer to use like-for-like skin grafts. Dorsal hand defects are best resurfaced with grafts taken from the medial or dorsal forearm (**Fig. 2**) and there are several donor sites for glabrous skin to cover palmar defects.[7,8] Regional flaps from the forearm leave conspicuous donor defects and result in significant color mismatch in dark-skinned individuals. These flaps should be reserved for dorsal hand defects because of the good color and texture match. Free fasciocutaneous flaps (eg, anterolateral thigh [ALT] and lateral arm) provide a reasonable color match with a relatively concealed donor site but tend to be bulky. Suprafascial flap elevation or staged debulking/liposuction may be necessary. Free

muscle flaps (eg, gracilis) provide good volume replacement in the setting of extensive soft tissue loss. Perforator-based propeller flaps probably offer the best compromise; they provide like-for-like replacement, are relatively easy to perform, and do not require sacrifice of a dominant vessel, and the donor site may be linearly closed in many instances.

## CLASSIFICATION OF SOFT TISSUE DEFECTS OF THE HAND

The authors categorize hand defects based on the following parameters:

- Surface
- Size
- Location

The defect may be located on the palmar, dorsal, or lateral (midaxial) surface of the hand or a combination of more than 1 surface. Because of

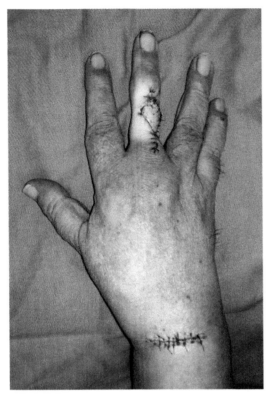

**Fig. 2.** Resurfacing small defects using like-for-like skin grafts. An elderly patient with advanced dementia sustained a dorsal finger infection after a cat bite. The resultant defect after débridement was resurfaced with a full-thickness skin graft obtained from the dorsum of the wrist. This site was chosen because both the defect and the donor site could be safely protected in a cast. The dorsal skin provides an excellent color and texture match, and the transverse skin-crease incision will heal with a concealed scar.

the unique properties of glabrous skin, the authors have simplified defect surfaces into dorsal and palmar defects. The relative size of the defect is more important than an absolute measurement. One surface of a single metacarpal has been described as a unit.[1] Small defects comprise a single surface of a metacarpal (eg, dorsal or palmar). Medium-sized defects involve 2 adjacent surfaces of a metacarpal (eg, dorsal and lateral) or contiguous surface of 2 adjacent metacarpals (eg, dorsal surfaces of index and middle metacarpals). Anything larger is considered a large defect and includes involvement of noncontiguous surfaces. Finally, the authors divide the hand into radial, central, and ulnar thirds based on location to aid in the choice of appropriate flaps. The radial third comprises the first metacarpal (thumb) and includes the thenar region and the first web space; the central third spans the second and third metacarpals (index and middle fingers); and the ulnar third

includes the fourth and fifth metacarpals (ring and small fingers). Additional factors in decision making are summarized in **Box 1**.

# FORMULATING RECONSTRUCTIVE STRATEGY BASED ON CLASSIFICATION
## Surface (Dorsal and Palmar)

The dorsum of the hand excluding the digits measures approximately 10 cm wide by 12 cm long. Dorsal soft tissue defects commonly are associated with injury to the tendons, bones, and joints and frequently require a flap. The laxity of dorsal skin makes it suitable for local flaps, based on a random pattern of vascularization, an axial pedicle, or a perforator. It is uncommon to encounter injuries that result in loss of the entire palmar skin. The skin is thick and soft tissue defects usually have a healthy subcutaneous bed, which takes a split-thickness skin graft. Glabrous skin is also unique for the reasons discussed earlier and in limited supply, with the only other source the plantar surface of the foot. Skin over the thenar subunit is mobile, whereas the skin over the central triangular and metacarpal subunits has minimal laxity. Consequently, most of the local palmar flaps arise from the thenar and radial midpalmar regions.

| Box 1 |
|---|
| **Considerations in soft tissue reconstruction of the hand** |

Defect characteristics

- Size
- Depth
- Location
- Finger/thumb involvement
- Additional tissues involved, for example, bone, tendon, and nerve

Technical considerations

- Level of difficulty
- Available resources

Patient factors

- Hand dominance
- Occupation and functional demands
- Preexisting illnesses, for example, diabetes, peripheral vascular disease, and renal impairment
- Compliance to postoperative rehabilitation plan
- Cosmetic concerns, preferences, and expectations

## Size (Small, Medium, and Large)

The reconstructive options available for the hand include healing by secondary intention, skin grafts, local random pattern flaps, pedicled perforator-based flaps, pedicled axial pattern flaps, pedicled distant flaps, and free flaps. Small defects may be amenable to healing by secondary intention or skin grafting (palmar defects). The other options include random pattern local flaps like rotation or transposition (dorsal defects). In general, perforator-based flaps are suitable for small defects and some medium-sized defects, axial pattern flaps are suitable for medium-sized effects and some large defects, and distant pedicled or free flaps are suitable for large defects.

## Location (Radial, Central, and Ulnar)

**Tables 1** and **2** summarize the options for reconstructions of soft tissue defects of the hand based on the surface, size, and location of the defect. Reconstructive options are discussed.

## PEDICLED PERFORATOR-BASED LOCAL FLAPS

These options are only viable if the zone of injury is limited and the blood supply to the skin adjacent to the defect is maintained. Ideally, the reconstructive surgeon should perform the initial débridement(s) for several reasons. First, it is crucial that any skin

**Table 1**
**Options for dorsal hand defects**

| Small Defects (1 Unit) | Medium Defects (2 Units) | Large Defects (More Than 2 Units) |
|---|---|---|
| Skin grafts | Radial defects | Distant |
| • Medial forearm | • RAP flap | • Groin/ abdominal flap |
| • Groin | • Reverse RFF | |
| Local flaps | • Extended RFF | Free |
| • Random pattern flap | Central defects | • ALT flap |
| Radial defects | • PIA flap | • Medial sural artery perforator flap |
| • FDMA flap | • Extended PIA flap | |
| • RAP flap | Ulnar defects | |
| Central defects | • UAP flap | • Dorsalis pedis flap |
| • Dorsal metacarpal artery perforator flap | | • RFF |
| • PIA flap | | • Lateral arm flap |
| Ulnar defects | | |
| • UAP flap | | |

*Abbreviations:* RAP, Radial artery perforator; UAP, Ulnar artery perforator.

**Table 2**
**Options for volar hand defects**

| Small Defects (1 Unit) | Medium Defects (2 Units) | Large Defects (More Than 2 Units) |
|---|---|---|
| Secondary intention | Preferred options | Distant |
| Skin grafts | • Medialis pedis free flap | • Groin/ abdominal flap |
| • Palm (hypothenar, skin creases) | • MPA free flap | Free |
| Radial and central defects | Alternatives | • ALT flap |
| • Reverse thenar perforator flap | • RAP flap (radial defects) | • Medial sural artery perforator flap |
| • Radial midpalmar island flap | • UAP flap (ulnar defects) | • Dorsalis pedis flap |
| • Volar glabrous palm flap | | • RFF |
| Ulnar defects | | • Lateral arm flap |
| • Ulnar palmar perforator flap | | |

*Abbreviations:* RAP, Radial artery perforator; UAP, Ulnar artery perforator.

extensions to explore adjacent neurovascular structures, tendon or bone do not damage the adjacent perforators. Second, the adjacent skin must be inspected carefully for degloving because such injuries are likely to compromise the perforators. Third, digital blocks should be avoided because they may damage the perforators, in particular the veins. Finally, the reconstructive surgeon may look for sizable perforators in the vicinity during the initial wound débridement, although the authors do not recommend any further vessel dissection because of the risk of vasospasm. Some of the common perforator-based pedicled laps suitable for hand reconstruction include

1. First dorsal metacarpal artery (FDMA) flap: this is a good choice for small defects of the thumb and first web space.[9] The FDMA arises from the deep branch of the radial artery and it reliably perfuses the dorsal skin up to the middle of the proximal phalanx of the index finger. The flap may be raised as an island or with a tail of skin from the dorsum of the first web space. It is important that the FDMA is retained in a broad strip of fascia and not skeletonized during flap elevation, and inclusion of a cutaneous vein minimizes the risk of flap congestion.

2. Dorsal metacarpal artery perforator flap: the dorsal metacarpal artery perforator (Quaba) flap offers a straightforward option for small defects over metacarpals, the web spaces, and the proximal phalanges.[10] The cutaneous perforators of the dorsal metacarpal artery arise at the level of the metacarpal neck in the second to fourth intermetacarpal spaces, just distal to the juncturae tendinum. The skin over the dorsum of the hand is thin and pliable and provides an excellent match for resurfacing dorsal hand and finger defects. The flap can reliably resurface defects up to the middle of the proximal phalanx and the donor defect can be closed linearly in most cases. A curved elliptical design can be used to obtain more distal reach when the flap is rotated and straightened. Finally, the authors avoid tunneling the flap under an intact skin bridge.

3. Radial artery perforator (RAP) flap: Timmons[11] described the distribution of cutaneous perforators arising from the radial artery in 1986. A majority of these congregate around the radial styloid.[12,13] Koshima and colleagues[14] demonstrated the use of an adipofascial flap based on these perforators for reconstruction of dorsal hand defects. The optimal dimensions of the RAP flap are 12 cm by 4 cm although flaps up to 18 cm in length have been described.[3,12]

The authors prefer to use the RAP to resurface small to medium-sized defects on the radial surface of the hand, particularly on the dorsum because of the good color and texture match (**Fig. 3**). The lateral antebrachial cutaneous nerve can be included to provide a sensate flap. Chang and colleagues[12] advocated ligation of the cephalic vein at the base of the flap because a patent vein caused significant flap congestion and compromised viability. The RAP flap does not reliably reach beyond the MPJ and alternative options should be selected for concomitant coverage of digital defects.[15]

4. Ulnar artery perforator (UAP) flap: Becker and Gilbert[16] described the ulnar flap based on a dorsal branch of the ulnar artery, passing deep to the flexor carpi ulnaris (FCU) muscle. This flap is a good choice for small to medium-sized defects involving the ulnar side of the hand and wrist. The volar (radial) incision is made first and suprafascial dissection continued ulnarly until the FCU tendon is identified. The dissection is then continued subfascially while the FCU tendon is retracted radially. The ulnar artery is identified, and a suitable perforator is selected. Reliable perforators from the ulnar artery may be found 4 to 6 cm proximal to the pisiform.[3,17] Mathy and colleagues[18] studied the entire course of the ulnar

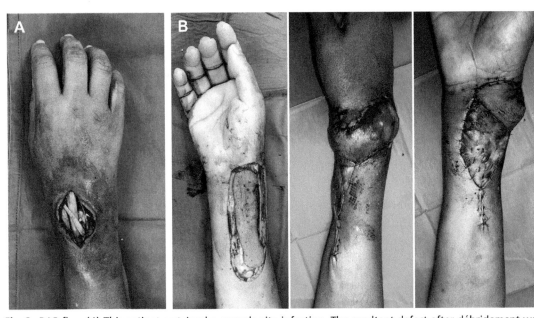

**Fig. 3.** RAP flap. (*A*) This patient sustained a cannula-site infection. The resultant defect after débridement was over the dorsum of the wrist and proximal hand, with exposed wrist and finger extensor tendons. (*B*) An RAP flap was used to resurface the defect (*left*). The donor defect was covered with a hand-meshed split-thickness skin graft. There was superficial epidermolysis of the distal part of the flap (*center*). The RAP provides a good match for dorsal hand/wrist defects and preserves the radial artery. The donor site, however, is conspicuous (*right*).

artery and reported that 94% of forearms had at least 1 sizable (>0.5-mm) cutaneous perforator within 3 cm of the midpoint of a line connecting the medial epicondyle and pisiform. All forearms had at least 1 perforator within 6 cm of the midpoint. In their series, 6% of flaps had perforators originating from an anomalous superficial ulnar artery. Any of these perforators can therefore be incorporated in flaps to resurface more proximal forearm defects. The advantages of this flap over the RAP flap are the more concealed incision and relatively hairless skin in this part of the forearm. Skin grafts used to cover larger donor defects tend to heal better because the grafts are applied over muscle rather than tendons/paratenon in the case of a RAP flap (**Fig. 4**).

5. Glabrous skin perforators flaps: small radial and central defects can be resurfaced with perforator flaps arising from the thenar region. They have been variously named the radial mid-palmar island flap,[19] reverse thenar perforator flap,[20,21] and the volar glabrous palmar flap.[22] These flaps measure, on average, 5 cm by 2 cm and rely on the laxity of the thenar skin. There is a confluence of arteries at the thenar region, where the superficial palmar arch meets the superficial palmar branch of the radial artery, the radialis indices artery, and the princeps pollicis artery.[19,20] Perforators arising from this confluence form the basis of propeller or reverse-flow flaps. Alternatively, a free flap may be harvested based on the superficial palmar branch of the radial artery itself. Small

ulnar defects (eg, over the hypothenar border) usually do not result in exposure of critical structures and are amenable to skin grafting or healing by secondary intention. In selected cases, the ulnar palmar perforator flap can be used to resurface palmar defects measuring approximately 2 cm by 6 cm.[23] The flap is based on a septocutaneous perforator from the ulnar digital artery to the small finger, emerging between the hypothenar muscles at the level of the metacarpal neck.

## PEDICLED AXIAL PATTERN FLAPS
### Radial Forearm Flap

The RFF or the adipofascial RFF can be used for small to medium-sized defects over the radial and central compartments.[6] Since its first description as a free flap in 1978, the RFF has remained one of the most versatile flaps in reconstructive surgery.[24] The RFF used for resurfacing hand defects is essentially a reverse-flow flap and relies on a patent ulnar artery–radial artery communication in the hand. The RFF is relatively easy to raise and reliable and provides thin, pliable skin for soft tissue resurfacing. An extended pedicle may be obtained if the superficial branch of the radial artery is ligated and the pivot point is based on the deep branch of the radial artery, just before it dives volarly around the base of the thumb metacarpal. The extended RFF can be used to extend the reach of the flap to resurface defects over the web spaces and MPJ (**Fig. 5**). The main drawbacks of this flap

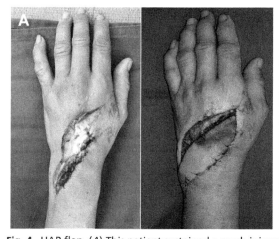
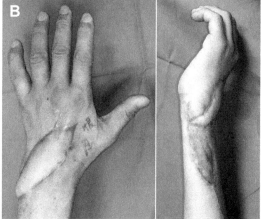

**Fig. 4.** UAP flap. (*A*) This patient sustained a crush injury from factory machinery, and the result is an untidy dorsal wound with an area of full-thickness skin burn. The underlying extensor tendons were disrupted (*left*). All unhealthy skin was excised and the extensor tendons were repaired. A UAP flap was used to cover the resultant defect. The flap was partially inset at the initial stage; nevertheless, there is epidermolysis of the tip (*right*). (*B*) The final outcome is aesthetically pleasing with good color and texture match (*left*). The skin grafted donor site is concealed and not easily visible (*right*).

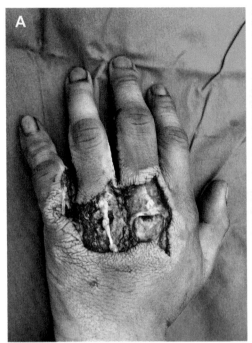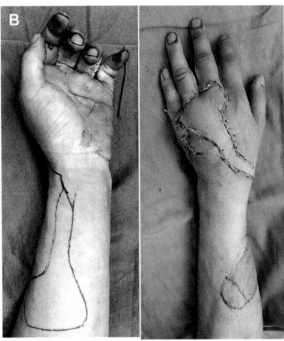

**Fig. 5.** Reverse RFF. (*A*) A motor vehicle accident resulted in a composite defect of the dorsum of the hand involving loss of extensor tendons, partial loss of MPJ surfaces, and a comminuted fracture of the small finger proximal phalanx. There was extensive particulate contamination and a radical débridement was performed. (*B*) Soft tissue reconstruction was achieved using an extended RFF (*left*) and the donor site was covered using a split-thickness skin graft. Bone and tendon grafting were deferred to a later stage because of the extensive initial contamination. The flap provides good color and texture match, but the donor site is conspicuous. Hand-meshing the skin graft results in a more uniform and pleasing appearance (*right*).

are sacrifice of a major vessel to the hand, a poor color match—especially for the palmar surface of the hand, and a cosmetically unappealing donor site. The cosmetically unappealing donor site can be addressed with the use of a reversed adipofascial RFF and skin grafting, with primary closure of the donor site.[25] This is not recommended, however, if delayed procedures are planned, for example, bone grafting and tendon reconstruction.

### Posterior Interosseous Artery Flap

The PIA flap was described by Angrigiani and Zancolli and is a versatile flap that does not require sacrifice of a major artery.[26,27] The reverse-flow PIA flap relies on a patent communication between the anterior interosseous artery (AIA) and PIA at the level of the carpus and is ideal for defects over the central and ulnar parts of the dorsum of the hand (**Fig. 6**). The pivot point of the flap is 2 cm proximal to the distal radioulnar joint, where the communicating branch from the AIA emerges through the interosseous membrane to meet the PIA. A line

connecting the lateral epicondyle and the distal radioulnar joint denotes the axis of the flap. The authors recommend making the ulnar incision first and identifying the extensor carpi ulnaris (ECU) tendon. The extensor digiti minimi (EDM) tendon is identified next and gentle traction with a tendon hook can be used to confirm its action on the small finger. The communicating perforator between the AIA and PIA is identified in the interval between the EDM (fifth extensor compartment) and ECU (sixth extensor compartment). The authors make it a point to identify this perforator before proceeding with the rest of flap harvest because the carpal communication and/or the distal PIA may be absent in approximately 5% of the population.[27–29] A large cutaneous perforator from the PIA (the so-called median cutaneous branch) is found approximately midway along the axis, and this part is incorporated into the flap design.[27] The proximal (safe) limit of the flap is at a point 6 cm distal to the lateral epicondyle and the PIA is ligated here, proximal to the emergence of the medial perforator. More proximal dissection requires separation of the motor branch of the PIA nerve to the

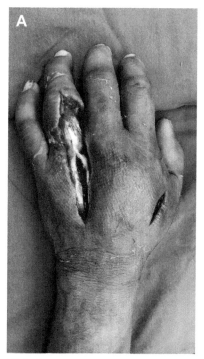
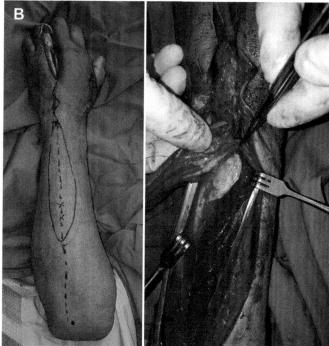
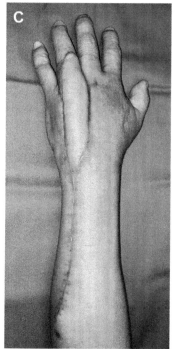

**Fig. 6.** PIA flap. (*A*) A dorsal defect of the hand due to infection was resurfaced using a PIA flap. (*B*) The proximal end of the flap is designed to include the large median perforator (*left*). The carpal communicating branch (indicated with forceps) is first identified distally, between the ECU and EDM tendons (*right*). Flap dissection then proceeds from distal to proximal, starting with the ulnar incision first. A standard PIA flap without an extended pedicle safely permits coverage of the MPJs and proximal phalanges of the digits. (*C*) The outcome is aesthetically pleasing, the donor site was closed linearly, and no major vessel had to be sacrificed.

ECU from the flap pedicle and, in circumstances where the artery lies deep to the nerve branch, the latter has to be sacrificed.[30] The donor defect can be closed linearly in flaps measuring 3 cm to 4 cm in width. Zaidenberg and colleagues[31] demonstrated an "extended PIA flap" based on the communication between the PIA and dorsal intercarpal arch. The more distal pivot point allows the flap to cover the web spaces and digits.

## DISTANT PEDICLED FLAPS

The lower abdomen has several arteries emanating from the external iliac and superficial femoral arteries that can reliably be used for soft tissue coverage of the hand. These are the superficial circumflex iliac artery (SCIA), superficial inferior epigastric artery (SIEA), superficial external pudendal artery, deep inferior epigastric artery, and the paraumbilical perforators. Pedicled groin and hypogastric flaps have become the workhorse for soft tissue reconstruction of the hand and have been extensively described in the literature. Complex defects can be reconstructed using a combination of flaps (**Fig. 7**). These flaps are easy to raise and do not require microsurgical expertise or sacrifice of a major artery. The obvious drawback is having the hand strapped to the trunk for 2 weeks to 3 weeks in a dependent position and delaying rehabilitation.

Al-Qattan and Al-Qattan[32] recently reviewed the indications for these flaps in the microsurgical era and concluded that there remained specific situations where these flaps are strongly indicated. These include hand defects in small children, soft tissue coverage prior to toe transfers, high-voltage electrical burns with questionable patency of the major arteries, and multiple hand and digital defects.

There are specific design elements that can optimize patient comfort and clinical outcomes. The surgeon should bring the hand to the groin and work backwards. Chuang and colleagues[33] described a simple method of defining the safe boundaries of the groin flap. Sabapathy and Bajantri[34] highlighted some basic principles concerning flap design and inset: adequate débridement, keeping the base narrow and the pedicle long, thinning the distal end, and performing a robust inset. They did not advocate tubing the

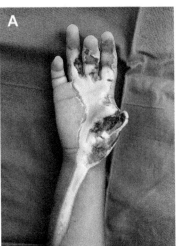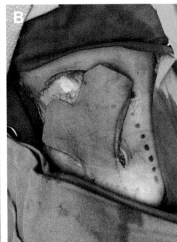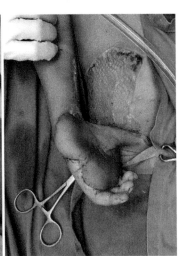

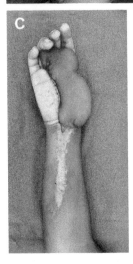

**Fig. 7.** Combined SCIA and SIEA flap in complex hand defects. (*A*) A severe crush-avulsion injury in a 3 year old. The child's hand was caught on a high-tension cable in an amusement park and the thumb; most of the thenar muscles and overlying skin were avulsed. There are full-thickness burns of the index, middle and ring fingers. There also was segmental losses of the flexor tendons and radial digital nerve of the ring finger. (*B*) After thorough débridement, flexor tendon and nerve grafting were performed. Soft tissue reconstruction was achieved using a large, composite flap based on the SCIA and SIEA (*left*). The SCIA component was designed to cover the palmar aspect and the SIEA flap was used to cover the thumb metacarpal and carpo-metacarpal joint (*right*). The limb of the SIEA flap was designed to be longer so it could wrap around the thumb stump. The flap base has been kept narrow and the differential lengths of each component allow the hand to rest comfortably by the side with some degree of mobility. The edges of the flap have been thinned and beveled, so that inset can be performed easily with good skin apposition. (*C*) Appearance after flap division. The groin/abdominal flap is a good indication in a young child where microsurgery is difficult. The flap provides a healthy soft tissue base for subsequent toe transfer while preserving vessels for microsurgery. A round of flap thinning can significantly reduce the bulk of the palmar tissue.

pedicle because well-vascularized tissue is wasted in the process. Bajantri and colleagues[35] also described a method of making backcuts to orientate the flap in an appropriate direction to cover dorsal, volar, and radial-sided and ulnar-sided defects. This allowed the hand to rest comfortably and permitted some degree of mobility. The essence of the concept lies in designing a flap with unequal limbs—designing a J shape instead of an inverted U shape.

## FREE FLAPS

Free flaps can be broadly divided into fasciocutaneous and muscle flaps, and there are numerous options available. The exact choice of flap depends on size of the defect, type of tissue (glabrous vs nonglabrous skin), whether volume replacement is necessary, the necessary pedicle length, and the need for additional/staged procedures (**Fig. 8**). These factors must be balanced with the aesthetic principles, discussed previously, and donor site considerations.

### *Flap Options for Dorsal Skin*

The free flap choices for resurfacing dorsal hand defects include RFF, lateral arm flap, ALT flap, medial sural artery perforator flap, and dorsalis pedis flap.[1,36–43] These flaps provide good color and texture match. The RFF, dorsalis pedis flap,

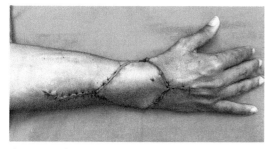

**Fig. 8.** Free lateral arm flap after resection of synovial sarcoma. This patient presented with a synovial sarcoma arising from the dorsum of the wrist. The tumor had fungated through the skin, and the resection required excision of skin and extensor tendons. Tendon transfers and grafting were performed, and the soft tissue defect was resurfaced using a free lateral arm flap from the opposite upper limb. The thin and pliable fasciocutaneous flap provided an excellent gliding plane for the underlying tendon grafts. The robust, well-vascularized tissue is resilient to subsequent radiotherapy and the relatively long pedicle allows the anastomosis to be performed outside the field of radiotherapy.

and medial sural artery perforator flap provide extremely thin and pliable tissue that is ideal for reconstruction of dorsal hand defects. Both the RFF and dorsalis pedis flap are limited, however, by the size of the defect and the corresponding donor defect. Although the foot is a concealed site, skin grafts applied here are more prone to ulceration. The medial sural artery perforator flap is technically challenging and the surgeon should be familiar with the surgical anatomy of this vascular system.[44] The ALT flap is a versatile flap, and large flaps may be taken with minimal donor site morbidity (**Fig. 9**). A long pedicle length may be obtained and a flow-through design can be used if revascularization is required.[45,46] A drawback to this flap is that the skin tends to be thick, particularly in women, and staged liposuction and/or debulking may be necessary.[47] A major factor in the choice of these flaps is surgeon preference and technical expertise.

### *Flap Options for Palmar Skin*

Glabrous skin is a valuable commodity and the plantar aspect of the foot is the only other site besides the hand where such tissue is available. Rodriguez-Vegas[48] provide an excellent review of the historical descriptions and vascular basis of free glabrous skin flaps from the plantar aspect of the foot. The posterior tibial artery divides into the medial and lateral plantar arteries just after it emerges from the tarsal tunnel, deep to the abductor hallucis muscle. The medial plantar artery (MPA) passes distally within a septum between the abductor hallucis and flexor digitorum brevis muscles and divides further into a lateral (superficial) and medial (deep) branch at the level of the talonavicular joint. Septocutaneous branches from the lateral (superficial) branch of the MPA are the basis of the medial plantar and MPA perforator flaps. Perforators from the medial (deep) branch of the MPA nourish the overlying skin that is the basis of the medialis pedis flap. The medialis pedis flap is thus more dorsal than the medial plantar flap. In their series, the flaps were used for resurfacing small to medium-sized palmar and digital defects. Flaps wider than 2 cm to 3 cm required skin grafting, and the majority (75%) of skin grafts took partially. This probably is related to the inevitable shear forces and moisture. An additional problem is the short arterial pedicle. These flaps are technically demanding and should be performed in units with strong microsurgical support.

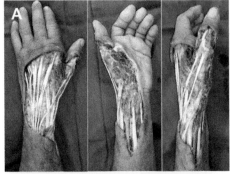

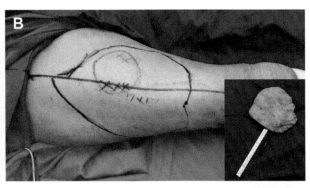

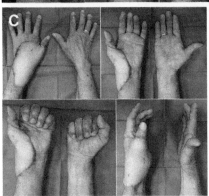

**Fig. 9.** Maintaining the aesthetics of the hand. (*A*) An extensive soft tissue defect of the hand from necrotizing fasciitis. There is loss of the entire dorsal skin and the defect extends to the thenar region and distal forearm. (*B*) A free ALT flap with a long pedicle (*inset*) was harvested from the contralateral thigh. (*C*) Final outcome. The flap was inset at the boundaries of the functional subunits—along the thenar and thumb interphalangeal creases and near the junction of the palmar and dorsal surfaces. The flap is not excessively bulky and there is a reasonable color match.

## SUMMARY

There are multiple options available for reconstruction of soft tissue defects of the hand. The main goal of reconstruction is to provide thin, pliable skin that permits mobility. The reconstructive strategy depends on the location and size of the defect, presence of concomitant digital defects, the need for staged procedures, and available resources. Providing an aesthetically pleasing outcome is increasingly becoming a priority, and traditional favorites, such as the RFF, are giving way to perforator-based flaps and selected free flaps. Distant flaps from the groin and lower abdomen continue to be relevant in the microsurgical era. Ultimately, the reconstructive surgeon should have a large armamentarium at his or her disposal so that a strategy can be tailored to patients' specific needs.

## REFERENCES

1. Ono S, Sebastin SJ, Ohi H, et al. Microsurgical flaps in repair and reconstruction of the hand. Hand Clin 2017;33(3):425–41.
2. Guimberteau JC, Delage JP, McGrouther DA, et al. The microvacuolar system: how connective tissue sliding works. J Hand Surg Eur Vol 2010;35(8): 614–22.
3. Ono S, Sebastin SJ, Yazaki N, et al. Clinical applications of perforator-based propeller flaps in upper limb soft tissue reconstruction. J Hand Surg Am 2011;36(5):853–63.
4. Summers BK, Siegle RJ. Facial cutaneous reconstructive surgery: general aesthetic principles. J Am Acad Dermatol 1993;29(5 Pt 1):669–81 [quiz: 682–3].
5. Rehim SA, Kowalski E, Chung KC. Enhancing aesthetic outcomes of soft-tissue coverage of the hand. Plast Reconstr Surg 2015;135(2): 413e–28e.
6. Page R, Chang J. Reconstruction of hand soft-tissue defects: alternatives to the radial forearm fasciocutaneous flap. J Hand Surg Am 2006;31(5): 847–56.
7. Milner CS, Thirkannad SM. Resurfacing glabrous skin defects in the hand: the thenar base donor site. Tech Hand Up Extrem Surg 2014;18(2): 89–91.
8. Tan RE, Ying CT Jr, Sean LW Jr, et al. Well-camouflaged skin graft donor sites in the hand. Tech Hand Up Extrem Surg 2015;19(4):153–6.
9. Foucher G, Braun JB. A new island flap transfer from the dorsum of the index to the thumb. Plast Reconstr Surg 1979;63(3):344–9.
10. Quaba AA, Davison PM. The distally-based dorsal hand flap. Br J Plast Surg 1990;43(1):28–39.

11. Timmons MJ. The vascular basis of the radial fore-arm flap. Plast Reconstr Surg 1986;77(1):80–92.

12. Chang SM, Hou CL, Zhang F, et al. Distally based radial forearm flap with preservation of the radial artery: anatomic, experimental, and clinical studies. Microsurgery 2003;23(4):328–37.

13. Saint-Cyr M, Mujadzic M, Wong C, et al. The radial artery pedicle perforator flap: vascular analysis and clinical implications. Plast Reconstr Surg 2010; 125(5):1469–78.

14. Koshima I, Moriguchi T, Etoh H, et al. The radial artery perforator-based adipofascial flap for dorsal hand coverage. Ann Plast Surg 1995;35(5):474–9.

15. Ho AM, Chang J. Radial artery perforator flap. J Hand Surg Am 2010;35(2):308–11.

16. Becker C, Gilbert A. The ulnar flap. Handchir Mikro-chir Plast Chir 1988;20(4):180–3.

17. Georgescu AV, Matei I, Ardelean F, et al. Micro-surgical nonmicrovascular flaps in forearm and hand reconstruction. Microsurgery 2007;27(5): 384–94.

18. Mathy JA, Moaveni Z, Tan ST. Perforator anatomy of the ulnar forearm fasciocutaneous flap. J Plast Reconstr Aesthet Surg 2012;65(8):1076–82.

19. Kim KS, Hwang JH. Radial midpalmar island flap. Plast Reconstr Surg 2005;116(5):1332–9.

20. Seyhan T. Reverse thenar perforator flap for volar hand reconstruction. J Plast Reconstr Aesthet Surg 2009;62(10):1309–16.

21. Tapan M, Igde M, Yildirim AR, et al. Reverse thenar perforator flap for large palmar and digital defects. J Hand Surg Am 2018;43(10):956.e1-e6.

22. Orbay JL, Rosen JG, Khouri RK, et al. The glabrous palmar flap: the new free or reversed pedicled palmar fasciocutaneous flap for volar hand reconstruction. Tech Hand Up Extrem Surg 2009;13(3): 145–50.

23. Hao PD, Zhuang YH, Zheng HP, et al. The ulnar palmar perforator flap: anatomical study and clinical application. J Plast Reconstr Aesthet Surg 2014; 67(5):600–6.

24. Soutar DS, Scheker LR, Tanner NS, et al. The radial forearm flap: a versatile method for intra-oral reconstruction. Br J Plast Surg 1983;36(1):1–8.

25. Jin YT, Guan WX, Shi TM, et al. Reversed island fore-arm fascial flap in hand surgery. Ann Plast Surg 1985;15(4):340–7.

26. Zancolli EA, Angrigiani C. Posterior interosseous is-land forearm flap. J Hand Surg Br 1988;13(2):130–5.

27. Angrigiani C, Grilli D, Dominikow D, et al. Posterior interosseous reverse forearm flap: experience with 80 consecutive cases. Plast Reconstr Surg 1993; 92(2):285–93.

28. Buchler U, Frey HP. Retrograde posterior inteross-eous flap. J Hand Surg Am 1991;16(2):283–92.

29. Penteado CV, Masquelet AC, Chevrel JP. The anatomic basis of the fascio-cutaneous flap of the posterior interosseous artery. Surg Radiol Anat 1986;8(4):209–15.

30. Keogh A, Graham DJ, Tan B. Posterior interosseous artery pedicle flap: an anatomical study of the relationship between the posterior interosseous nerve and artery. J Hand Surg Eur Vol 2018;43(10): 1050–3.

31. Zaidenberg EE, Farias-Cisneros E, Pastrana MJ, et al. Extended posterior interosseous artery flap: anatomical and clinical study. J Hand Surg Am 2017;42(3):182–9.

32. Al-Qattan MM, Al-Qattan AM. Defining the indications of pedicled groin and abdominal flaps in hand reconstruction in the current microsurgery era. J Hand Surg Am 2016;41(9):917–27.

33. Chuang DC, Colony LH, Chen HC, et al. Groin flap design and versatility. Plast Reconstr Surg 1989; 84(1):100–7.

34. Sabapathy SR, Bajantri B. Indications, selection, and use of distant pedicled flap for upper limb reconstruction. Hand Clin 2014;30(2):185–99, vi.

35. Bajantri B, Latheef L, Sabapathy SR. Tips to orient pedicled groin flap for hand defects. Tech Hand Up Extrem Surg 2013;17(2):68–71.

36. Wang HD, Alonso-Escalante JC, Cho BH, et al. Versatility of free cutaneous flaps for upper extremity soft tissue reconstruction. J Hand Microsurg 2017; 9(2):58–66.

37. Meky M, Safoury Y. Composite anterolateral thigh perforator flaps in the management of complex hand injuries. J Hand Surg Eur Vol 2013;38(4): 366–70.

38. Adani R, Tarallo L, Marcoccio I, et al. Hand reconstruction using the thin anterolateral thigh flap. Plast Reconstr Surg 2005;116(2):467–73 [discussion: 474–7].

39. Giessler GA, Schmidt AB, Germann G, et al. The role of fabricated chimeric free flaps in reconstruction of devastating hand and forearm injuries. J Reconstr Microsurg 2011;27(9):567–73.

40. Caroli A, Adani R, Castagnetti C, et al. Dorsalis pe-dis flap with vascularized extensor tendons for dorsal hand reconstruction. Plast Reconstr Surg 1993; 92(7):1326–30.

41. Lin CH, Lin CH, Lin YT, et al. The medial sural artery porforator flap: a versatile donor site for hand reconstruction. J Trauma 2011;70(3):736–43.

42. Xie RG, Gu JH, Gong YP, et al. Medial sural artery perforator flap for repair of the hand. J Hand Surg Eur Vol 2007;32(5):512–7.

43. Jeevaratnam JA, Nikkhah D, Nugent NF, et al. The medial sural artery perforator flap and its application in electrical injury to the hand. J Plast Reconstr Aesthet Surg 2014;67(11):1591–4.

44. Wong MZ, Wong CH, Tan BK, et al. Surgical anatomy of the medial sural artery perforator flap. J Reconstr Microsurg 2012;28(8):555–60.

45. Zhan Y, Fu G, Zhou X, et al. Emergency repair of upper extremity large soft tissue and vascular injuries with flow-through anterolateral thigh free flaps. Int J Surg 2017;48:53–8.

46. Qing L, Wu P, Liang J, et al. Use of flow-through anterolateral thigh perforator flaps in reconstruction of complex extremity defects. J Reconstr Microsurg 2015;31(8):571–8.

47. Lin TS. One-stage debulking procedure after flap reconstruction for degloving injury of the hand. J Plast Reconstr Aesthet Surg 2016;69(5):646–51.

48. Rodriguez-Vegas M. Medialis pedis flap in the reconstruction of palmar skin defects of the digits: clarifying the anatomy of the medial plantar artery. Ann Plast Surg 2014;72(5):542–52.

# Thumb Basal Joint Arthritis

Brent B. Pickrell, MD, Kyle R. Eberlin, MD*

## KEYWORDS

- Basal joint arthritis • CMC arthritis • Trapezial-metacarpal joint • Osteoarthritis • Trapeziectomy
- Ligament reconstruction tendon interposition

## KEY POINTS

- Thumb basal joint arthritis is a common condition that may be treated with both nonoperative and operative modalities.
- Nonoperative treatment modalities include splinting, corticosteroid injections, and behavioral modification with hand therapy.
- Options for surgical intervention include arthroscopic debridement, trapeziectomy alone, trapeziectomy with ligament reconstruction and tendon interposition, trapeziectomy with tightrope suspension, extension osteotomy, and arthrodesis, although high-level evidence is currently lacking to support one surgical treatment over another.

## INTRODUCTION

Degenerative arthritis of the thumb carpometacarpal (CMC) joint is a common condition that can result in pain, progressive deformity, weakness, and loss of motion. It can be a cause of functional disability, particularly in postmenopausal women,[1] and is a frequently noted radiologic finding that seems to correlate with advanced age and female gender.[2] The age-adjusted prevalence of thumb CMC arthritis is 7% for men and 15% for women.[3] Radiographically, it has been estimated to affect up to 36% of postmenopausal women.[4,5]

Despite the ubiquitous nature of thumb CMC arthritis, not all patients with radiographic changes are symptomatic and present for evaluation by a hand surgeon. In fact, most patients with arthritic changes at the thumb CMC joint are able to adapt their activities and do not undergo intervention.

In some individuals, however, nonoperative modalities are unsuccessful in mitigating symptoms. Surgical interventions for thumb CMC arthritis are among the most common procedures performed by US hand surgeons, with only carpal tunnel and trigger finger release being more common.[6] The goals of treatment include pain relief, maintenance of thumb motion, and provision of joint stability.

## PATHOPHYSIOLOGY

Because of the common nature of this condition, there has been a focus on elucidating the etiology of the disease process. Many prior reports implicate the anterior oblique ligament in the pathophysiology of this condition; however, some contemporary anatomic studies indicate that the pathomechanics may involve the dorsoradial ligament.[7,8] Clifton and colleagues[9] suggested a possible role for the peptide hormone relaxin to explain female predilection, although this mechanism is still not well understood.

Regardless of the cause, patients develop subluxation of the thumb metacarpal on the trapezium[10] and progressive erosive changes of the trapeziometacarpal joint, resulting in wear and progressive deterioration of the articular cartilage. Over time, thumb mechanics are altered and there can be hyperextension of the metacarpophalangeal (MP) joint, resulting in further pain and instability.

Disclosures: Dr B.B. Pickrell has no disclosures. Dr K.R. Eberlin is a consultant for AxoGen and Integra.
Division of Plastic and Reconstructive Surgery, Harvard Medical School, Massachusetts General Hospital, Wang Building, 55 Fruit Street, Boston, MA 02114, USA
* Corresponding author.
E-mail address: keberlin@mgh.harvard.edu

Clin Plastic Surg 46 (2019) 407–413
https://doi.org/10.1016/j.cps.2019.02.010

plasticsurgery.theclinics.com

## DIAGNOSIS

The diagnosis of thumb CMC arthritis is made primarily based on history and physical examination and is further supported by radiographic imaging.[1] Patients typically present with a gradual, insidious onset of progressively worsening pain at the base of the thumb at the CMC joint. They may describe pain with pinching and gripping maneuvers and/or difficulty turning keys, opening jars, or gripping door knobs. Symptoms should be differentiated from first extensor compartment tenosynovitis (de Quervain disease) and stenosing tenosynovitis of the thumb (trigger thumb).

On examination, there is often point tenderness over the thumb CMC joint. Axial grind test is positive if there is pain on axial compression and rotation of the thumb metacarpal. This test has a 97% specificity but only 30% sensitivity.[11] A more sensitive test may be the "traction-shift" test in which the metacarpal is passively subluxed and then relocated, eliciting pain with this motion (67% sensitivity, 100% specificity).[11] The senior investigator typically uses both maneuvers during physical examination of patients with suspected CMC arthritis.

With progressive disease, examination findings include a dorsoradial prominence of the base of the thumb metacarpal caused by dorsal subluxation: the "shoulder sign."[10] In addition, the thumb may develop an adduction deformity with compensatory hyperextension of the MP joint and flexion of the interphalangeal joint: the characteristic "Z deformity."[1] Pinch and grip strength are often diminished.[1]

Radiographic evaluation includes posteroanterior, lateral, and oblique views of the hand to visualize the CMC joint. The Robert view[12] may be helpful, as it allows visualization of all 4 trapezial articulations; the thumb is positioned with the dorsal side of the hand flat on the plate with pronation of the wrist. The Lewis modification[13–15] of the Robert view angles 15° proximally and is preferred by some investigators.[16] Advanced imaging is rarely performed. In 1973, Eaton and Littler[17] devised a widely accepted radiographic staging system for thumb CMC arthritis (**Table 1**). However, this classification system has been recently challenged due to suboptimal interobserver reliability.[18]

## TREATMENT
### Nonoperative Management

Treatment for CMC arthritis of the thumb often begins with nonoperative management, particularly

**Table 1**
**Eaton classification of thumb carpometacarpal arthritis**

| Eaton Stage | Radiographic Characteristics |
|---|---|
| I | Normal or slightly widened trapeziometacarpal joint; trapeziometacarpal subluxation up to one-third of the articular surface; normal articular contours |
| II | Decreased trapeziometacarpal joint space; trapeziometacarpal subluxation up to one-third of the articular surface; osteophytes or loose bodies <2 mm |
| III | Decreased trapeziometacarpal joint space; trapeziometacarpal subluxation more than one-third of the articular surface; osteophytes or loose bodies ≥2 mm; subchondral cysts or sclerosis |
| IV | Involvement of the scaphotrapezial joint or less commonly the trapezio-trapezoid or trapeziometacarpal joint of the index |

(*From* Bakri K, Moran SL. Thumb carpometacarpal arthritis. Plast Reconstr Surg 2015;135:508–20; with permission.)

in patients with mild or moderate symptoms and/or early-stage radiographic disease. Nonoperative management options include activity modification, oral analgesics, provision of orthoses, strengthening/flexibility exercises, and corticosteroid injections.

### Orthoses
Splinting is a common first-line treatment for many patients. The goals of splinting for CMC arthritis are to increase stability and reduce mechanical stress, thereby decreasing pain and improving function. Orthoses have been shown to provide modest pain relief for CMC arthritis in several prior studies,[19–21] but results may take up to 12 months to fully manifest.[22] A systematic review published in 2015 concluded that orthoses can provide pain relief but do not seem to alter function, strength, or dexterity.[23] Recently, Becker and colleagues[19] showed that Neoprene orthoses may be more comfortable, as effective, and cheaper than customized thermoplastic splints. Similarly, a review by Egan and Brousseau[24] concluded that most splints are equivalent in terms of comfort, pain relief, or function. Patients may wear orthoses either at nighttime only or as needed during the day.

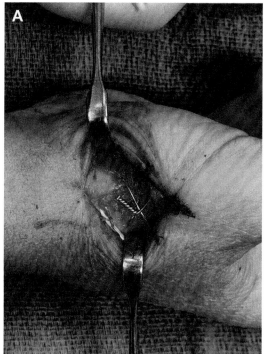 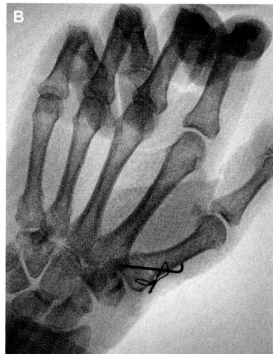

**Fig. 1.** (*A, B*) After performing an apex volar osteotomy, the osteotomized segments are stabilized with a 20-gauge steel wire passed through drill holes made in the proximal and distal portions of the osteotomized metacarpal. The wires are then twist-tied to compress the surfaces together. (*Courtesy of* Neal Chen, MD, Massachusetts General Hospital.)

## Oral analgesics

Oral analgesics (eg, nonsteroidal antiinflammatory drugs) are commonly used by patients and can be supplemented with topical Diclofenac gel, which has been shown in a double-blind randomized control trial (RCT)[25] to reduce pain by 40% in hand osteoarthritis. These medications may provide pain relief but do not alter the natural history of disease (ie, articular changes). Older patients and those with renal dysfunction should be cautioned about the prolonged use of NSAIDs.

## Injections

Corticosteroid injections may provide short-term pain relief for patients with early CMC arthritis.[26,27] Injecting 2.5 to 40 mg of triamcinolone with or without local anesthetic is common practice and may be effective.[1] Despite its use for early stage arthritis, an RCT in 2004 showed no benefit from intraarticular steroid injection in moderate to severe CMC arthritis compared with placebo injection.[28] There is significant practice variation with regard to steroid injections; some surgeons use them regularly, whereas others use them infrequently in the care of patients with CMC arthritis.

Hyaluronic acid injections may also be effective and aim to restore the reduced viscoelasticity

of synovial fluid in the joint space.[29] A recent systematic review[23] found evidence for pain relief from both steroid and hyaluronate injections and noted that most studies found hyaluronate to be more effective and longer-lasting than steroid injections.

## Operative Treatment

Many surgical options are available for patients who remain symptomatic despite nonoperative management. Surgical options include extension osteotomy, CMC arthroscopy with debridement, trapeziectomy alone, trapeziectomy with ligament reconstruction and tendon interposition (LRTI), trapeziectomy with tightrope suspension, CMC arthrodesis, and implant arthroplasty. However, there is little high-level evidence to favor one operation over another.[30]

### Extension osteotomy

An osteotomy of the thumb metacarpal may decrease attritional wear of the CMC joint. This is done by performing a 30-degree metacarpal closing wedge extension osteotomy (**Fig. 1**), which can inhibit dorsoradial subluxation and alter the force distribution to unload the volar segment of the CMC joint.[31] Although it does not surgically alter the trapeziometacarpal joint, it has been shown to be successful in improving symptoms.[32–34] Chou and colleagues[32] found high satisfaction rates and low pain levels, as well as similar pinch strength and thumb radial abduction compared with contralateral untreated thumbs. At 2-year follow-up, Tomaino[34] reported increased grip and pinch strength in patients with Eaton stage I disease and greater than 90% patient satisfaction. Hobby and colleagues[33] reported long-term pain relief (mean 6.8 years) in 80% of patients undergoing this technique.

## Carpometacarpal arthroscopy with debridement

Another surgical option for early stage CMC arthritis that has recently gained popularity is CMC arthroscopy with debridement and synovectomy. Arthroscopy avoids the need for a larger incision over the CMC joint with less soft tissue dissection, offering the theoretic benefit of a minimally invasive approach with limited morbidity and quicker recovery. In this technique, first described by Menon[35] and Berger,[36] a 1.9-mm-diameter arthroscope is placed through the 1-R (radial) and 1-U (ulnar) portals. Synovectomy is performed with a 2-mm shaver. The distal trapezium is debrided with a 2.9-mm arthroscopic bur, removing 2 mm of distal trapezium and 1 to 2 mm of the thumb metacarpal base. Depending on the patient's demands and stage of disease, various adjunctive arthroscopic procedures can be considered, including capsuloligamentous shrinkage, suture button suspensionplasty, or ligament reconstruction.[37]

Both medium- and long-term outcomes for arthroscopic techniques have been reported and seem to be similar to those of other treatment modalities. Wong and Ho[37] reviewed their experience with debridement and synovectomy alone in 65 patients with predominantly Eaton stage II/III disease and found that excellent to good pain relief occurred in 44.7% of patients in an average follow-up of 7 years. However, there was only minimal improvement in strength. Culp and Rekant[38] performed 24 cases of arthroscopic debridement, shrinkage, and partial/complete trapeziectomy and reported good to excellent outcomes in 88%. They concluded that arthroscopic debridement and synovectomy was best in Eaton I/II disease. Hofmeister and colleagues[39] reported favorable long-term results on 18 thumbs at 7.6-year follow-up using arthroscopic shrinkage, trapeziectomy, and Kirchner wire fixation. A subjective improvement in pain, pinch activities, strength, and range of motion (ROM) was noted in all patients, and no patient had further surgery on his/her thumb.

## Trapeziectomy alone

Surgical excision of the trapezium was first described by Gervis in 1947[16] and remains a common component of many surgical techniques for the treatment of CMC arthritis.[1] With this technique, the trapezium is excised in its entirety and the joint space is maintained through the development of hematoma. A Cochrane review published in 2009 indicated that trapeziectomy alone was associated with fewer complications than trapeziectomy with LRTI, while providing similar functional outcomes with regard to improvement in pain, grip, and pinch strength.[40] Other studies have indicated equivalency of trapeziectomy alone compared with trapeziectomy with LRTI, and it is unknown if further benefit is conferred through the addition of adjunctive techniques other than trapeziectomy alone.

## Trapeziectomy with ligament reconstruction and tendon interposition

First described by Burton and Pellegrini,[41] trapeziectomy with LRTI was designed to reconstruct the anterior oblique ligament of the thumb CMC joint in order to maintain the length of the thumb metacarpal to prevent subsidence. This is the most common operation performed for CMC arthritis in the United States and is considered by many to be the standard for surgical intervention.[42,43] In this procedure, a trapeziectomy is performed and either half or all of the flexor carpi radialis (FCR) tendon is woven through the base of the thumb metacarpal in an oblique orientation to provide support and reconstruct the beak ligament (**Fig. 2**). Suspensionplasty with the abductor pollicis longus has also been performed with good results.[44]

Yuan and colleagues[42] found an increasing trend in the utilization of trapeziectomy with LRTI between 2001 (84%) and 2010 (90%). Female sex was significantly associated with LRTI, and women were less likely to undergo trapeziectomy alone (odds ratio 0.49). In addition, the investigators noted that 95% of surgeons perform only 1 type of surgical procedure, and among those, 93% perform only trapeziectomy with LRTI. Despite widespread surgeon preference in the literature, there is no conclusive evidence to indicate superiority of trapeziectomy with LRTI over simple trapeziectomy, ligament reconstruction, or tendon interposition.[1] Nonetheless, this technique is technically straightforward and generally has reliable results.

## Trapeziectomy with tightrope suspensionplasty

An alternative technique to address the length and suspension of the thumb metacarpal is the

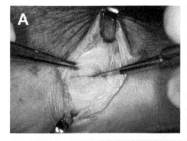
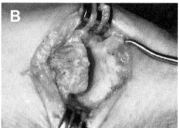
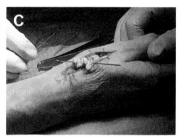
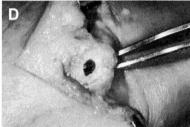
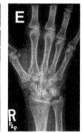

**Fig. 2.** (A) A longitudinal capsulotomy is made between extensor pollicis longus muscle and extensor pollicis brevis tendons to expose the thumb CMC joint. (B) The trapezium is then removed en block or piecemeal. (C) The flexor carpi radialis tendon is harvested proximally and then delivered distally. (D) The tendon is passed through a bone tunnel made at the base of the first metacarpal. (E) At 1-year postoperative. (*Courtesy of* Jesse Jupiter, MD, Massachusetts General Hospital.)

tightrope suspensionplasty. This technique is similar to others described in which trapeziectomy is first performed, either arthroscopically or open. Next, an incision is made on the dorsal hand, just ulnar to base of the index metacarpal. A 0.045-in guidewire with integrated retriever loop is then passed obliquely from the base of the thumb metacarpal to the facet at the radial base of the index metacarpal. The suture from the mini TightRope system (Arthrex, Naples, FL) is then passed from an ulnar to radial direction through the 2 drill holes made with the guidewire.[45] The tightrope suspension acts to resist migration of the thumb metacarpal into the space remaining after trapeziectomy. Other purported benefits include decreased operative time, a possible decrease in recovery time, limited dissection, and sparing of the FCR muscle tendon.[45]

Roman and colleagues[45] found that patients with Eaton III/IV osteoarthritis undergoing trapeziectomy and suture suspension had increased thumb strength and ROM with complete relief of pain. Yao and colleagues[46,47] similarly published reassuring data at both 2- and 5-year follow-ups without significant complications.

### Arthrodesis
Arthrodesis is an alternative to other surgical treatments for patients with higher physical demands.[7] Although this technique is most often used for younger patients, older and less physically active patients may benefit as well.[43,48] Hattori and colleagues[48] found that arthrodesis was equally effective for improving DASH scores and grip strength in older and younger patients, with the exception of improved pinch strength in younger patients. Recent modifications of traditional arthrodesis techniques have been described. Harston and colleagues[49] reported a V-shaped osteotomy at the base of the thumb metacarpal with an 83% fusion rate, significant improvement in disability scores, and no significant complications. Kazmers and colleagues[50] reported a locking cage plate construct in 14 patients and compared it with 22 patients undergoing LRTI. The modified arthrodesis showed 25% greater pinch strength as well as similar range of motion compared with LRTI.

Not all patients benefit from arthrodesis. A 2016 study indicated that in women older than 40 years with Eaton stage II or III disease, arthrodesis was inferior to trapeziectomy with LRTI.[51] In a recent RCT, arthrodesis was found to result in significantly more complications compared with trapeziectomy with LRTI.[52]

### Implant arthroplasty
Prosthetic arthroplasty of the trapezium has been used to treat CMC arthritis. Implant arthroplasty seeks to preserve joint biomechanics, avoid metacarpal subsidence, and provide immediate stability.[53] Current available options include silicone, Artelon, Stablyx, metallic, and pyrolytic carbon implants. Vitale and colleagues[53] provide a comprehensive summary of the various implants and their evolution. Overall, functional outcomes data are mixed with an increased complication rate and cost associated with implants. Many implants suffer from extrusion, inflammatory reactions, loosening, and failure that may require revision surgery.[53] At present, long-term data are limited and current studies do not suggest that implant

arthroplasty is superior to trapeziectomy. Complication rates have limited widespread acceptance of this technique.

## SUMMARY

Thumb CMC arthritis is a common condition treated by hand surgeons. Most patients are treated without surgery, but those with persistent and recalcitrant symptoms affecting quality of life may benefit from surgical intervention. There are myriad surgical options, and the best option depends on the patient's goals and functional demands, surgeon experience, and patient preference.

## REFERENCES

1. Bakri K, Moran SL. Thumb carpometacarpal arthritis. Plast Reconstr Surg 2015;135:508–20.
2. Becker SJE, Briet JP, Hageman MGJS, et al. Death, Taxes, and trapeziometacarpal arthrosis. Clin Orthop Relat Res 2013;471(12):3738–44.
3. Haara MM, Heliovaara M, Kroger H, et al. Osteoarthritis in the carpometacarpal joint of the thumb. Prevalence and associations with disability and mortality. J Bone Joint Surg Am 2004;86(7):1452–7.
4. Dahaghin S, Bierma-Zeinstra SMA, Ginai AZ, et al. Prevalence and pattern of radiographic hand osteoarthritis and association with pain and disability (the Rotterdam study). Ann Rheum Dis 2005;64(5):682–7.
5. Sonne-Holm S, Jacobsen S. Osteoarthritis of the first carpometacarpal joint: a study of radiology and clinical epidemiology. Results from the Copenhagen Osteoarthritis Study. Osteoarthritis Cartilage 2006;14(5):496–500.
6. Veltre DR, Yakavonis M, Curry EJ, et al. Regional variations of Medicare physician payments for hand surgery procedures in the United States. Hand (N Y) 2017.
7. Maes-Clavier C, Bellemere P, Gabrion A, et al. Anatomical study of the ligamentous attachments and articular surfaces of the trapeziometacarpal joint. Consequences on surgical management of its osteoarthrosis. Chir Main 2014;33:118–23.
8. Lin JD, Karl JW, Strauch RJ. Trapeziometacarpal joint stability: the evolving importance of the dorsal ligaments. Clin Orthop Relat Res 2014;472:1138–45.
9. Clifton KB, Rodner C, Wolf JM. Detection of relaxin receptor in the dorsoradial ligament, synovium, and articular cartilage of the trapeziometacarpal joint. J Orthop Res 2014;32:1061–7.
10. Moskowitz RW. Osteoarthritis: diagnosis and medical/surgical management. Philadelphia: Wolters Kluwer/Lippincott Williams & Wilkins; 2007.
11. Choa RM, Parvizi N, Giele HP. A prospective case-control study to compare the sensitivity and specificity of the grind and traction-shift (subluxation-relocation) clinical tests in osteoarthritis of the thumb carpometacarpal joint. J Hand Surg Eur Vol 2014;39:282–5.
12. Robert P. Bulletins et memoires de la Societe de Radiologie Medicale de France 1936;24:687–90.
13. Lewis S. New angles on the radiographic examination of the hand—III. Radiogr Today 1988;54:47–8.
14. Ballinger P, Frank E, Merrill V. Merrill's atlas of radiographic positions & radiologic procedures. 10th edition. St Louis (MO): Elsevier; 2003. p. 108–9.
15. Ladd AL. The Robert's view: a historical and clinical perspective. Clin Orthop Relat Res 2014;472:1097–100.
16. Gervis WH. Osteo-arthritis of the trapezio-metacarpal joint treated by excision of the trapezium. Proc R Soc Med 1947;40:492.
17. Eaton RG, Littler JW. Ligament reconstruction for the painful thumb carpometacarpal joint. J Bone Joint Surg Am 1973;55:1655–66.
18. Berger AJ, Momeni A, Ladd AL. Intra- and interobserver reliability of the Eaton classification for trapeziometacarpal arthritis: a systematic review. Clin Orthop Relat Res 2014;472:1155–9.
19. Becker SJ, Bot AG, Curley SE, et al. A prospective randomized comparison of neoprene vs thermoplast hand-based thumb spica splinting for trapeziometacarpal arthrosis. Osteoarthritis Cartilage 2013;21:668–75.
20. Weiss S, LaStayo P, Mills A, et al. Prospective analysis of splinting the first carpometacarpal joint: an objective, subjective, and radiographic assessment. J Hand Ther 2000;13:218–26.
21. Weiss S, Lastayo P, Mills A, et al. Splinting the degenerative basal joint: custom-made or prefabricated neoprene? J Hand Ther 2004;17:401–6.
22. Rannou F, Dimet J, Boutron I, et al. Splint for base-of-thumb osteoarthritis. A randomized trial. Ann Intern Med 2009;150:661–9.
23. Spaans AJ, van Minnen LP, Kon M, et al. Conservative treatment of thumb base osteoarthritis: a systematic review. J Hand Surg Am 2015;40(1):16–21.
24. Egan MY, Brousseau L. Splinting for osteoarthritis of the carpometacarpal joint: a review of the evidence. Am J Occup Ther 2007;61:70–8.
25. Altman RD, Dreiser RL, Fisher CL, et al. Diclofenac sodium gel in patients with primary hand osteoarthritis: a randomized, double-blind, placebo-controlled trial. J Rheumatol 2009;36:1991–9.
26. Joshi R. Intraarticular corticosteroid injection for first carpometacarpal osteoarthritis. J Rheumatol 2005;32:1305–6.
27. Dieppe PA. Are intra-articular steroid injections useful for the treatment of the osteoarthritis joint? Br J Rheumatol 1991;30:199.
28. Meenagh GK, Patton J, Kynes C, et al. A randomised controlled trial of intra-articular corticosteroid

injection of the carpometacarpal joint of the thumb in osteoarthritis. Ann Rheum Dis 2004;63:1260–3.

29. Peyron JG. A new approach to the treatment of osteoarthritis: viscosupplementation. Osteoarthritis Cartilage 1993;1(2):85–7.

30. Wajon A, Vinycomb T, Carr E, et al. Surgery for thumb (trapeziometacarpal joint) osteoarthritis. Cochrane Database Syst Rev 2015;(2):CD004631.

31. Tomaino MM. Basal metacarpal osteotomy for osteoarthritis of the thumb. J Hand Surg Am 2011;36: 1076–9.

32. Chou FH, Irrgang JJ, Goitz RJ. Long term follow-up of first metacarpal extension osteotomy for early CMC arthritis. Hand 2014;9:178–83.

33. Hobby JL, Lyall HA, Meggitt BF. First metacarpal osteotomy for trapeziometacarpal osteoarthritis. J Bone Joint Surg Br 1998;80:508–12.

34. Tomaino MM. Treatment of Eaton stage 1 trapeziometacarpal disease with thumb metacarpal extension osteotomy. J Hand Surg Am 2000;25:1100–6.

35. Menon J. Arthroscopic management of trapeziometacarpal joint arthritis of the thumb. Arthroscopy 1996;12(5):581–7.

36. Berger RA. A technique for arthroscopic evaluation of the first carpometacarpal joint. J Hand Surg Am 1997;22(6):1077–80.

37. Wong CWY, Ho PC. Arthroscopic management of thumb carpometacarpal joint arthritis. Hand Clin 2017;33:795–812.

38. Culp RW, Rekant MS. The role of arthroscopy in evaluating and treating trapeziometacarpal disease. Hand Clin 2001;17:315–9.

39. Hofmeister EP, Leak RS, Culp RW, et al. Arthroscopic hemitrapeziectomy for first carpometacarpal arthritis: results at 7-year follow-up. Hand (N Y) 2009;4:24–8.

40. Wajon A, Carr E, Edmunds I, et al. Surgery for thumb (trapeziometacarpal joint) osteoarthritis. Cochrane Database Syst Rev 2009;(7):CD004631.

41. Burton RI, Pellegrini VD Jr. Surgical management of basal joint arthritis of the thumb: Part II. Ligament reconstruction with tendon interposition arthroplasty. J Hand Surg Am 1986;11:324–32.

42. Yuan F, Aliu O, Chung KC, et al. Evidence-based practice in the surgical treatment of thumb carpometacarpal joint arthritis. J Hand Surg Am 2017; 42(2):104–12.

43. Wolf JM, Delaronde S. Current trends in nonoperative and operative treatment of trapeziometacarpal osteoarthritis: a survey of US hand surgeons. J Hand Surg Am 2012;37:77–82.

44. Soejima A, Hanamura T, Kikuta T, et al. Suspensionplasty with the abductor pollicus longus tendon for osteoarthritis in the carpometacarpal joint of the thumb. J Hand Surg Am 2006;31(3):425–8.

45. Roman PB, Linnell JD, Moore JB. Trapeziectomy arthroplasty with suture suspension: short- to medium-term outcomes from a Single-surgeon experience. J Hand Surg Am 2016;41(1):34–9.

46. Yao J, Song Y. Suture-button suspensionplasty for thumb carpometacarpal arthritis: a minimum 2-year follow-up. J Hand Surg Am 2013;38(6):1161–5.

47. Yao J, Cheah AE. Mean 5-year follow-up for suture button suspensionplasty in the treatment of thumb carpometacarpal joint osteoarthritis. J Hand Surg Am 2017;42(7):569.e1-11.

48. Hattori Y, Doi K, Dormitorio B, et al. Arthrodesis for primary osteoarthritis of the trapeziometacarpal joint in elderly patients. J Hand Surg Am 2016;41: 753–9.

49. Harston A, Manon-Matos Y, McGill S, et al. The follow-up of trapeziometacarpal arthrodesis using V-shaped osteotomy for osteoarthritis of the first carpometacarpal joint. Tech Hand Up Extrem Surg 2015;19:18–22.

50. Kazmers NH, Hippensteel KJ, Calfee RP, et al. Locking plate arthrodesis compares favorably with LRTI for thumb trapeziometacarpal arthrosis: early outcomes from a longitudinal cohort study. HSS J 2017;13:54–60.

51. Spekreijse KR, Selles RW, Kedilioglu MA, et al. Trapeziometacarpal arthrodesis or trapeziectomy with ligament reconstruction in primary trapeziometacarpal osteoarthritis: a 5-year follow-up. J Hand Surg Am 2016;41(9):910–6.

52. Vermeulen GM, Brink SM, Slijper H, et al. Trapeziometacarpal arthrodesis or trapeziectomy with ligament reconstruction in primary trapeziometacarpal osteoarthritis: a randomized controlled trial. J Bone Joint Surg Am 2014;96:726–33.

53. Vitale MA, Taylor F, Ross M, et al. Trapezium prosthetic arthroplasty (silicone, Artelon, metal, and pyrocarbon). Hand Clin 2013;29:37–55.

# Phalangeal and Metacarpal Fractures

Amir H. Taghinia, MD, MPH, MBA[a,b,]*, Simon G. Talbot, MD[b,c]

## KEYWORDS

- Phalangeal • Metacarpal • Fracture • Fixation • Hand

## KEY POINTS

- Most hand fractures can be treated nonoperatively, although operative treatment remains an important option for select cases.
- Recent operative techniques improve outcomes by reducing soft tissue trauma and facilitating early motion.
- As treatment options evolve, the principles of hand fracture care remain unchanged, requiring the surgeon to carefully balance stability against early motion.

## INTRODUCTION

In most cases, hand fractures can be treated nonoperatively with satisfactory functional and aesthetic outcomes. Starting approximately 50 years ago, the advent of advanced imaging, implants, and a better understanding of fracture healing ignited more operative approaches. However, clinicians soon realized that wide-open exposure and implant application (while promising rigid fixation) came at a high cost: soft tissue injury; disruption of local healing biology; and functional morbidity such as pain, infection, adhesions, and stiffness. New high-quality evidence demonstrates that nonoperative treatment of some displaced hand fractures results in equivalent functional and patient-reported outcomes as those repaired operatively. Hence, the pendulum has swung back with more reliance on nonoperative treatment and minimally invasive percutaneous options. Individualized open repair remains a critical adjunct in a small subset of fractures, whereas wide-awake anesthesia has obviated some operative risks.

## DIAGNOSIS

History, examination, and plain radiographic imaging form the cornerstone of diagnosis. The mechanism of injury should corroborate the nature and degree of injury, or else suspicion should be raised about tumor, infection, or abuse. The clinician should assess digital alignment during motion: malalignment perpendicular to the plane of motion is poorly tolerated (**Fig. 1**). Radiographic examination with 3 standard views is sufficient and necessary for diagnosing most hand fractures. Computed tomography can be helpful in severely comminuted or intraarticular fractures to better delineate anatomy.

## TREATMENT PRINCIPLES AND GENERAL CONSIDERATIONS

The clinician should treat the patient, not the radiograph or the fracture. Fractures are best approached in a holistic manner, taking into account the particulars of the bone and soft tissue injury and rehabilitation, along with the medical, social, and psychological factors of the patient.

Disclosure Statement: The authors have nothing to disclose.
[a] Department of Plastic and Oral Surgery, Boston Children's Hospital, 300 Longwood Avenue, Enders 1, Boston 02115, MA, USA; [b] Harvard Medical School, Boston, MA, USA; [c] Division of Plastic Surgery, Brigham and Women's Hospital, 75 Francis Street, Boston 02115, MA, USA
* Corresponding author. Department of Plastic and Oral Surgery, Boston Children's Hospital, 300 Longwood Avenue, Enders 1, Boston, MA 02115.
E-mail address: amir.taghinia@childrens.harvard.edu

Clin Plastic Surg 46 (2019) 415–423
https://doi.org/10.1016/j.cps.2019.02.011
0094-1298/19/© 2019 Elsevier Inc. All rights reserved.

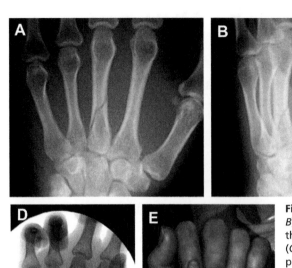
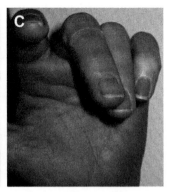
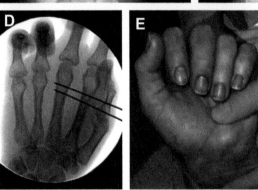

**Fig. 1.** A seemingly innocuous metacarpal fracture (*A*, *B*) can cause significant rotatory malalignment. Note that scissoring is maximum at midcomposite flexion (*C*). Intraoperative reduction and transmetacarpal pinning is performed (*D*) with improved alignment (*E*).

The goal is to restore preinjury locomotor function via bony alignment and stabilization followed by timely rehabilitation. The main requirement for bony healing—stability—is often in direct conflict with the main requirement for function—early motion. Balancing these competing interests to obtain satisfactory healing and function underlies the basic tenets of fracture care.

Many hand fractures can be treated nonoperatively. In most cases, apparently significant displacement on a magnified radiograph can heal with minimal to no functional sequelae. However, even nonoperative treatment poses risks (**Table 1**).

Surgical management may be indicated for irreducible or unstable fractures, multiple or open fractures, displaced intraarticular fractures, and some fractures associated with soft tissue injuries. Surgery may be done percutaneously or via an open approach. Methods of fixation include Kirschner wires, plates, screws, dynamic traction devices, and external fixators. Plates and screws provide rigidity (**Fig. 2**), whereas the other methods provide stability; postoperative motion should be titrated commensurate to the level of stability. One should balance the advantage of increasing mechanical stability (eg, plates and screws) against the additional harm of surgical trauma (soft tissue injury,

stripping of periosteum, extensor tendon adhesions). Plate fixation of metacarpal and phalangeal fractures risks significant complications[1] and may provide no major advantage in long-term function.[2,3] The literature is sparse on the latter issue, because widely heterogeneous presentations often prevent direct comparison and treatment bias abounds.

Open digital fractures can be temporarily irrigated in the emergency department, the skin closed, splint applied, and fracture fixation delayed for a few days. A recent, large database analysis of 3506 patients with metacarpal, proximal phalangeal, and middle phalangeal fractures showed that patients are not at greater risk for infection based on the diagnosis of open fracture alone.[4] Furthermore, open fractures taken to the operating room more than 1 day after presenting did not have a higher incidence of infection.

## EXTRAARTICULAR FRACTURES

The treatment of extraarticular metacarpal and phalangeal fractures has undergone a recent change toward conservative or less invasive approaches. Multiple investigators have advocated acceptance of mild deformity to avoid the risks

**Table 1**
**Common risks of fracture treatment**

| Nonoperative Risks | Operative Risks |
|---|---|
| Mal-union and nonunion | Mal-union and nonunion |
| Stiffness due to prolonged immobilization | Stiffness due to adhesions |
| Pressure skin necrosis | Hardware extrusion, breakage, or loosening |
| Muscle ischemia from tightness | Infection |

of surgical intervention for metacarpal fractures, particularly of the fifth metacarpal neck (Boxer fracture).[5–10] The acceptable degree of angulation in metacarpal neck fractures has been determined by expert opinion. Measuring angles in fifth metacarpal neck fractures is a standard technique, and it seems to influence the decision for surgery. Tosti and colleagues[11] showed that surgeons who were shown radiographs of fifth metacarpal neck fractures with measured angulation were more likely to recommend surgery. Nevertheless, a Cochrane review found no good evidence that more significant mal-union causes worse

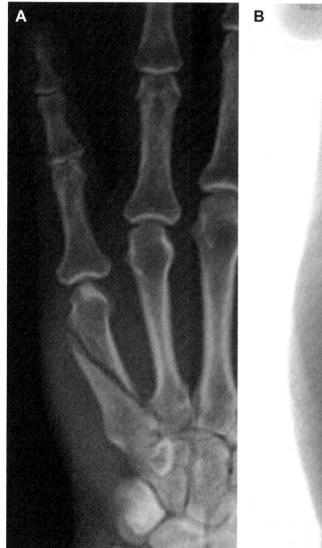
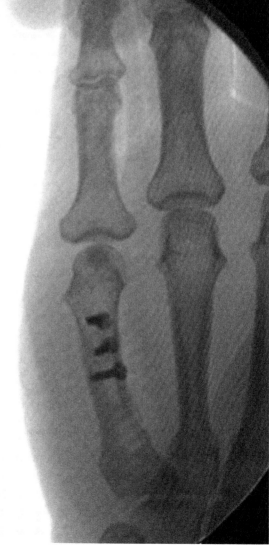

**Fig. 2.** Leg screws provide rigid fixation for long oblique or spiral fractures (*A*, *B*) and allow early motion. Screws perpendicular to the fracture line may be placed in multiple planes.

hand function or unacceptable deformity.[12] A randomized, multicenter trial showed no difference in functional outcomes of fifth metacarpal neck fractures treated with soft wrap/buddy taping versus reduction and casting.[13] The investigators noted that patients treated with soft wrap or buddy taping must be willing to accept loss of the metacarpal head prominence, although satisfaction with appearance was not different between the groups. Regardless, attempts at reduction without definitive fixation may not even be effective. Pace and colleagues[14] compared fifth digit metacarpal neck fractures with and without attempted reduction and immobilization and found no difference in fracture angle between the 2 groups at final follow-up.

Lastly, in a large multicenter randomized trial, Sletten and colleagues[15] compared conservative treatment without fracture reduction (n = 43) with closed reduction and bouquet pinning (n = 42) for fifth digit metacarpal neck fractures between 30 and 50 degrees of angulation. At 1 year they found no statistical difference in QuickDASH score, pain, satisfaction, range of motion, grip strength, or quality of life between the 2 groups. The operative group had higher satisfaction with hand appearance but longer sick leave and more complications. The summary of these recent findings suggests that moderately angulated (30–50 degrees) fifth metacarpal neck fractures should be treated conservatively, perhaps with little to no immobilization, as long as the patient accepts a change in appearance of the hand. For fractures with a greater degree of angulation, reduction and operative fixation is recommended.

To balance the competing interests of early motion versus stability and avoid open treatment, del Piñal and colleagues[16] presented results of intramedullary fixation of hand fractures using cannulated headless compression screws. The screws are inserted retrograde via a small arthrotomy of the joint distal to the fracture (**Fig. 3**), and patients start motion immediately. All of the 69 fractures in the study united and patients returned to full function within 2.5 months. Other investigators confirmed feasibility in smaller studies.[17–19] The technique does not work well for long oblique fractures or those with cortical discontinuity. Callus formation was prominent in some fractures and absent in others, indicating a mixture of rigid and dynamic stability. Cadaveric studies have confirmed that intramedullary fixation is biomechanically weaker than plating but stronger than K-wire fixation.[20,21] One concern is potential long-term complications from the articular defect

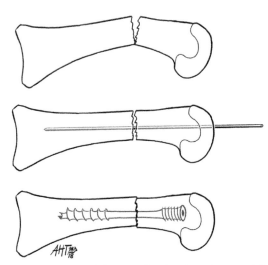

**Fig. 3.** Metacarpal fracture fixed with an intramedullary headless compression screw to minimize soft tissue dissection and allow early motion.

created in the metacarpal or phalangeal head with screw insertion. However, a single hole represents a minor portion of the total surface area, and it is located dorsally, away from the most load-bearing area of the articular surface.[22]

In keeping with the theme of simplifying hand fracture care, additional contemporary operative concepts include single pin for proximal phalangeal fractures,[23] transarticular pinning of proximal phalangeal fractures,[24] using only 2 (vs 3) lag screws in oblique fractures,[25] abandoning lag screws altogether in favor of (non-lagged) interfragmentary screws,[26] and lastly, using only local anesthesia for fracture fixation (see later discussion).

## INTRAARTICULAR FRACTURES

Mallet fractures have been treated in different ways. Wehbe and Schneider[27] proposed that almost all mallet fractures can be treated conservatively, ignoring joint subluxation and size/displacement of the bone fragment; however this has not been universally accepted. Conservative management with splinting alone is typically quoted for closed injuries involving less than one-third of the articular surface and without distal interphalangeal joint (DIP) joint subluxation. Studies support isolated immobilization of only the DIP joint.[28,29] Many different splints have been advocated with no clear winner.[30] The most important determinant of nonoperative treatment outcome seems to be patient compliance.

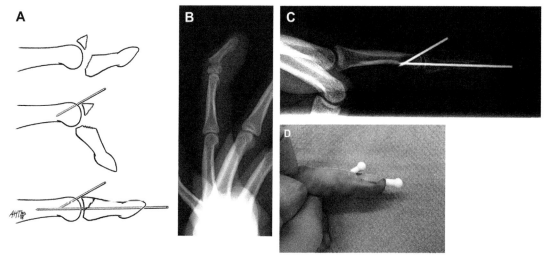

**Fig. 4.** Mallet fracture reduced and fixed with an extension blocking k-wire (*A*). Extension blocking wires can also help stabilize multi-fragmented mallet injuries (*B–D*).

Operative management of mallet fractures may include DIP pinning alone, extension block pinning (**Fig. 4**), compression pinning, or open reduction and internal fixation with screws, tension bands, or pull-through wires, and no technique is necessarily superior. A recent multicenter study showed no significant differences in the functional outcomes of palmarly subluxed mallet fractures treated with K-wire fixation and extension block pinning, K-wires used as joysticks, or interfragmentary mini screws.[31]

Proximal interphalangeal (PIP) joint fracture/dislocations pose one of the more challenging clinical scenarios in hand surgery. The PIP joint's inherent tendency for stiffness and the risk of posttraumatic osteoarthritis create a difficult scenario in which the benefits of reconstructive precision weigh heavily against the damage of soft tissue dissection. The more of the volar base of the middle phalanx is involved, the more dorsal subluxation occurs. A recent biomechanical study showed stability of the joint with 20% volar defects of the middle phalangeal base and the threshold for stability seemed to be around 40%.[32] There is substantial interobserver agreement among surgeons for assessment of articular fracture characteristics (gap, step, subluxation, or dislocation) and the recommendation to operate or not.[33] However, the recommendation for the type of operation is more variable with only fair interobserver agreement. This finding is not surprising, given the myriad of different treatment options that exist, with none showing clear superiority (**Table 2**).[33–35]

Dynamic traction has become a more common option in recent years, particularly for comminuted PIP joint fracture dislocations (**Fig. 5**). This follows from the realization that an anatomic PIP joint reduction is not a prerequisite for good function. However, by using pins and rubber bands (several constructs have been published) to hold the joint to length while reducing fracture fragments via ligamentotaxis, concentric articular congruity can be achieved.[36,37] This allows fracture healing while keeping the joint mobile.

Another technique gaining traction in recent years is the use of the hemihamate arthroplasty for resurfacing of the volar lip of the middle phalanx at the PIP joint. This technique is useful for severely comminuted fractures in which an articular surface cannot be recreated locally. It requires shotgunning the PIP joint through a volar approach, harvesting a portion of the hamate from its distal articular surface, transferring a custom-cut graft, and using the ridge between the fourth and fifth metacarpal bases to approximate the articular surface of the middle phalanx to recreate joint congruity.[36] This technically demanding procedure can be applied to acute and chronic cases and excellent

| Table 2 Options for treatment of proximal interphalangeal joint fracture/dislocations | |
|---|---|
| Traditional Techniques | Contemporary Additional Techniques |
| Extension block pinning Volar plate arthroplasty | Volar plating Dynamic or static traction devices Hemihamate arthroplasty |

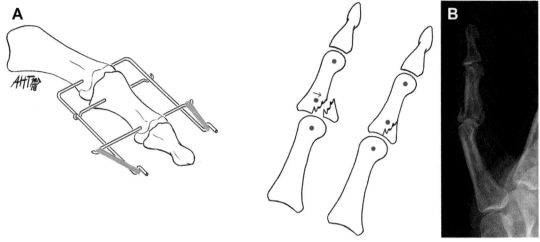

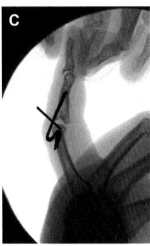

**Fig. 5.** Dynamic external fixator holds the PIP joint to length and allows motion while healing. This is especially useful for comminuted fractures where internal fixation may be impossible. Several different types of constructs exist using pins and rubber bands, including the one shown diagrammatically (*A*) and that shown in plain films (*B, C*). Red *arrow* (*A*) indicates the necessary direction of translation.

results have been reported with minimal donor site morbidity.[35,38]

## WIDE-AWAKE LOCAL ANESTHESIA

The wide-awake local anesthesia technique has been advocated in treatment of many routine hand conditions including carpal tunnel release, flexor tendon repair, and fracture fixation.[39–41] Local anesthesia with epinephrine is infiltrated in the surgical site[42] and allowed 25 minutes[43] to provide analgesia and vasoconstriction (**Fig. 6**). The open procedure is then performed without a tourniquet and without any other anesthesia. The advantage of this technique is that sedatives are not required, thus avoiding preanesthetic evaluation, expediting postoperative recovery, and decreasing costs. Furthermore, fracture stability and rotational alignment can be tested directly by having the patient move the digit.

The disadvantages of this technique are that the patient needs to be compliant and able to withstand multiple injections. In addition, the surgical field is not as bloodless as under tourniquet control. Digital necrosis caused by epinephrine seems to be inaccurate dogma[44,45] and has not been a problem.

## SUMMARY

The management of phalangeal and metacarpal fractures continues to evolve. Nonoperative or less invasive techniques, limiting the need for soft tissue dissection and resultant stiffness, continue to be developed and become more popular. The competing forces of fracture stability to optimize healing and early mobilization to optimize function need careful balancing. As imaging, equipment, and techniques improve,

**A** **B**

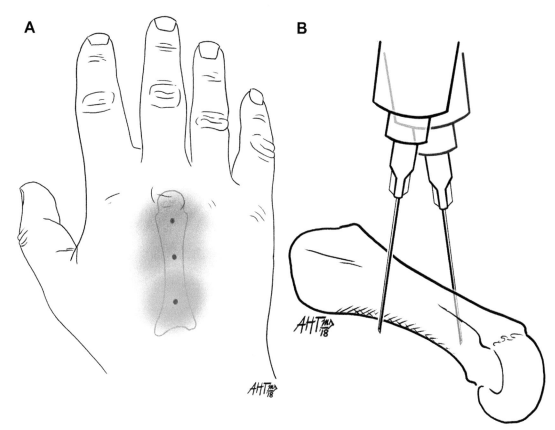

**Fig. 6.** The hand can be anesthetized before metacarpal surgery (*A*) with injection of local anesthesia starting proximally (*green dot*) and advancing distally with 2 additional injections (*purple* and *pink dots*). A field effect can be obtained by pivoting the needle and injecting on both sides of the metacarpal (*B*).

hand surgeons can tailor individualized care to the unique needs of each patient.

## REFERENCES

1. Page SM, Stern PJ. Complications and range of motion following plate fixation of metacarpal and phalangeal fractures. J Hand Surg Am 1998;23(5): 827–32.
2. Pandey R, Soni N, Bhayana H, et al. Hand function outcome in closed small bone fractures treated by open reduction and internal fixation by mini plate or closed crossed pinning: a randomized controlled trial. Musculoskelet Surg 2018. [Epub ahead of print].
3. Facca S, Ramdhian R, Pelissier A, et al. Fifth metacarpal neck fracture fixation: locking plate versus K-wire? Orthop Traumatol Surg Res 2010;96(5): 506–12.
4. Minhas SV, Catalano LW. Comparison of open and closed hand fractures and the effect of urgent operative intervention. J Hand Surg Am 2019;44(1):65. e1-7.
5. Neumeister MW, Webb K, McKenna K. Non-surgical management of metacarpal fractures. Clin Plast Surg 2014;41(3):451–61.
6. Kollitz KM, Hammert WC, Vedder NB, et al. Metacarpal fractures: treatment and complications. Hand (N Y) 2014;9(1):16–23.
7. Westbrook AP, Davis TR, Armstrong D, et al. The clinical significance of malunion of fractures of the neck and shaft of the little finger metacarpal. J Hand Surg Eur Vol 2008;33(6):732–9.
8. Tang JB, Blazar PE, Giddins G, et al. Overview of indications, preferred methods and technical tips for hand fractures from around the world. J Hand Surg Eur Vol 2015;40(1):88–97.
9. Giddins GEB. The non-operative management of hand fractures. J Hand Surg Eur Vol 2015;40(1): 33–41.
10. Sahu A, Gujral SS, Batra S, et al. The current practice of the management of little finger metacarpal fractures–a review of the literature and results of a survey conducted among upper limb surgeons in the United Kingdom. Hand Surg 2012;17(1):55–63.
11. Tosti R, Ilyas AM, Mellema JJ, et al. Interobserver variability in the treatment of little finger metacarpal

neck fractures. J Hand Surg Am 2014;39(9): 1722–7.

12. Poolman RW, Goslings JC, Lee JB, et al. Conservative treatment for closed fifth (small finger) metacarpal neck fractures. Cochrane Database Syst Rev 2005;(3):CD003210.

13. van Aaken J, Fusetti C, Luchina S, et al. Fifth metacarpal neck fractures treated with soft wrap/buddy taping compared to reduction and casting: results of a prospective, multicenter, randomized trial. Arch Orthop Trauma Surg 2016;136(1):135–42.

14. Pace GI, Gendelberg D, Taylor KF, et al. The effect of closed reduction of small finger metacarpal neck fractures on the ultimate angular deformity. J Hand Surg Am 2015;40(8):1582–5.

15. Sletten IN, Hellund JC, Olsen B, et al. Conservative treatment has comparable outcome with bouquet pinning of little finger metacarpal neck fractures: a multicentre randomized controlled study of 85 patients. J Hand Surg Eur Vol 2015; 40(1):76–83.

16. del Piñal F, Moraleda E, Rúas JS, et al. Minimally invasive fixation of fractures of the phalanges and metacarpals with intramedullary cannulated headless compression screws. J Hand Surg Am 2015; 40(4):692–700.

17. Doarn MC, Nydick JA, Williams BD, et al. Retrograde headless intramedullary screw fixation for displaced fifth metacarpal neck and shaft fractures: short term results. Hand (N Y) 2015;10(2):314–8.

18. Ruchelsman DE, Puri S, Feinberg-Zadek N, et al. Clinical outcomes of limited-open retrograde intramedullary headless screw fixation of metacarpal fractures. J Hand Surg Am 2014;39(12):2390–5.

19. Tobert DG, Klausmeyer M, Mudgal CS, et al. Intramedullary fixation of metacarpal fractures using headless compression screws. J Hand Microsurg 2016;8(3):134–9.

20. Melamed E, Hinds RM, Gottschalk MB, et al. Comparison of dorsal plate fixation versus intramedullary headless screw fixation of unstable metacarpal shaft fractures: a biomechanical study. Hand (N Y) 2016; 11(4):421–6.

21. Jones CM, Padegimas EM, Weikert N, et al. Headless screw fixation of metacarpal neck fractures: a mechanical comparative analysis. Hand (N Y) 2017. [Epub ahead of print].

22. ten Berg PWL, Mudgal CS, Leibman MI, et al. Quantitative 3-dimensional CT analyses of intramedullary headless screw fixation for metacarpal neck fractures. J Hand Surg Am 2013;38(2):322–30.e2.

23. Shewring DJ, Trickett RW, Smith A, et al. Fractures at the junction of diaphysis and metaphysis of the proximal phalanges in adults. J Hand Surg Eur Vol 2018;43(5):506–12.

24. Saied AR, Sabet Jahromi M. Treatment of proximal phalanx fractures: transarticular pinning the metacarpophalangeal joint or cross pinning from the base of the proximal phalanx-a prospective study. Eur J Trauma Emerg Surg 2018. [Epub ahead of print].

25. Zelken JA, Hayes AG, Parks BG, et al. Two versus 3 lag screws for fixation of long oblique proximal phalanx fractures of the fingers: a cadaver study. J Hand Surg Am 2015;40(6):1124–9.

26. Nicklin S, Ingram S, Gianoutsos MP, et al. In vitro comparison of lagged and nonlagged screw fixation of metacarpal fractures in cadavers. J Hand Surg Am 2008;33(10):1732–6.

27. Wehbé MA, Schneider LH. Mallet fractures. J Bone Joint Surg Am 1984;66(5):658–69.

28. Bendre AA, Hartigan BJ, Kalainov DM, et al. Mallet finger. J Am Acad Orthop Surg 2005; 13(5):336–44.

29. Smit JM, et al. Treatment options for mallet finger: a review. Plast Reconstr Surg 2010; 126(5):1624–9.

30. Handoll HHG, Vaghela MV. Interventions for treating mallet finger injuries. Cochrane Database Syst Rev 2004;(3):CD004574.

31. Lucchina S, Badia A, Dornean V, et al. Unstable mallet fractures: a comparison between three different techniques in a multicenter study. Chin J Traumatol 2010;13(4):195–200.

32. Tyser AR, Tsai MA, Parks BG, et al. Stability of acute dorsal fracture dislocations of the proximal interphalangeal joint: a biomechanical study. J Hand Surg Am 2014;39(1):13–8.

33. Janssen SJ, Molleman J, Guitton TG, et al. What middle phalanx base fracture characteristics are most reliable and useful for surgical decision-making? Clin Orthop Relat Res 2015;473(12):3943–50.

34. McAuliffe JA. Dorsal fracture dislocation of the proximal interphalangeal joint. J Hand Surg Am 2008; 33(10):1885–8.

35. Gonzalez RM, Hammert WC. Dorsal fracture-dislocations of the proximal interphalangeal joint. J Hand Surg Am 2015;40(12):2453–5.

36. Caggiano NM, Harper CM, Rozental TD, et al. Management of proximal interphalangeal joint fracture dislocations. Hand Clin 2018;34(2):149–65.

37. Morgan JP, Gordon DA, Klug MS, et al. Dynamic digital traction for unstable comminuted intra-articular fracture-dislocations of the proximal interphalangeal joint. J Hand Surg Am 1995;20(4):565–73.

38. McAuliffe JA. Hemi-hamate autograft for the treatment of unstable dorsal fracture dislocation of the proximal interphalangeal joint. J Hand Surg Am 2009;34(10):1890–4.

39. Bezuhly M, Sparkes GL, Higgins A, et al. Immediate thumb extension following extensor indicis proprius-to-extensor pollicis longus tendon transfer using the wide-awake approach. Plast Reconstr Surg 2007; 119(5):1507–12.

40. Lalonde DH, Martin AL. Wide-awake flexor tendon repair and early tendon mobilization in zones 1 and 2. Hand Clin 2013;29(2):207–13.

41. Xing SG, Tang JB. Surgical treatment, hardware removal, and the wide-awake approach for metacarpal fractures. Clin Plast Surg 2014;41(3):463–80.

42. Lalonde DH, Wong A. Dosage of local anesthesia in wide awake hand surgery. J Hand Surg Am 2013; 38(10):2025–8.

43. McKee DE, Lalonde DH, Thoma A, et al. Optimal time delay between epinephrine injection and

incision to minimize bleeding. Plast Reconstr Surg 2013;131(4):811–4.

44. Thomson CJ, Lalonde DH, Denkler KA, et al. A critical look at the evidence for and against elective epinephrine use in the finger. Plast Reconstr Surg 2007;119(1):260–6.

45. Fitzcharles-Bowe C, Denkler K, Lalonde D. Finger injection with high-dose (1:1,000) epinephrine: does it cause finger necrosis and should it be treated? Hand (N Y) 2007; 2(1):5–11.

# Pediatric Hand and Wrist Fractures

Janice C.Y. Liao, MBBS, MRCS[a], Alphonsus K.S. Chong, MBBS, FAMS[a,b],*

## KEYWORDS

- Pediatric hand fractures • Physeal injuries • Seymour fractures • Phalangeal neck fractures
- Metacarpal fractures • Scaphoid fractures • Distal radius fractures

## KEY POINTS

- Closed fractures with no clinical malrotation or scissoring generally have a favorable outcome with conservative management.
- The possibility of a Seymour fracture should be considered in pediatric fingertip injuries. A true lateral radiograph facilitates diagnosis and the condition should be treated as an open fracture.
- Conservative treatment of Al Qattan type II phalangeal neck fractures is associated with remodeling of sagittal malalignment and translation.
- Patients with clinical signs of carpal fractures and normal radiographs should be immobilized. Patients with persistent pain at review after 10 days to 14 days with a normal repeat radiograph should have an MRI done.
- Sporting injuries can occur through high-energy trauma or repeated stress. Chronic wrist pain in gymnast or finger pain in climbers should be assessed radiographically for stress related physeal injuries. Conservative treatment with splinting and complete rest from training a usually sufficient.

## EPIDEMIOLOGY

Hand and wrist fractures have been consistently reported as among the most common fractures in children.[1–3] They are 3 times more common in boys and peak in the teenage years (**Fig. 1**).[4] Forearm fractures compromise the largest proportion of fractures.[1] In the hand, the proximal phalanx and the fifth ray are the most commonly affected bone and digit, respectively (**Fig. 2**).[4] Distal phalangeal fractures tend to occur in toddlers starting to explore the world with their hands, making them susceptible to fingertip crush injuries from slammed doors. With increasing age, the distribution of fractures moves proximally, with median ages of 12 years for proximal phalanx

fractures and 15 years for metacarpal fractures. This distribution corresponds to the increasing body weight and participation in sporting activities during the teenage years.

## CONSIDERATIONS IN THE PEDIATRIC POPULATION

Epidemiologic studies generally use 17 years or 18 years of age as the limit for pediatric fractures. The unique considerations in the management of pediatric hand fractures, however, apply to children with open physes with the potential to remodel. In addition, the ability of a child to participate and cooperate in the management may

Disclosure: The authors have nothing to disclose.
a Department of Hand and Reconstructive Microsurgery, University Orthopaedics Hand and Reconstructive Microsurgery Cluster, National University Health System, 1E, Kent Ridge Road, Singapore 119228;
b Department of Orthopaedic Surgery, Yong Loo Lin School of Medicine, National University of Singapore, Singapore
* Corresponding author. Department of Hand and Reconstructive Microsurgery, University Orthopaedics Hand and Reconstructive Microsurgery Cluster, National University Health System, 1E, Kent Ridge Road, NUHS Tower Block, Level 11, Singapore 119228.
E-mail address: doscksa@nus.edu.sg

Clin Plastic Surg 46 (2019) 425–436
https://doi.org/10.1016/j.cps.2019.02.012
0094-1298/19/© 2019 The Authors. Published by Elsevier Inc. This is an open access article under the CC BY-NC-ND license (http://creativecommons.org/licenses/by-nc-nd/4.0/).

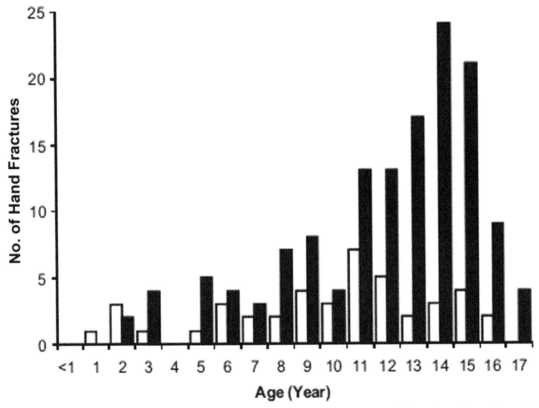

**Fig. 1.** The distribution of hand fractures by gender and age. White bars, girls; black bars, boys. (*From* Chew EM, Chong AK. Hand fractures in children: epidemiology and misdiagnosis in a tertiary referral hospital. J Hand Surg Am 2012;37(8):1686; with permission.)

affect the surgical indications and rehabilitation protocols.

### Physis

In the pediatric population, fractures tend to occur through the physis because it is weaker than the surrounding bone and ligament. With a high healing potential, closed reduction needs to be done early. If delayed, percutaneous intrafocal pins may be required to aid reduction.[5] Most pediatric hand fractures can be treated nonsurgically due to the remarkable potential of the physis to remodel. This remodeling occurs most reliably in the line of motion (flexion-extension), less in the coronal plane, and least in clinical malrotation and scissoring. Growth arrest occurs in 5% to 10% of cases in patients with physeal fractures.[6] It is rare after pediatric hand fractures, and length discrepancy has fewer functional implications compared with the larger long bones, especially in the lower limbs.[7] Nevertheless, it is important to counsel patients and their parents of the potential sequelae of physeal injury, including

shortening, angular deformity, and joint surface incongruity.[8]

### Surgical Considerations

Open reduction of a dislocated physis should be performed after 1 or 2 failed attempts at closed reduction to minimize further injury to the physis. Intraoperatively, the physis should be handled atraumatically. Implants are not required for stable fractures postreduction. If a fracture remains unstable, the choice of implants should be physeal-friendly. Kirschner wires used should be the smallest size that provides adequate stability. Placement needs to be planned carefully to avoid multiple passes through the physis.

### Compliance with Treatment

Cast immobilization is the treatment of choice in nonsurgical treatment of pediatric fractures due to fear of noncompliance. Compliance can vary greatly, and may not always correlate with the age of the child. Treatment should be

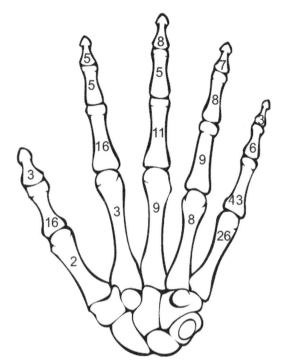

**Fig. 2.** The distribution of hand fractures by bone and ray. (*From* Chew EM, Chong AK. Hand fractures in children: epidemiology and misdiagnosis in a tertiary referral hospital. J Hand Surg Am 2012;37(8):1686; with permission.)

individualized and the ability of the child to cooperate can be gauged from discussion with the parents and involvement of the child in the management. In a sensible and cooperative child, splint immobilization can be considered to improve comfort and compliance with treatment. The authors have had good clinical results with splinting in appropriate patients.

## PHALANGEAL FRACTURES
### Distal Phalanx

#### Nail bed injuries and tuft fractures

Tuft fractures usually result from a crush injury, most commonly from a door.[9] These injuries often are associated with nail bed injuries and pulp lacerations (**Fig. 3**). When the nail is intact and adherent, the authors recommend nonoperative treatment regardless of hematoma size, presence of fracture, or injury mechanism. There is no significant difference in cosmetic outcome between operative treatment and conservative treatment.[10] Injuries with disruption of the nail plate are treated with nail plate removal, débridement and irrigation, and nail bed repair. Nail replacement in the pediatric population has been shown to increase morbidity, including delayed wound healing and infection.[11] The authors recommend nail replacement only in injuries involving the proximal nail fold to prevent the risk of synonychia and in fractures requiring an external splint. Nail bed repairs are commonly done with absorbable sutures (**Fig. 4**). Medical adhesives have been shown to achieve good outcome in terms of pain and appearance.[12] The use of medical adhesives significantly reduces the operative time, which is helpful in the pediatric population.

#### Seymour fractures

Seymour fractures are transepiphyseal Salter-Harris fracture (SH) type I or SH type II fractures of the distal phalanx with associated nail bed injury. It occurs in younger patients, with an average age of 8.7 years.[13] The nail bed injury is often not apparent because the nail bed is avulsed proximally and interposed between the fracture site to preventing successful closed reduction. Clinically, patients may present with a

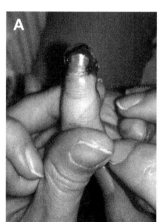
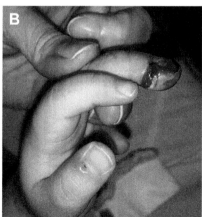
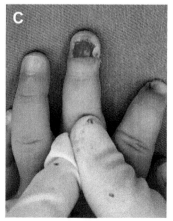

**Fig. 3.** (*A, B*) Two-year-old patient with nail bed injury, pulp laceration, and tuft fracture sustained from a crush injury. (*C*) After nail plate removal and nail bed repair with Vicryl 6-0 sutures.

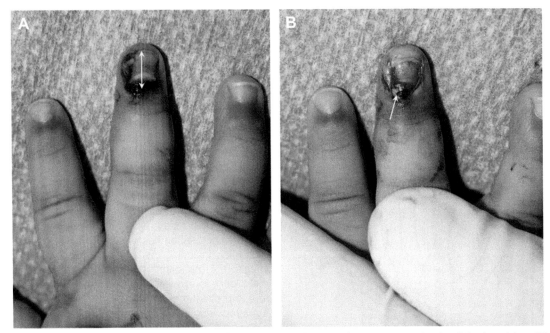

**Fig. 4.** (*A*) The appearance of a longer nail plate (*white double arrow*) suggests proximal nail bed avulsion. (*B*) After nail plate removal, nail bed was found to be interposed between the fracture site (*white arrow*).

pseudomallet deformity, with proximal nail plate sitting above the eponychium, which makes the nail plate appear longer (see **Fig. 4**). It is essential to be suspicious and always obtain true postero-anterior and lateral radiographs of the injured finger to confirm the diagnosis. Radiographs may show obvious displacement through the fracture or more subtle dorsal displacement of the epiphysis (**Fig. 5**). The authors use and recommend the principles of open fracture management (**Box 1**) (see **Fig. 5**). Missed diagnosis and delayed treatment are associated with increased risk of osteomyelitis and nail plate deformities.[13]

**Bony mallet**

There is paucity of literature on bony mallet in the pediatric population, and treatment is largely based on adults. In contrast to Seymour fractures, mallet fractures occur predominantly in patients older than 12 years of age.[15] Axial injury with forced flexion of an extended distal interphalangeal joint (DIPJ) results in avulsion of terminal tendon, with a fragment of epiphysis recognized as an SH type III or SH type IV fracture. In adult mallet fractures, there are studies to support both conservative and surgical treatment.[16] For nonoperative treatment, compliance with splint

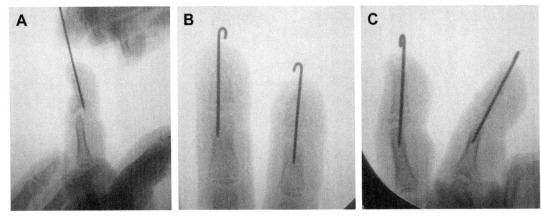

**Fig. 5.** (*A*) Lateral radiograph showing dorsal displacement of the epiphysis in a Seymour fracture. The Kirschner wire was used to aid the reduction. (*B, C*) Fracture reduced and DIPJ transfixed.

maybe feasible because patients tend to be older. The splint can be reinforced with a boxing glove dressing, but the skin needs to be checked regularly. Surgical indications are listed in **Box 2**. Good clinical and radiological outcomes with minimal complications in 51 pediatric mallet fractures, both acute and chronic, have been reported.[17]

## Middle and Proximal Phalanx

### Phalangeal neck fractures

Phalangeal neck fractures are unique to the pediatric population, accounting for 13% of pediatric finger fractures.[18] These fractures typically present with an apex volar angulation with dorsal displacement of the phalangeal head (**Fig. 6**). They are inherently unstable and believed to have poor remodeling potential due to the increased distance from the physis.[19] These fractures are classified by Al Qattan into type I undisplaced, type II displaced with some bone-to-bone contact, and type III displaced with no bone-to-bone contact.[14] Troublesome phalangeal neck fractures are associated with poor prognostic factors and result in an unsatisfactory outcome despite surgical treatment (**Box 3**).[20] Although surgical treatment of type II fractures has been common practice,[5,14] several reports have shown remarkable remodeling of phalangeal neck fractures with nonoperative treatment. In 8 patients who were treated nonoperatively for phalangeal neck fracture malunion, fractures

were remodeled with correction in the sagittal plane from 30° to 0° and coronal plane from 10° to 5°.[21] Sagittal translation also corrected from 58% at injury to 0% at final follow-up. All patients achieved functional range of motion and only 2 reported cosmetic deformities in the coronal plane. In the authors' institution, type II fractures without scissoring or obvious coronal deformity are treated nonoperatively. A recent review of these patients showed that there was significant improvement in the sagittal angulation and translation (see **Fig. 6**). It is imperative, however, to follow-up these patients with repeat radiographs. The authors treated a 4-year-old patient with a type II fracture, which converted to a type III fracture 2 weeks postinjury in a cast requiring closed reduction and percutaneous pinning (**Fig. 7**).

### Proximal phalangeal extraoctave fractures

SH type II fractures of the proximal phalanx are the most common hand fractures.[4] The fifth ray is most commonly injured from a hyperabduction injury, also known as an extraoctave fracture. This fracture typically result in an apex volar and radial deformity (**Fig. 8**). Due to the extraoctave fracture proximity to the physis, remarkable remodeling takes place and surgical treatment is rarely required. In the authors' center, approximately 25% of patients who presented to the Emergency Department with an extraoctave fracture underwent manipulation and reduction in the emergency department either by the emergency physicians or hand surgery residents. Only 2% of the patients with clinical malrotation and/or scissoring underwent surgery. Deformity should be assessed with fingers in midflexion because malrotation or scissoring easily can be missed with fingers in extension (**Fig. 9**). Close reduction and percutaneous pinning is the preferred surgical treatment. Although good cosmetic and functional recovery is expected at 1 year postsurgery, there is an initial 5% complication rate of infection, pin site complications, malunion, and stiffness.[22]

## METACARPAL FRACTURES

Metacarpal fractures are common in children, with 80% involving the fifth metacarpal neck.[18] The median age of children sustaining metacarpal fracture is 15 years, which is nearing skeletal maturity.[4] Therefore, the management of these fractures is similar to that in the adult population. The key indications for surgical treatment are clinical malrotation and scissoring. Associated fight bite injuries also must be excluded. Various acceptable apex dorsal angulation has been reported. In general, the tolerance for angulation increases from index

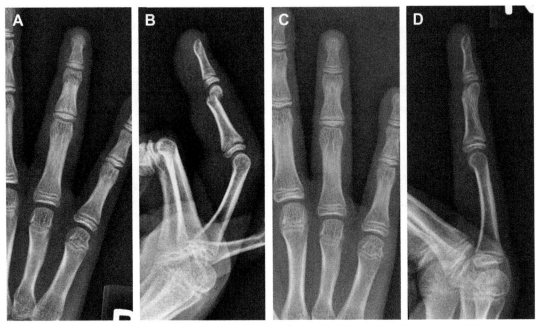

**Fig. 6.** Radiographs of a 12-year-old patient with right ring finger phalangeal neck fracture. (*A, B*) Residual apex volar angulation and dorsal displacement post closed reduction. (*C, D*) Significant remodeling at 3 months after injury.

finger to little finger and in younger patients with higher potential for remodeling. An acceptable degree of 10°, 20°, 30°, or 40° angulation in the index through the small finger metacarpals is a reasonable guide.[23] The authors have had good clinical results treating most pediatric metacarpal neck fractures nonoperatively. A recent randomized controlled trial showed that a hand-based thermoplastic splint improved early range of motion and grip strength with no significant difference in complications and noncompliance compared with the ulnar gutter plaster splint.[24]

## CARPAL FRACTURES

Carpal fractures are uncommon in children but can be difficult to diagnose due to nonspecific clinical symptoms and incomplete ossification

---

**Box 3**
**Poor prognostic factors for phalangeal neck fractures**

- Vascular compromise
- Partial amputation
- Comminution of the phalangeal head
- Concomitant epiphyseal fracture
- All Al-Qattan Type III fractures

---

of the carpal bones. Similar to adults, scaphoid fractures are the most common followed by capitate fractures.[25] Other carpal fractures are rare. Carpal fractures often result from high-energy trauma. In a review of pediatric all-terrain vehicles injuries, 32 hand fractures were composed of 15 metacarpal, 10 phalanx, 3 scaphoid, and 1 perilunate fracture dislocations and 1 pisiform, 1 hamate, and 1 triquetrum fractures.[26] Another series looking at 61 children with suspected carpal fractures found 14 scaphoid fractures, 4 capitate fractures, 3 triquetral fractures, and 1 trapezoid bone bruising.[27] The authors recommend immobilization of all patients with clinical signs of carpal fractures even with normal radiographs. Patients with persistent pain during review at 10 days to 14 days postinjury and a normal repeat radiograph should have an MRI done (**Fig. 10**). Nonoperative treatment with cast immobilization has a high-success union rate, with mean healing time of 56 days with no complications.[27]

### Acute Scaphoid Fractures

Scaphoid fractures are the most common carpal fractures in children, with an increasing incidence in the past 2 decades. A recent epidemiology study quoted an incidence of 11 per 100,000 per annum.[28] The average age of incidence in boys was 12.2 years and in girls was 10.3 years.

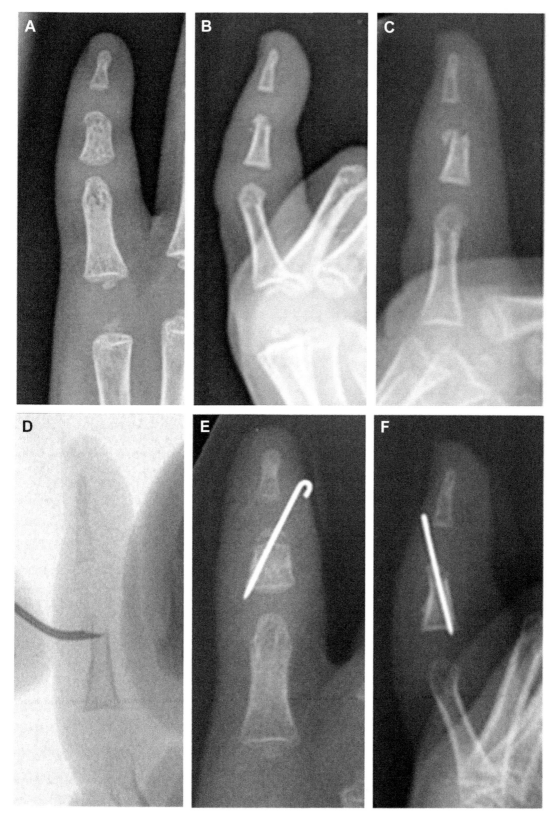

**Fig. 7.** (*A, B*) The initial radiographs for a 4-year-old patient with left little finger phalangeal neck fracture. (*C*) At 2 weeks showing fracture displacement with significant dorsal angulation and epiphyseal dissociation with bayonet deformity. (*D, E, F*) Close reduction was performed with the aid of intrafocal elevation using a 23-gauge needle and fixed with a 0.7-mm Kirschner wire.

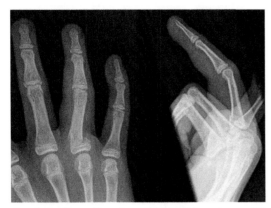

**Fig. 8.** Radiographs of a 12-year-old patient with right ring finger proximal phalanx base fracture with apex radial angulation (*Left* is PA view, *Right* is lateral view).

No scaphoid fractures were observed in boys below the age of 11 years and in girls below the age of 9 years. Historically, pediatric scaphoid fractures tend to occur at the distal pole and generally heal well. Recent analysis showed that increasing body mass index produces a fracture pattern similar to the adult population, with waist fractures the most common followed by distal pole fractures and proximal pole fractures.[29] Cast immobilization of acute scaphoid fracture has been shown to achieve union rates of more than 90% in the pediatric and adolescent populations.[29] The duration of immobilization depends on the fracture location, displacement, and chronicity. Waist fractures require longer immobilization with radiological healing between 5 weeks and 16 weeks compared with distal pole fractures, which take 4 weeks to 8 weeks.[30] The authors recommend assessing patients at 4 weeks to 6 weeks for clinical and radiological healing and to continue with casting or splinting for another 4 weeks to 6 weeks if fracture has not united. If fracture union still cannot be confirmed at 12 weeks, a CT scan can be done to assess fracture healing.

## Chronic Scaphoid Fractures/Nonunion

Natural history of scaphoid nonunion in the pediatric population is not well understood. Dorsal intercalated segment instability deformity does not necessarily occur after nonunion and may not be corrected with surgical fixation of the scaphoid.[30] Pediatric scaphoid nonunion, however, has not been reported to progress to scaphoid nonunion advanced collapse. A 23% union rate has been reported for chronic scaphoid fractures (defined as presentation >6 weeks from injury) treated with casting. The authors treated a 16-year-old patient who opted for conservative treatment of his scaphoid fracture, which eventually united after 3 years (**Fig. 11**). All chronic fractures or nonunions treated with surgical fixation with or without bone graft achieved a union rate of 95%.[31]

## Capitate Fractures

Pediatric capitate fractures are not well studied. The capitate is the first carpal bone to ossify, rendering it more plastic and possibly more vulnerable to fracture compared with other carpal bones. A review of 53 patients with capitates fractures compared 43 adult patients to 10 pediatric patients under 16 years of age.[25] The mean age of the pediatric population was 13 years. In children, isolated fractures were more common, whereas in adults, carpal fractures were more commonly associated with perilunate greater arc injury. Only 2 of 10 patients were treated surgically. One developed a nonunion requiring revision surgery. All pediatric patients achieved functional range of

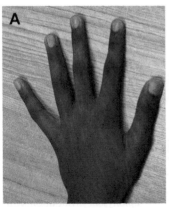
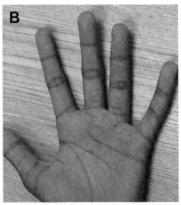
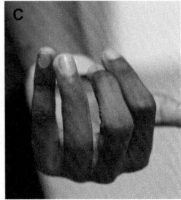

**Fig. 9.** (*A, B*) Left ring finger appears normal in full extension. (*C*) Malrotation and scissoring are evident only in midflexion of the fingers (*Left*: dorsal view; *Middle*: palmar view; *Right*: midflexion view).

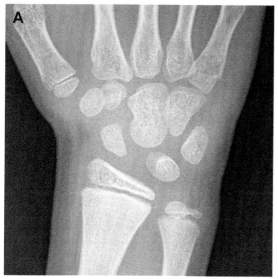 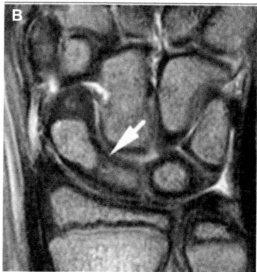

**Fig. 10.** (*A*) Radiograph of a 9-year-old boy with right thumb and wrist pain after a fall with tenderness in the anatomic snuffbox showed incomplete enchondral ossification of the scaphoid. (*B*) MRI showed an undisplaced scaphoid waist fracture (*arrow*). Tip of arrow denotes the fracture site. (*Courtesy of* Dr Foo Tun Lin, Raffles Hospital, Singapore.)

motion at latest follow-up, in contrast to 48% in adults.

## DISTAL RADIUS FRACTURES

Distal radius fractures are the most common pediatric fractures, comprising 20% of all pediatric fractures.[32] They are more common in boys and peak in the teenage years.[33] A majority of pediatric distal radius fractures are torus fractures resulting from a compression force with buckling of the concave side. Greenstick fractures occur from a bending force with unicortical break of the convex side. These fractures are inherently stable and can be treated with a short period of immobilization with a cast or splint and with no difference in outcome.[34]

Bicortical metaphyseal fractures often are displaced and are treated with closed reduction and cast immobilization if the alignment is unacceptable. Varying radiological parameters defining an acceptable alignment have been reported.[35] In general, remodeling potential is higher closer to the physis, in the plane of motion and with more remaining years of growth. The authors prefer a short arm cast because it has been shown as effective as a long arm cast in maintaining reduction, with better ability to perform activities of daily living and fewer days of missed school.[36] Although one-third of the distal radius fractures requiring close reduction resulted in late redisplacement, equivalent clinical outcome has been reported for distal radius fractures treated with closed

reduction and cast immobilization versus initial pin fixation.[37]

The treatment principles of transphyseal fractures are similar to those of metaphyseal fractures, with additional considerations to minimize physeal trauma. Reduction maneuvers should be performed gently, with adequate analgesia and with multiple attempts avoided. The overall risk of physeal arrest has been reported to be 4%.[36] Fractures with less than 15° of angulation and up to 1 cm of shortening have been reported to fully remodel with no functional impairment.[38]

## SPORTING INJURIES

Increased participation in sports and at a higher level in conjunction with heavier weight of the patients contribute to increasing sporting injuries in the teenage population. Pediatric hand and wrist fractures can occur acutely, through sports that result in high-energy trauma, or chronically, through repeated stress injury. The rates of acute hand/wrist injuries have been reported to be the highest in football, followed by similar rates in softball, wrestling, basketball, and hockey. Injuries occur from contact with another player, contact with a playing apparatus, or contact with the playing surface.[38] All-terrain vehicles also have been reported to be associated with high incidence of upper extremity fractures, including rare carpal fractures, such as perilunate fracture dislocation and pisiform, hamate, and triquetral fractures.[26] The recent emerging hoverboard has been

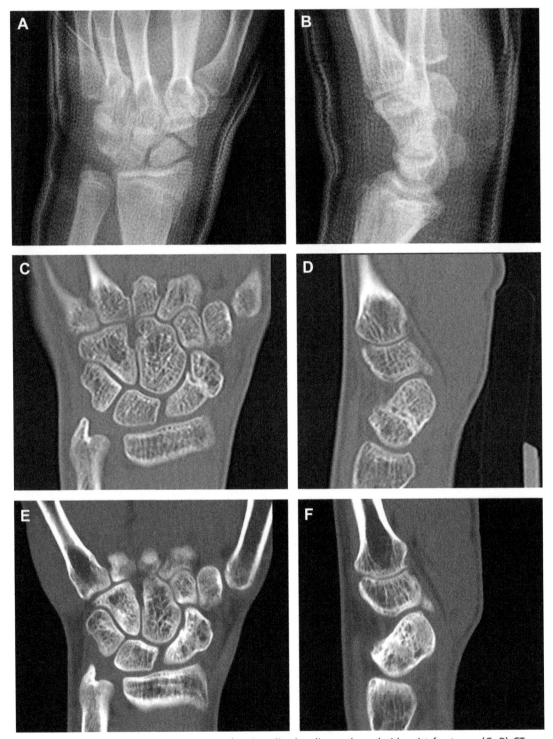

**Fig. 11.** (*A, B*) Radiographs on presentation showing distal radius and scaphoid waist fractures. (*C, D*) CT scan done at 1 year postinjury showing scaphoid waist nonunion. (*E, F*) Repeat scan done at 3 years postinjury showing fracture union.

reported to cause more upper extremity fractures than other childhood recreational activities.[39,40]

Unlike acute fractures from sporting injuries, repeated stress injuries often are overlooked. Chronic wrist pain is commonly seen in gymnastics and other sports that involve repeated loading across the distal radius physis. Patients report dorsal wrist pain aggravated by

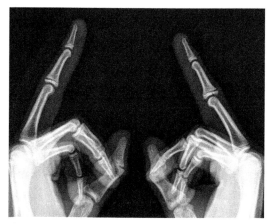

**Fig. 12.** A teenage rock climber with bilateral middle finger middle phalanx SH type III fractures that healed with rest and immobilization (*left* and *right* lateral views respectively).

loading the wrist joint. Radiograph shows stress-related physeal injury, including widening and beaking of the physis, cystic changes of the metaphysis, and increased ulnar variance.[41] Treatment involves 4 weeks to 6 weeks of resting, splinting, and training modification. Another notable repeated stress injury is middle phalanx base epiphyseal fracture in elite adolescent climbers. This is usually an SH type III fracture involving the middle finger or ring finger and more often associated with crimp grip (**Fig. 12**).[42] In acute injuries, a majority of patients achieve excellent results with nonoperative treatment involving complete rest from climbing and gentle active range of motion until fracture healing.[42] Recovery in delayed presentations with chronic nonunion is less predictable, with risks of osteonecrosis with resultant pain, permanent deformity and stiffness.[43]

## SUMMARY

Pediatric hand and wrist fractures are common. Distal fractures like Seymour fractures and phalangeal neck fractures occur more commonly in younger patients and are unique to the pediatric population. Proximal fractures like metacarpal fractures tend to occur in teenage years, with increasing body weight and participation in sporting activities, and have more resemblance to adult fractures. Understanding of the physeal anatomy and carpal ossification is important in the accurate diagnosis of pediatric fractures. Consideration of the physeal biology and compliance with treatment are central to the management of these fractures. A majority have a favorable outcome with nonoperative treatment.

Operative treatment should be considered in patients with clinical malrotation and scissoring, open fractures, and significant fracture displacement. Physeal-friendly surgical approaches and implants should be used to minimize the sequelae of physeal injury.

## REFERENCES

1. Chung KC, Spilson SV. The frequency and epidemiology of hand and forearm fractures in the United States. J Hand Surg Am 2001;26(5):908–15.
2. Hastings H 2nd, Simmons BP. Hand fractures in children. A statistical analysis. Clin Orthop Relat Res 1984;188:120–30.
3. Worlock PH, Stower MJ. The incidence and pattern of hand fractures in children. J Hand Surg Br 1986;11(2):198–200.
4. Chew EM, Chong AK. Hand fractures in children: epidemiology and misdiagnosis in a tertiary referral hospital. J Hand Surg Am 2012;37(8):1684–8.
5. Matzon JL, Cornwall R. A stepwise algorithm for surgical treatment of type II displaced pediatric phalangeal neck fractures. J Hand Surg Am 2014;39(3): 467–73.
6. Dabash S, Prabhakar G, Potter E, et al. Management of growth arrest: current practice and future directions. J Clin Orthop Trauma 2018;9(Suppl 1): S58–66.
7. Culp RW, Osgood JC. Posttraumatic physeal bar formation in the digit of a child: a case report. J Hand Surg Am 1993;18(2):322–4.
8. Shapiro F. Epiphyseal growth plate fracture-separations: a pathophysiologic approach. Orthopedics 1982;5(6):720–36.
9. Satku M, Puhaindran ME, Chong AK. Characteristics of fingertip injuries in children in Singapore. Hand Surg 2015;20(3):410–4.
10. Roser SE, Gellman H. Comparison of nail bed repair versus nail trephination for subungual hematomas in children. J Hand Surg Am 1999;24(6):1166–70.
11. Miranda BH, Vokshi I, Milroy CJ. Pediatric nailbed repair study: nail replacement increases morbidity. Plast Reconstr Surg 2012;129(2):394e–6e.
12. Edwards S, Parkinson L. Is fixing pediatric nail bed injuries with medical adhesives as effective as suturing?: a review of the literature. Pediatr Emerg Care 2019;35(1):75–7.
13. Reyes BA, Ho CA. The high risk of infection with delayed treatment of open seymour fractures: salter-harris I/II or juxta-epiphyseal fractures of the distal phalanx with associated nailbed laceration. J Pediatr Orthop 2017;37(4):247–53.
14. Al-Qattan MM. Extra-articular transverse fractures of the base of the distal phalanx (Seymour's fracture) in children and adults. J Hand Surg Br 2001;26(3): 201–6.

15. Lankachandra M, Wells CR, Cheng CJ, et al. Complications of distal phalanx fractures in children. J Hand Surg Am 2017;42(7):574.e1-e6.

16. Wehbe MA, Schneider LH. Mallet fractures. J Bone Joint Surg Am 1984;66(5):658–69.

17. Reddy M, Ho CA. Comparison of percutaneous reduction and pin fixation in acute and chronic pediatric mallet fractures. J Pediatr Orthop 2019;39(3): 146–52.

18. Mahabir RC, Kazemi AR, Cannon WG, et al. Pediatric hand fractures: a review. Pediatr Emerg Care 2001;17(3):153–6.

19. Green DP. Hand injuries in children. Pediatr Clin North Am 1977;24(4):903–18.

20. Al-Qattan MM, Al-Munif DS, AlHammad AK, et al. The outcome of management of "troublesome" vs "non-troublesome" phalangeal neck fractures in children less than 2 years of age. J Plast Surg Hand Surg 2016;50(2):93–101.

21. Puckett BN, Gaston RG, Peljovich AE, et al. Remodeling potential of phalangeal distal condylar malunions in children. J Hand Surg Am 2012;37(1): 34–41.

22. Boyer JS, London DA, Stepan JG, et al. Pediatric proximal phalanx fractures: outcomes and complications after the surgical treatment of displaced fractures. J Pediatr Orthop 2015;35(3):219–23.

23. Cornwall R. Finger metacarpal fractures and dislocations in children. Hand Clin 2006;22(1):1–10.

24. Davison PG, Boudreau N, Burrows R, et al. Forearm-based ulnar gutter versus hand-based thermoplastic splint for pediatric metacarpal neck fractures: a blinded, randomized trial. Plast Reconstr Surg 2016;137(3):908–16.

25. Kadar A, Morsy M, Sur YJ, et al. Capitate fractures: a review of 53 patients. J Hand Surg Am 2016;41(10): e359–66.

26. Shannon SF, Hernandez NM, Sems SA, et al. Pediatric orthopaedic trauma and associated injuries of snowmobile, ATV, and dirtbike accidents: a 19-year experience at a level 1 pediatric trauma center. J Pediatr Orthop 2018;38(8):403–9.

27. Eckert K, Trobs RB, Schweiger B, et al. Diagnostically approach to pediatric carpal fractures: a retrospective analysis. Z Orthop Unfall 2016;154(1):43–9 [in German].

28. Ahmed I, Ashton F, Tay WK, et al. The pediatric fracture of the scaphoid in patients aged 13 years and under: an epidemiological study. J Pediatr Orthop 2014;34(2):150–4.

29. Gholson JJ, Bae DS, Zurakowski D, et al. Scaphoid fractures in children and adolescents: contemporary injury patterns and factors influencing time to union. J Bone Joint Surg Am 2011;93(13):1210–9.

30. Nellans KW, Chung KC. Pediatric hand fractures. Hand Clin 2013;29(4):569–78.

31. Jauregui JJ, Seger EW, Hesham K, et al. Operative management for pediatric and adolescent scaphoid nonunions: a meta-analysis. J Pediatr Orthop 2019; 39(2):e130–3.

32. Cheng JC, Shen WY. Limb fracture pattern in different pediatric age groups: a study of 3,350 children. J Orthop Trauma 1993;7(1):15–22.

33. Shah NS, Buzas D, Zinberg EM. Epidemiologic dynamics contributing to pediatric wrist fractures in the United States. Hand (N Y) 2015;10(2):266–71.

34. Boutis K, Willan A, Babyn P, et al. Cast versus splint in children with minimally angulated fractures of the distal radius: a randomized controlled trial. CMAJ 2010;182(14):1507–12.

35. Pretell Mazzini J, Rodriguez Martin J. Paediatric forearm and distal radius fractures: risk factors and re-displacement–role of casting indices. Int Orthop 2010;34(3):407–12.

36. Bae DS. Pediatric distal radius and forearm fractures. J Hand Surg Am 2008;33(10):1911–23.

37. Miller BS, Taylor B, Widmann RF, et al. Cast immobilization versus percutaneous pin fixation of displaced distal radius fractures in children: a prospective, randomized study. J Pediatr Orthop 2005;25(4):490–4.

38. Do TT, Strub WM, Foad SL, et al. Reduction versus remodeling in pediatric distal forearm fractures: a preliminary cost analysis. J Pediatr Orthop B 2003; 12(2):109–15.

39. Donnally CJ 3rd, Lawrie CM, Rush AJ 3rd, et al. The season of hoverboards: a case series of fractures. Pediatr Emerg Care 2017;33(5):325–8.

40. Kattan AE, AlShomer F, Alhujayri AK, et al. A case series of pediatric seymour fractures related to hoverboards: increasing trend with changing lifestyle. Int J Surg Case Rep 2017;38:57–60.

41. Mariscalco MW, Saluan P. Upper extremity injuries in the adolescent athlete. Sports Med Arthrosc Rev 2011;19(1):17–26.

42. Hochholzer T, Schoffl VR. Epiphyseal fractures of the finger middle joints in young sport climbers. Wilderness Environ Med 2005;16(3):139–42.

43. El-Sheikh Y, Lutter C, Schoeffl I, et al. Surgical management of proximal interphalangeal joint repetitive stress epiphyseal fracture nonunion in elite sport climbers. J Hand Surg Am 2018;43(6):572.e1–5.

# Injuries Around the Proximal Interphalangeal Joint

Ruth En Si Tan, MBBS,
Andre Eu Jin Cheah, MBBS, MMed, MBA*

### KEYWORDS

- Proximal interphalangeal joint • Fracture • Dislocation • Surgical fixation • Finger

### KEY POINTS

- Proximal interphalangeal joint (PIPJ) injuries should not be underestimated because they can lead to notable loss of hand function.
- Treatment of PIPJ injuries should focus on stable, concentric joint reduction to achieve early mobilization.
- Surgical treatment should be adopted only when the expected outcomes are better than that of nonsurgical treatment.

 Video content accompanies this article at http://www.plasticsurgery.theclinics.com.

## INTRODUCTION

The proximal interphalangeal joint (PIPJ) is the most frequently injured joint in the hand.[1] PIPJ injuries are challenging to treat due the joint's propensity for stiffness and late presentation, because it is not uncommon for these injuries to be dismissed at the initial presentation. With inadequate treatment, PIPJ injuries frequently lead to stiffness, deformity in the form of flexion contractures, and pain from premature degenerative arthritis. PIPJ injuries typically occur in young active individuals whose active lifestyles may be severely curtailed by a stiff and painful finger resulting in part from suboptimal treatment.

PIPJ injuries include

1. Ligamentous injuries: volar plate and/or collateral injuries
2. Intra-articular fractures

3. Subluxations or dislocations
4. A combination of the above

There are 3 main types of intra-articular fractures of the base of middle phalanx:

1. Dorsal fracture subluxations or dislocations
2. Volar fracture subluxations or dislocations
3. Pilon fractures

## ANATOMY, BIOMECHANICS, AND CLASSIFICATION

The primary stability of the PIPJ is provided by its bony articular surface, the proper and accessory collateral ligaments, and the volar plate. Secondary stability is afforded by the flexor and extensor tendons.

The fracture pattern at the base of the middle phalanx depends on the direction of the force

Disclosure statement: Neither of the authors has any funding sources or commercial or financial conflicts of interest to declare.
Department of Hand and Reconstructive Microsurgery, National University Health System, Level 11, Tower Block, 1E Kent Ridge Road, 119228, Singapore
* Corresponding author.
E-mail address: andre_cheah@nuhs.edu.sg

Clin Plastic Surg 46 (2019) 437–449
https://doi.org/10.1016/j.cps.2019.03.005
0094-1298/19/© 2019 The Authors. Published by Elsevier Inc. This is an open access article under the CC BY-NC-ND license (http://creativecommons.org/licenses/by-nc-nd/4.0/).

and position of the joint.[2] A combination of longitudinal load and either hyperextension or hyperflexion causes dorsal or volar fracture dislocations, respectively.[3,4] A predominantly axial load disrupts both the dorsal and volar cortices of the middle phalanx base, creating, by definition, a pilon fracture.

Fracture dislocations have been divided into stable, tenuous, and unstable categories.[3,5,6] Previous biomechanical studies showed that the volar plate is the primary passive restraint against PIPJ hyperextension forces,[7] whereas, more recently, Caravaggi and colleagues[8] have suggested that the loss of bony restraint plays a much larger role compared with the collateral ligaments. As the debate continues regarding how much articular involvement leads to instability and how much flexion is required to keep the joint reduced, there is a general consensus that between 30% and 50% of articular involvement renders joint stability tenuous whereas more than 50% articular involvement indicates joint instability.[3,5]

## EVALUATION

Initial assessment should include a thorough history, including chronicity and mechanism of injury. Physical examination should pay special attention to the stability of the PIPJ, with the use of local anesthesia if necessary. Lateral stability is tested in zero (for the proper collateral ligaments) and 30° of flexion (for the accessory collateral ligaments). Radiological assessment with anteroposterior and true lateral films is crucial to diagnosis of PIPJ injuries. When there is joint subluxation, a V sign is seen, which describes an asymmetric joint space seen on a true lateral radiograph[9] (**Fig. 1**).

Features to note on radiographs include[10]

1. Percentage of articular surface involvement
2. Articular step or gap
3. Comminution or fragmentation
4. Number of fracture fragments
5. Joint subluxation or dislocation

An estimate of the involved articular surface from plain radiographs enables classification of fractures according to their stability and serves as a guide to treatment. The degree of articular comminution[10] and size of fracture fragment, however, were found to be underestimated.[11] One possible reason suggested was that fractures entered the joint at varying angles that were difficult to assess with standard radiographs. Hence, oblique radiographs or advanced imaging may provide further insight into the severity of an injury. In pilon fractures, neither the initial degree of

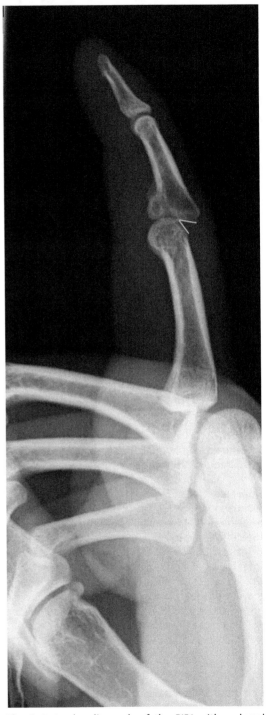

**Fig. 1.** Lateral radiograph of the PIPJ with a dorsal fracture subluxation demonstrating a V sign (*yellow lines*).

radiographic displacement nor any findings on CT help determine the need for surgery. Due to their configuration, pilon fractures are unstable and prone to collapse if not supported.

## GOALS OF TREATMENT

The main aim in treatment of PIPJ injuries is to achieve a stable joint for early mobilization.[3,12,13] This is important to prevent stiffness. Although anatomic restoration of the joint surface is a desirable goal, it is not the foremost priority.

Joint stability is achieved through[3,14–20]

1. Concentric joint reduction—this enables gliding motion of the joint without hinging, which occurs when there is joint subluxation.
2. Restoration of stabilizers—this may include both bony and soft tissue stabilizers of the PIPJ.

## TREATMENT OF PROXIMAL INTERPHALANGEAL JOINT COLLATERAL LIGAMENT INJURIES

Collateral ligament injuries of the PIPJ are common and may be classified into grades I, II and III injuries. More than 20° of deformity on the lateral stress test in extension indicates complete collateral ligament injury with involvement of at least 1 other secondary stabilizer, such as the volar plate, bony anatomy, or accessory collateral ligament.

Grades I and II injuries may be treated nonsurgically, with short-term immobilization in a splint followed by early buddy taping, whereas operative treatment may be considered for grade III injuries. This is still a topic of controversy, however, with some investigators advocating repair only if there is subluxation and closed reduction is not possible, whereas others report that surgical repair is necessary,[21] especially in young workers and athletes.[22–24]

Collateral ligaments typically fail proximally. If there is enough substance of the collateral ligament on the condyle of the proximal phalanx, it may be repaired directly. Otherwise, a microsuture anchor may be used. Lee and colleagues[25] found that operative repair of grade II radial collateral ligament injuries resulted in lower pain score, more rapid recovery of finger motion, and better appearance of the PIPJ compared with nonsurgical treatment at short-term follow-up.

Although conservative treatment may achieve goals of joint stability and range of motion (ROM), operative treatment carries the advantage of allowing earlier ROM and decreased swelling. Surgical intervention should be balanced against a patient's needs and risk of complications, such as skin irritation from the suture anchor knot.

## TREATMENT OF PROXIMAL INTERPHALANGEAL JOINT DISLOCATIONS

PIPJ dislocations are classified as dorsal, volar, lateral, or rotatory, depending on the position of the middle phalanx relative to the proximal phalanx.[26,27] Dorsal and lateral dislocations are the most common and usually can be reduced in a closed fashion. Lateral dislocations frequently have a dorsal component.[28] Volar and rotatory dislocations are rare injuries and are irreducible usually by closed methods due to interposition of soft tissue, which requires open reduction.

Suspicion is required for patients who report rotatory traction injury.[28] Puckering of the skin on clinical examination suggests soft tissue interposition.[27] Ultrasound or MRI facilitates assessment of the soft tissue injury involved.

### Closed Reduction

Closed reduction is attempted under local anesthesia. Dorsal and dorsolateral dislocations are reduced with gentle longitudinal traction accompanied by pressure on the base of the middle phalanx. This prevents entrapment of the collateral ligament or volar plate. Reduction of volar and rotatory dislocations is attempted with the metacarpophalangeal joint and PIPJ flexed to relax the entrapped extensor apparatus.[27]

### Open Reduction

Open reduction should be performed as soon as possible to avoid joint contracture, fibrosis, and adhesions. Dorsal dislocations commonly are dealt with via a volar or lateral approach. The volar plate may be interposed in the joint,[29] or the head of the proximal phalanx may penetrate volar soft tissues or flexor tendon in a buttonhole mechanism.[30,31]

Volar dislocations are more serious injuries. Reduction may be blocked due to entrapment of the volar plate,[32] central slip,[33] lateral band,[34] collateral ligaments,[35] or fracture fragment.[36] An axial compression force with rotational element brings the lateral band of the extensor tendon on the volar side of the head of the proximal phalanx and remains entrapped in the joint.[37] Open reduction usually is via a dorsal or lateral approach.

Repair of ruptured collateral ligaments with microsuture anchors is beneficial for early ROM, whereas volar plate avulsions are treated more commonly with extension block splinting or buddy taping. Repair of the central slip should be performed routinely to prevent boutonniere deformity.[26,27,38]

## TREATMENT OF PROXIMAL INTERPHALANGEAL JOINT FRACTURE DISLOCATIONS

Stable PIPJ injuries are commonly treated nonsurgically, with extension block splinting or buddy taping. There is no universally accepted treatment, however, of unstable fracture dislocations of the PIPJ.[39] In a survey of surgeons using lateral radiographs of the PIPJ, Janssen and colleagues[10] found that there was substantial agreement when deciding for operative versus nonoperative treatment, but there was variation regarding which surgical technique to use for the same fracture. Articular step or gap greater than 2 mm and joint subluxation or dislocation were associated most strongly with a decision for operative treatment.

Myriad surgical treatment options have been described for unstable PIPJ injuries. Mean PIPJ ROM using various approaches has been reported to be approximately 80°, and there is little difference between the efficacy of these methods.[40] If operative treatment is chosen, the outcomes of the chosen procedure should match or be better than that expected of conservative treatment. **Table 1** summarizes the indications of current treatment options.

### Pinning

The advantage of the pinning method is its simplicity and ability to maintain an extension block angle more securely compared with a splint.[41] Newington and colleagues[42] suggested that accurate anatomic reduction of the fracture itself is not required, provided a congruous and concentric reduction of the PIPJ is achieved—this is the main goal of percutaneous pinning. An anatomically imperfect joint surface associated with radiological degenerative changes may still have a good clinical outcome and may not always affect the ROM.[42-45] Complications include recurrent subluxation and pin track infection.[46]

### Extension block pinning

First described by Inoue and Tamura,[47] extension block pinning involves closed reduction of the dorsal fracture dislocation and drilling of a

**Table 1**
**Current practices in treatment of proximal interphalangeal joint fracture dislocations**

| Method | Indications | Contraindications | Typically Used for Chronic Injuries |
|---|---|---|---|
| Percutaneous pinning<br>  Extension block<br>  Across the PIPJ | Can be used when a quick and simple method is desired or if soft tissue is unstable prohibiting an open approach | Fractures involving the dorsal cortex of the middle phalanx base | No |
| Interfragmentary screw | Large fragments | Severe comminution | No |
| Plate and screws<br>  Volar plate<br>    With raft screws<br>    Buttress alone<br>  Dorsal plate<br>  Lateral plate | Large to comminuted fracture fragments<br>Pilon fractures<br>Comminuted fragments <50% of phalangeal base, which are too small for an interfragmentary screw<br>Pilon fractures<br>Volar fracture dislocations<br>Pilon fractures | For a pure buttress volar plate, there should not be a fracture involving the dorsal cortex of the middle phalanx base | No |
| External fixation | Comminuted volar, dorsal lip or pilon fractures of the middle phalanx base<br>Augmentation of other surgical methods | Concomitant fractures involving the proximal and middle phalanx | Yes |
| VPA<br>HHA | Large volar base defect<br>Comminuted volar lip fractures (not amenable to fixation) | Fractures involving the dorsal cortex of the middle phalanx base or proximal phalangeal head fracture<br>Preexisting PIPJ osteoarthritis | Yes<br>Yes |

Kirschner (K) wire into the distal, dorsal aspect of the proximal phalanx to block the terminal extension and prevent dorsal dislocation[41,46,48,49] (**Fig. 2**). Typically, a 1.2-mm or 1.4-mm K wire is inserted at an angle dorsal to the coronal plane through or beside the central slip into the distal dorsal aspect of the proximal phalanx.[46] Percutaneous intramedullary fracture reduction,[50] closed reduction and pinning of the volar fragment,[49] or open reduction and pinning of fragments[46] may be performed together with extension block pinning. Postoperatively, flexion of the PIPJ is allowed with extension limited by the K wire. The K wire is removed after an average of 3 weeks.[41,46]

### Pinning across the proximal interphalangeal joint

Another method of pinning involves transfixing of the PIPJ (see **Fig. 2**), using a K wire inserted from the dorsum of the base of the middle phalanx just distal to the central slip insertion and then passed proximally across the PIPJ joint into the proximal phalanx head with the PIPJ in 30° to 60° of flexion.[42,45,51] Postoperatively, the K wire is removed after 4 weeks[45] and active ROM of the PIPJ commenced thereafter.

Satisfactory outcomes have been reported despite the PIPJ being in slight dorsal subluxation, especially when the middle phalanx heals in a position that restores the concavity of the phalangeal base.[18,43,45,51,52] If the palmar fragment does not heal, the joint is more likely to hinge and not glide normally.

### Open Reduction and Internal Fixation

Open reduction and internal fixation (ORIF) ideally allows for anatomic reduction of the joint and articular fragments, while restoring stability with the crucial volar lip buttress and allowing early ROM. Reducing the articular surface (for example, a central depressed fragment) may prevent secondary osteoarthrosis[40] but is less crucial. Factors influencing the results after ORIF include patient age, size of palmar fragment, chronic cases, period of immobilization after surgery, and recurrence of subluxation. The most significant factor influencing PIPJ joint ROM after surgery is postoperative early motion, with a second factor patient age.[40]

Various methods of internal fixation have been described—dorsal and volar plating,[53,54] buttress plating,[40] hook plating,[55] and screw fixation from volar[19,51,56] and dorsal[57] approaches, After internal fixation, splint immobilization, extension block pinning, or an external fixator may be used to augment the fixation.[40] Techniques for fixation of small fragments include K wires,[20,22,58,59] miniscrews,[56,60,61] pull-out sutures with tension banding,[3,17] and a combination of these techniques (**Fig. 3**). The volar approach to the PIPJ commonly is used (Video 1).[62]

Interfragmentary screws are indicated for larger fracture fragments, whereas plate fixation is more suited to comminuted fragments.[63] Volar plate fixation uses the principle of buttressing to maintain fracture reduction, with screws to maintain the intra-articular surface.[53] The addition of a plate, as opposed to screw fixation alone, provides a wider surface to hold the fragments in reduction, especially smaller ones.[53,64] The proximal part of the plate can be fashioned into a hook and wrapped around the small fragments that remain attached to the volar plate, which reduces comminuted fragments (**Fig. 4**).[53] Placement of screws in the diaphysis of the middle

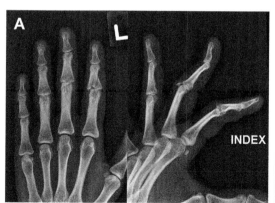
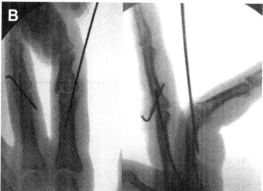

**Fig. 2.** PA (*left*) and lateral (*right*) radiographs of a patient who sustained a PIPJ dorsal fracture subluxation of the index finger and volar fracture dislocation of the middle finger (*A*) who underwent fixation of index finger with an extension block K wire, and fixation of middle finger with a K wire transfixing the PIPJ and percutaneous pinning of the dorsal lip fragment (*B*). The *left* and *right* panels show the PA and lateral radiographs respectively.

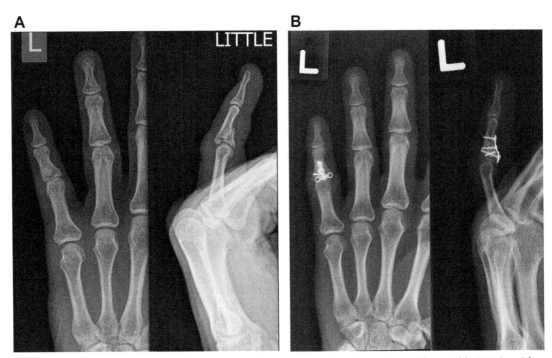

**Fig. 3.** PA and lateral radiographs on the *right* and *left* pane respectively of a patient with unstable PIPJ dorsal fracture subluxation with a centrally depressed fragment. (*B*) PA and lateral radiographs shown in the *right* and *left* panel respectively of the same patient underwent ORIR with combination of miniscrew fixation and volar plating.

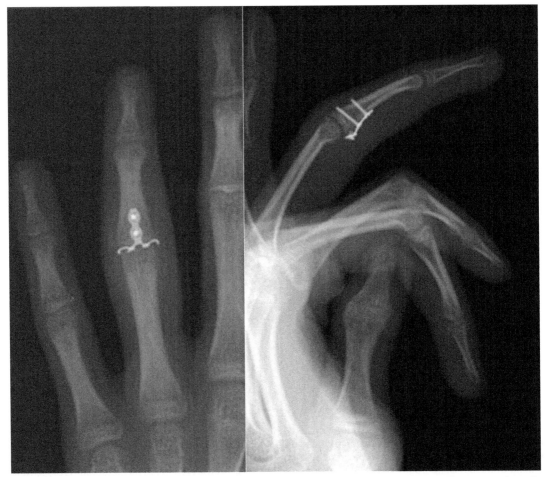

**Fig. 4.** PA and lateral radiographs on the *left* and *right* panels respectively demonstrating the usage of a volar hook plate technique.

phalanx distally adds to stability without affecting the viability of the fracture fragments; the subchondral screws provide structural support for centrally depressed fragments, which have been reduced.[53,54] The availability of smaller implants in recent years has facilitated this technique of ORIF.[64] Foo and colleagues[63] demonstrated that a plate and screw construct showed the greater resistance to displacement and implant failure compared with interfragmentary screws or a buttress plate alone. Flexion contracture due to flexor tendon adhesion after palmar plating can occur[40,53,54] and may necessitate secondary surgery for implant removal and tenolysis.

## External Fixation

Many types of external fixators have been described, including static[65] or dynamic.[2,16,66–77]

Dynamic distraction external fixation makes use of ligamentotaxis through distraction to obtain and maintain fracture reduction. Static external fixators have fallen out of fashion in favor of dynamic ones that allowed early active motion to achieve better clinical outcomes.[72] An ideal external fixator maintains congruent joint surfaces, reduces the fracture by ligamentotaxis, is low profile, prevents compression forces, and allows immediate active motion.[2] The distraction is based off a transverse wire through the axis of the PIPJ rotation in the head of the proximal phalanx (**Fig. 5**).

A biomechanical study found that less traction is required to keep the joint reduced with increased flexion of the PIPJ.[6] Importantly, the investigators found that with the PIPJ in full extension, no amount of force could keep the joint reduced in unstable dorsal fracture dislocations. Hence, an optimal PIPJ flexion angle of 20° was suggested to maintain joint reduction while minimizing risk of flexion contracture. For unstable dorsal fracture dislocations, modalities that do not restore the bony volar lip (such as splint and external fixation) need to have an element of dorsal blocking in their design. Otherwise, there is persistent subluxation when the PIPJ is in full extension. In contrast, when internal fixation restores the bony volar lip of the middle phalanx, extension blocking is not required because the bony buttress maintains reduction of the joint.[6]

## Volar Plate Arthroplasty

Originally described by Eaton and Malerich[18] in 1980 for treatment of acute and chronic PIPJ dorsal fracture dislocations up to 2 years after injury, volar plate arthroplasty (VPA) aims to resurface the fractured surface of the middle phalanx base

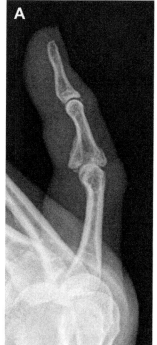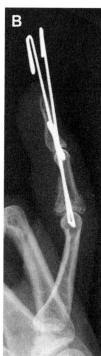

**Fig. 5.** (A) Radiographs of a patient who sustained a pilon fracture. (B) Distraction external fixation enabled restoration of joint congruity. (*Courtesy of Sandeep J Sebastin.*)

with the volar plate while providing a restraint to dorsal subluxation. Interposition of other types of soft tissue into the PIPJ has been described, including fat, tendon, and periosteum.[78]

The PIPJ is exposed via a shotgun approach after mobilization of the neurovascular bundles. The volar plate is incised along its most lateral (from the collaterals) and distal margins (from the base of the middle phalanx), creating a flap that is as broad and long as possible.[79] The volar plate is attached to the most dorsal part of the articular defect after fashioning of a trough. This trough should be perpendicular to the long axis of the middle phalanx to prevent angular deformity and asymmetric collapse.[18] Sutures are attached to radial and ulnar sides of the volar plate and passed as a pull-out suture over the dorsum of the middle phalanx. There should be smooth articular contour from the base of the middle phalanx to the volar plate.

Complications include angular deformities,[18,79,80] flexion contracture of PIPJ and distal interphalangeal joint (DIPJ),[4,80] pin and wire tract infections, redisplacement, and recurrent subluxation.[4,9,80] VPA has a tendency for flexion deformity, which increases with an increasing defect in the middle phalanx palmar base as the volar plate is advanced further into the joint.[81] Mild flexion contractures of the DIPJ 10° to 20° are common and expected, but more severe flexion contractures can occur if the joint is immobilized in excessive flexion or if the volar plate is insufficiently mobilized.[81]

### Hemi-Hamate Replacement Arthroplasty

Hemi-hamate replacement arthroplasty (HHA) has several characteristics that fulfill the treatment goals of PIPJ dorsal fracture dislocations.[81] It provides a stable bony palmar lip, enables early motion through rigid fixation, and restores native hyaline cartilage.

Originally described by Hastings[82,83] in 1999, with clinical results published in 2003, the hemi-hamate autograft reconstruction of the middle phalanx base is a technically challenging procedure that aims to restore joint congruity by replacing the damaged volar lip of the middle phalanx. The configuration of the hamate (dimensions, central ridge, and bicondylar facets) mimics the base of the middle phalanx volar lip. Reconstruction of the articular surface can be difficult in comminuted fractures, hence the usefulness of a graft.[39] It is more technically demanding than ORIF. Consequently, it may be reasonable to first attempt ORIF and then proceed to HHA when excessive comminution precludes ORIF.

Radiographs of a young patient with a malunited right middle finger PIPJ dorsal fracture dislocation are shown in **Fig. 6**. After shot-gunning the joint with the PIPJ hyperextended, the extent of volar lip involvement is assessed (**Fig. 7**) and removed to create a recipient site for the hemi-hamate graft (**Fig. 8**). The size of the graft required is measured in 3 planes. An incision is made over the fourth and fifth carpometacarpal joints in the same hand (**Fig. 9**) and a graft of appropriate size is harvested from the dorsal distal part of the hamate (**Fig. 10**). After harvesting, the graft is further contoured to match the recipient site accurately. The graft then is fixed with at least 2 lag screws (**Figs. 11** and **12**). The volar plate is repaired.

Most investigators recommend early active motion (between 1 day and 2 weeks)[39,82–86] with an extension block splint to prevent tendon adhesion and joint contracture. Subsequently, patients are allowed full active ROM of the joint after radiographic graft union. It has been recommended to wait 4 months before active loads are placed on joint.[39]

Overall complication rate was 35%, of which osteoarthritis is a major concern and reported as a radiological finding in up to 50% of the cases.[82,84,85] Possible reasons for this include denervation and poor vascularization, to which Rozen and colleagues[87] proposed a vascularized hemi-hamate free flap. Other complications

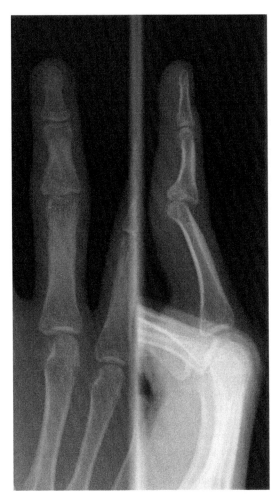

**Fig. 6.** PA and lateral radiographs in the *left* and *right* panes respectively of a patient with malunited PIPJ dorsal fracture dislocation. (*Courtesy of* Mark E Puhaindran.)

include PIPJ joint contracture (present in up to 10% of patients) and graft resorption. Donor site morbidity generally is low.

### Volar Fracture Dislocations

Volar fracture dislocations are associated with a dorsal lip or central slip fracture, with or without disrupting of the central slip and/or collateral ligaments. They are far less common than dorsal fracture dislocations and usually have worse outcomes with a delay to treatment due to failure of early diagnosis.[88] These injuries can range from complete dislocation of the PIPJ with disruption of the intra-articular surface to mild subluxation with a small dorsal lip fragment. With attenuation of the central slip, these injuries can progress to a boutonniere deformity.

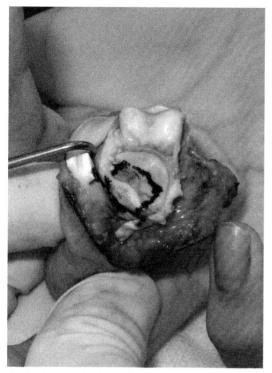

**Fig. 7.** Area of the involved middle phalanx base with unhealthy cartilage marked out (*purple line*). (*Courtesy of* Mark E Puhaindran.)

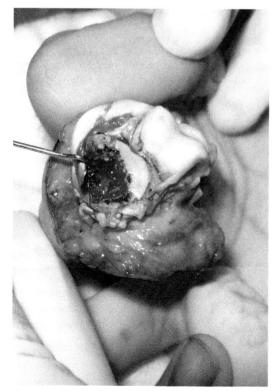

**Fig. 8.** Recipient site for hemi-hamate graft prepared using K-wire drill holes and osteotomes. (*Courtesy of* Mark E Puhaindran.)

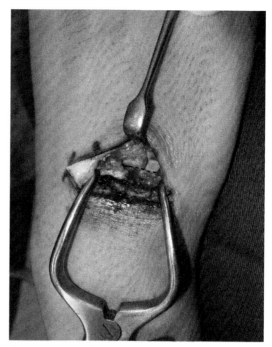

**Fig. 9.** Harvest of the hemi-hamate autograft (fourth and fifth CMCJ joint line is marked on the figure with a dotted line). (*Courtesy of* Mark E Puhaindran.)

Although there currently is no classification to describe or guide treatment, strategies follow the same principles as dorsal fracture dislocations with focus on early ROM. These include splinting in extension, closed reduction, and percutaneous

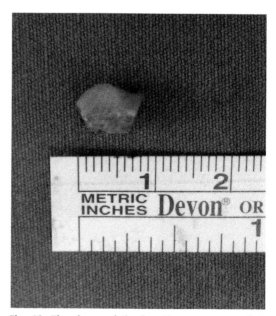

**Fig. 10.** The shape of the hemi-hamate autograft is similar to the base of the middle phalanx. (*Courtesy of* Mark E Puhaindran.)

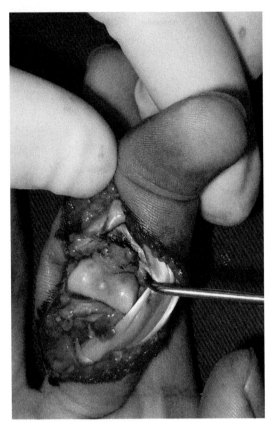

**Fig. 11.** Fixation was performed with 2 screws. (*Courtesy of* Mark E Puhaindran.)

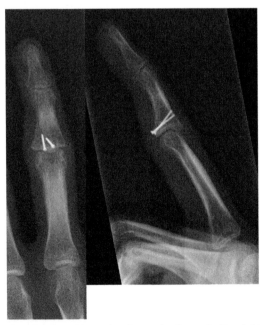

**Fig. 12.** PA and lateral radiographs shown in the *right* and *left* panels respectively demonstrating union of the hemi-hamate autograft and restoration of the PIPJ joint surface. (*Courtesy of* Mark E Puhaindran.)

pinning,[88,89] K-wire transfixion of the PIPJ,[88] external fixation,[89] miniplate or hook plate fixation,[55,90] screw fixation,[89,91] loop wire,[92] and reverse HHA.[93]

## DELAYED TREATMENT

Treatment may be delayed if a patient does not seek immediate medical attention. These injuries are difficult to treat because malunion at the articular surface may have already set in and can impair outcomes. In general, fracture dislocations more than 3 weeks to 6 weeks old[13,39,94] are considered chronic.

VPA, HHA, dynamic distraction external fixator, and silicon or pyrocarbon arthroplasties may be used for treatment of chronic injuries. VPA and HHA, however, require an intact dorsal base of middle phalanx and may not be used for pilon fractures.[13] Shen and colleagues[13] reported treatment outcomes of DFD in 10 patients treated with dynamic distraction external fixation—performed at least 21 days after injury with good outcomes. Remodeling of the fracture occurs resulting in a concentric PIPJ articular surface with good function and painless ROM. Incomplete remodeling also may occur but does not impair function or cause pain. The key is early active ROM and edema control.

## SUPPLEMENTARY DATA

Supplementary data related to this article can be found online at https://doi.org/10.1016/j.cps. 2019.03.005.

## REFERENCES

1. Williams CS. Proximal interphalangeal joint fracture dislocations: stable and unstable. Hand Clin 2012; 28(3):409–16, xi.
2. Hastings H 2nd, Ernst JM. Dynamic external fixation for fractures of the proximal interphalangeal joint. Hand Clin 1993;9(4):659–74.
3. Kiefhaber TR, Stern PJ. Fracture dislocations of the proximal interphalangeal joint. J Hand Surg Am 1998;23(3):368–80.
4. Durham-Smith G, McCarten GM. Volar plate arthroplasty for closed proximal interphalangeal joint injuries. J Hand Surg Br 1992;17(4):422–8.
5. Tyser AR, Tsai MA, Parks BG, et al. Stability of acute dorsal fracture dislocations of the proximal interphalangeal joint: a biomechanical study. J Hand Surg Am 2014;39(1):13–8.
6. Cheah AE, Foo TL, Liao JC, et al. Post-reduction stability of the proximal interphalangeal joint after dorsal fracture dislocation-A cadaveric study. J Hand Surg Asian Pac Vol 2016;21(3):382–7.

7. Bowers WH, Wolf JW Jr, Nehil JL, et al. The proximal interphalangeal joint volar plate. I. An anatomical and biomechanical study. J Hand Surg Am 1980; 5(1):79–88.

8. Caravaggi P, Shamian B, Uko L, et al. In vitro kinematics of the proximal interphalangeal joint in the finger after progressive disruption of the main supporting structures. Hand (N Y) 2015;10(3):425–32.

9. Bilos ZJ, Vender MI, Bonavolonta M, et al. Fracture subluxation of proximal interphalangeal joint treated by palmar plate advancement. J Hand Surg Am 1994;19(2):189–95.

10. Janssen SJ, Molleman J, Guitton TG, et al. What middle phalanx base fracture characteristics are most reliable and useful for surgical decision-making? Clin Orthop Relat Res 2015;473(12):3943–50.

11. Donovan DS, Podolnick JD, Reizner W, et al. Accuracy and reliability of radiographic estimation of volar lip fragment size in PIP dorsal fracture-dislocations. Hand (N Y) 2018. 1558944718777831. [Epub ahead of print].

12. Haase SC, Chung KC. Current concepts in treatment of fracture-dislocations of the proximal interphalangeal joint. Plast Reconstr Surg 2014;134(6): 1246–57.

13. Shen XF, Mi JY, Rui YJ, et al. Delayed treatment of unstable proximal interphalangeal joint fracture-dislocations with a dynamic external fixator. Injury 2015;46(10):1938–44.

14. Glickel SZ, Barron OA. Proximal interphalangeal joint fracture dislocations. Hand Clin 2000;16(3): 333–44.

15. Hastings H 2nd, Carroll C. Treatment of closed articular fractures of the metacarpophalangeal and proximal interphalangeal joints. Hand Clin 1988;4(3): 503–27.

16. Krakauer JD, Stern PJ. Hinged device for fractures involving the proximal interphalangeal joint. Clin Orthop Relat Res 1996;327:29–37.

17. Deitch MA, Kiefhaber TR, Comisar BR, et al. Dorsal fracture dislocations of the proximal interphalangeal joint: surgical complications and long-term results. J Hand Surg Am 1999;24(5):914–23.

18. Eaton RG, Malerich MM. Volar plate arthroplasty of the proximal interphalangeal joint: a review of ten years' experience. J Hand Surg Am 1980;5(3): 260–8.

19. Grant I, Berger AC, Tham SK. Internal fixation of unstable fracture dislocations of the proximal interphalangeal joint. J Hand Surg Br 2005;30(5):492–8.

20. Wilson JN, Rowland SA. Fracture-dislocation of the proximal interphalangeal joint of the finger. J Bone Joint Surg Am 1966;48(3):493–502.

21. Redler I, Williams JT. Rupture of a collateral ligament of the proximal interphalangeal joint of the fingers. Analysis of eighteen cases. J Bone Joint Surg Am 1967;49(2):322–6.

22. McCue FC, Honner R, Johnson MC, et al. Athletic injuries of the proximal interphalangeal joint requiring surgical treatment. J Bone Joint Surg Am 1970; 52(5):937–56.

23. Kato N, Nemoto K, Nakajima H, et al. Primary repair of the collateral ligament of the proximal interphalangeal joint using a suture anchor. Scand J Plast Reconstr Surg Hand Surg 2003;37(2):117–20.

24. Kato H, Minami A, Takahara M, et al. Surgical repair of acute collateral ligament injuries in digits with the Mitek bone suture anchor. J Hand Surg Br 1999; 24(1):70–5.

25. Lee SJ, Lee JH, Hwang IC, et al. Clinical outcomes of operative repair of complete rupture of the proximal interphalangeal joint collateral ligament: comparison with non-operative treatment. Acta Orthop Traumatol Turc 2017;51(1):44–8.

26. Freiberg A, Pollard BA, Macdonald MR, et al. Management of proximal interphalangeal joint injuries. Hand Clin 2006;22(3):235–42.

27. Boden RA, Srinivasan MS. Rotational dislocation of the proximal interphalangeal joint of the finger. J Bone Joint Surg Br 2008;90(3):385–6.

28. Frueh FS, Vogel P, Honigmann P. Irreducible dislocations of the proximal interphalangeal joint: algorithm for open reduction and soft-tissue repair. Plast Reconstr Surg Glob Open 2018;6(5):e1729.

29. Green SM, Posner MA. Irreducible dorsal dislocations of the proximal interphalangeal joint. J Hand Surg Am 1985;10(1):85–7.

30. Kung J, Touliopolis S, Caligiuri D. Irreducible dislocation of the proximal interphalangeal joint of a finger. J Hand Surg Br 1998;23(2):252.

31. Kjeldal I. Irreducible compound dorsal dislocations of the proximal interphalangeal joint of the finger. J Hand Surg Br 1986;11(1):49–50.

32. Oni OO. Irreducible buttonhole dislocation of the proximal interphalangeal joint of the finger (a case report). J Hand Surg Br 1985;10(1):100.

33. Posner MA, Wilenski M. Irreducible volar dislocation of the proximal interphalangeal joint of a finger caused by interposition of the intact central slip: a case report. J Bone Joint Surg Am 1978;60(1): 133–4.

34. Johnson FG, Greene MH. Another cause of irreducible dislocation of the proximal interphalangeal joint of a finger. J Bone Joint Surg Am 1966;48(3):542–4.

35. Cheung JP, Tse WL, Ho PC. Irreducible volar subluxation of the proximal interphalangeal joint due to radial collateral ligament interposition: case report and review of literature. Hand Surg 2015;20(1):153–7.

36. Whipple TL, Evans JP, Urbaniak JR. Irreducible dislocation of a finger joint in a child. A case report. J Bone Joint Surg Am 1980;62(5):832–3.

37. Peimer CA, Sullivan DJ, Wild DR. Palmar dislocation of the proximal interphalangeal joint. J Hand Surg Am 1984;9a(1):39–48.

38. Schernberg F, Elzein F, Gillier P, et al. Dislocations of the proximal interphalangeal joints of the long fingers. Anatomo-clinical study and therapeutic results. Ann Chir Main 1982;1(1):18–28.

39. Burnier M, Awada T, Marin Braun F, et al. Treatment of unstable proximal interphalangeal joint fractures with hemi-hamate osteochondral autografts. J Hand Surg Eur Vol 2017;42(2):188–93.

40. Watanabe K, Kino Y, Yajima H. Factors affecting the functional results of open reduction and internal fixation for fracture-dislocations of the proximal interphalangeal joint. Hand Surg 2015;20(1):107–14.

41. Maalla R, Youssef M, Ben Jdidia G, et al. Extension-block pinning for fracture-dislocation of the proximal interphalangeal joint. Orthop Traumatol Surg Res 2012;98(5):559–63.

42. Newington DP, Davis TR, Barton NJ. The treatment of dorsal fracture-dislocation of the proximal interphalangeal joint by closed reduction and Kirschner wire fixation: a 16-year follow up. J Hand Surg Br 2001;26(6):537–40.

43. Dionysian E, Eaton RG. The long-term outcome of volar plate arthroplasty of the proximal interphalangeal joint. J Hand Surg Am 2000;25(3):429–37.

44. Duteille F, Pasquier P, Lim A, et al. Treatment of complex interphalangeal joint fractures with dynamic external traction: a series of 20 cases. Plast Reconstr Surg 2003;111(5):1623–9.

45. de Haseth KB, Neuhaus V, Mudgal CS. Dorsal fracture-dislocations of the proximal interphalangeal joint: evaluation of closed reduction and percutaneous Kirschner wire pinning. Hand (N Y) 2015;10(1):88–93.

46. Waris E, Mattila S, Sillat T, et al. Extension block pinning for unstable proximal interphalangeal joint dorsal fracture dislocations. J Hand Surg Am 2016;41(2):196–202.

47. Inoue G, Tamura Y. Treatment of fracture-dislocation of the proximal interphalangeal joint using extension-block Kirschner wire. Ann Chir Main Memb Super 1991;10(6):564–8.

48. Viegas SF. Extension block pinning for proximal interphalangeal joint fracture dislocations: preliminary report of a new technique. J Hand Surg Am 1992;17(5):896–901.

49. Vitale MA, White NJ, Strauch RJ. A percutaneous technique to treat unstable dorsal fracture-dislocations of the proximal interphalangeal joint. J Hand Surg Am 2011;36(9):1453–9.

50. Waris E, Alanen V. Percutaneous, intramedullary fracture reduction and extension block pinning for dorsal proximal interphalangeal fracture-dislocations. J Hand Surg Am 2010;35(12):2046–52.

51. Aladin A, Davis TR. Dorsal fracture-dislocation of the proximal interphalangeal joint: a comparative study of percutaneous Kirschner wire fixation versus open reduction and internal fixation. J Hand Surg Br 2005;30(2):120–8.

52. Weiss AP. Cerclage fixation for fracture dislocation of the proximal interphalangeal joint. Clin Orthop Relat Res 1996;327:21–8.

53. Cheah AE, Tan DM, Chong AK, et al. Volar plating for unstable proximal interphalangeal joint dorsal fracture-dislocations. J Hand Surg Am 2012;37(1):28–33.

54. Ikeda M, Kobayashi Y, Saito I, et al. Open reduction and internal fixation for dorsal fracture dislocations of the proximal interphalangeal joint using a mini-plate. Tech Hand Up Extrem Surg 2011;15(4):219–24.

55. Kang GC, Yam A, Phoon ES, et al. The hook plate technique for fixation of phalangeal avulsion fractures. J Bone Joint Surg Am 2012;94(11):e72.

56. Hamilton SC, Stern PJ, Fassler PR, et al. Mini-screw fixation for the treatment of proximal interphalangeal joint dorsal fracture-dislocations. J Hand Surg Am 2006;31(8):1349–54.

57. Lee JY, Teoh LC. Dorsal fracture dislocations of the proximal interphalangeal joint treated by open reduction and interfragmentary screw fixation: indications, approaches and results. J Hand Surg Br 2006;31(2):138–46.

58. Lahav A, Teplitz GA, McCormack RR Jr. Percutaneous reduction and Kirschner-wire fixation of impacted intra-articular fractures and volar lip fractures of the proximal interphalangeal joint. Am J Orthop (Belle Mead NJ) 2005;34(2):62–5.

59. Eglseder WA, Jeter EC. Open reduction and internal fixation of proximal interphalangeal joint fracture-subluxations. Contemp Orthop 1992;24(1):45–50.

60. Green A, Smith J, Redding M, et al. Acute open reduction and rigid internal fixation of proximal interphalangeal joint fracture dislocation. J Hand Surg Am 1992;17(3):512–7.

61. Lee JY, Teoh LC, Seah VW. Extending the reach of the heterodigital arterialized flap by cross-finger transfer. Plast Reconstr Surg 2006;117(7):2320–8.

62. Cheah AE, Yao J. Surgical approaches to the proximal interphalangeal joint. J Hand Surg Am 2016;41(2):294–305.

63. Foo GL, Ramruttun AK, Cheah AE, et al. Biomechanics of internal fixation modalities for middle phalangeal base fracture dislocation. J Hand Surg Asian Pac Vol 2017;22(1):14–7.

64. Chew WY, Cheah AE. Volar plate and screw fixation for dorsal fracture-dislocation of the proximal interphalangeal joint: case report. J Hand Surg Am 2010;35(6):928–30.

65. Gaul JS Jr, Rosenberg SN. Fracture-dislocation of the middle phalanx at the proximal interphalangeal joint: repair with a simple intradigital traction-fixation device. Am J Orthop (Belle Mead NJ) 1998;27(10):682–8.

66. Agee JM. Unstable fracture dislocations of the proximal interphalangeal joint. Treatment with the force couple splint. Clin Orthop Relat Res 1987;214: 101–12.

67. Allison DM. Results in the treatment of fractures around the proximal interphalangeal joint with a pin and rubber traction system. J Hand Surg Br 1998; 23(5):700–1.

68. Bain GI, Mehta JA, Heptinstall RJ, et al. Dynamic external fixation for injuries of the proximal interphalangeal joint. J Bone Joint Surg Br 1998;80(6): 1014–9.

69. Deshmukh NV, Sonanis SV, Stothard J. Neglected volar dislocations of the interphalangeal joint. Hand Surg 2004;9(1):71–5.

70. Inanami H, Ninomiya S, Okutsu I, et al. Dynamic external finger fixator for fracture dislocation of the proximal interphalangeal joint. J Hand Surg Am 1993;18(1):160–4.

71. Majumder S, Peck F, Watson JS, et al. Lessons learned from the management of complex intraarticular fractures at the base of the middle phalanges of fingers. J Hand Surg Br 2003;28(6): 559–65.

72. Morgan JP, Gordon DA, Klug MS, et al. Dynamic digital traction for unstable comminuted intraarticular fracture-dislocations of the proximal interphalangeal joint. J Hand Surg Am 1995;20(4): 565–73.

73. Schenck RR. Classification of fractures and dislocations of the proximal interphalangeal joint. Hand Clin 1994;10(2):179–85.

74. Suzuki Y, Matsunaga T, Sato S, et al. The pins and rubbers traction system for treatment of comminuted intraarticular fractures and fracture-dislocations in the hand. J Hand Surg Br 1994;19(1):98–107.

75. de Soras X, de Mourgues P, Guinard D, et al. Pins and rubbers traction system. J Hand Surg Br 1997;22(6):730–5.

76. Hynes MC, Giddins GE. Dynamic external fixation for pilon fractures of the interphalangeal joints. J Hand Surg Br 2001;26(2):122–4.

77. Khan W, Fahmy N. The S-Quattro in the management of acute intraarticular phalangeal fractures of the hand. J Hand Surg Br 2006;31(1):79–92.

78. Ellis PR, Tsai TM. Management of the traumatized joint of the finger. Clin Plast Surg 1989;16(3):457–73.

79. Blazar PE, Robbe R, Lawton JN. Treatment of dorsal fracture/dislocations of the proximal interphalangeal joint by volar plate arthroplasty. Tech Hand Up Extrem Surg 2001;5(3):148–52.

80. Malerich MM, Eaton RG. The volar plate reconstruction for fracture-dislocation of the proximal interphalangeal joint. Hand Clin 1994;10(2):251–60.

81. Tyser AR, Tsai MA, Parks BG, et al. Biomechanical characteristics of hemi-hamate reconstruction versus volar plate arthroplasty in the treatment of dorsal fracture dislocations of the proximal interphalangeal joint. J Hand Surg Am 2015;40(2):329–32.

82. Calfee RP, Kiefhaber TR, Sommerkamp TG, et al. Hemi-hamate arthroplasty provides functional reconstruction of acute and chronic proximal interphalangeal fracture-dislocations. J Hand Surg Am 2009;34(7):1232–41.

83. Williams RM, Kiefhaber TR, Sommerkamp TG, et al. Treatment of unstable dorsal proximal interphalangeal fracture/dislocations using a hemi-hamate autograft. J Hand Surg Am 2003;28(5):856–65.

84. Afendras G, Abramo A, Mrkonjic A, et al. Hemi-hamate osteochondral transplantation in proximal interphalangeal dorsal fracture dislocations: a minimum 4 year follow-up in eight patients. J Hand Surg Eur Vol 2010;35(8):627–31.

85. Yang DS, Lee SK, Kim KJ, et al. Modified hemihamate arthroplasty technique for treatment of acute proximal interphalangeal joint fracture-dislocations. Ann Plast Surg 2014;72(4):411–6.

86. Korambayil PM, Francis A. Hemi-hamate arthroplasty for pilon fractures of finger. Indian J Plast Surg 2011;44(3):458–66.

87. Rozen WM, Niumsawatt V, Ross R, et al. The vascular basis of the hemi-hamate osteochondral free flap. Part 1: vascular anatomy and clinical correlation. Surg Radiol Anat 2013;35(7):585–94.

88. Rosenstadt BE, Glickel SZ, Lane LB, et al. Palmar fracture dislocation of the proximal interphalangeal joint. J Hand Surg Am 1998;23(5):811–20.

89. Meyer ZI, Goldfarb CA, Calfee RP, et al. The central slip fracture: results of operative treatment of volar fracture subluxations/dislocations of the proximal interphalangeal joint. J Hand Surg Am 2017;42(7): 572.e1-6.

90. Doering TA, Greenberg AS, Tuckman DV. Dorsal plating for intra-articular middle phalangeal base fractures with volar instability. Hand (N Y) 2018. 1558944718777868. [Epub ahead of print].

91. Tekkis PP, Kessaris N, Gavalas M, et al. The role of mini-fragment screw fixation in volar dislocations of the proximal interphalangeal joint. Arch Orthop Trauma Surg 2001;121(1–2):121–2.

92. Zhang X, Yang L, Shao X, et al. Treatment of bony boutonniere deformity with a loop wire. J Hand Surg Am 2011;36(6):1080–5.

93. Sinclair VF, Karantana A, Muir L. Reverse hemi-hamate arthroplasty for volar fracture dislocation of the proximal interphalangeal joint of the finger. J Hand Surg Eur Vol 2017;42(2):199–200.

94. Ruland RT, Hogan CJ, Cannon DL, et al. Use of dynamic distraction external fixation for unstable fracture-dislocations of the proximal interphalangeal joint. J Hand Surg Am 2008;33(1):19–25.

# Treatment of Carpal Instability and Distal Radioulnar Joint Instability

David Meng Kiat Tan, MBBS (Singapore), MMED Surgery (Singapore)*,
Jin Xi Lim, MBBS (Singapore), MMED Surgery (Singapore)

## KEYWORDS

- Carpal instability • Scapholunate instability • Perilunate instability • Distal radioulnar joint instability

## KEY POINTS

- Carpal instability and distal radioulnar joint instability is said to be present when the wrist exhibits symptomatic malalingment, abnromal kinematics and is unable to bear loads.
- The different forms of carpal instability can be classified according to different stages. This correlates well with pathoanatomy and serves as a guide to treatment.
- Stress radiography and fluoroscopy can be used to aid in the diagnosis of dynamic carpal instabilities whilst arthroscopy offers the most accurate assessment of these conditions.
- Distal radioulnar joint instability can result from injuries to the triangular fibrocartilage complex, an abnormal joint architecture or alterations in the radioulnar relationship from forearm fractures and malunion.
- The treatment of distal radioulnar joint instability without arthritis should address the TFCC and/or the bony relationship of the joint. When arthritis has developed, a salvage procedure is indicated.

 Video content accompanies this article at http://www.plasticsurgery.theclinics.com.

## CARPAL INSTABILITY

Carpal instability can occur after trauma, remotely after trauma, and sometimes without trauma. The 3 most important conditions are scapholunate instability, lunotriquetral instability, and perilunate instability complex. The carpus is considered unstable if it exhibits symptomatic malalignment, is not able to bear loads, and does not have normal kinematics during any portion of its arc of motion.[1]

### Classification

Although a majority of carpal instabilities arise from trauma, there are 6 important categories to consider when analyzing carpal instability[2] (**Table 1**). There are 4 patterns of instability that have been described by various investigators[3-5] and are widely accepted (**Fig. 1**).

Carpal instability dissociative (CID) refers to instability within a row of carpal bones, such as scaphoid fractures or scapholunate dissociation in the proximal row. Carpal instability nondissociative (CIND) is instability between rows either at the radiocarpal joint (eg, radiocarpal fracture dislocations) or midcarpal joint (eg, midcarpal instability). Carpal instability combined/complex (CIC) is a combination of CID and CIND, such as perilunate dislocations (PLDs). Carpal instability adaptive

Disclosures: The authors have nothing to disclose.
Department of Hand and Reconstructive Microsurgery, National University Hospital Singapore, 1E Kent Ridge Road, Tower Block, Level 11, Singapore 119228, Singapore
* Corresponding author.
*E-mail address:* david_mk_tan@nuhs.edu.sg

Clin Plastic Surg 46 (2019) 451–468
https://doi.org/10.1016/j.cps.2019.03.006

**Table 1**
**Analysis of carpal instability**

| Category I—Chronicity | Category II—Constancy | Category III—Etiology | Category IV—Location | Category V—Direction | Category VI—Pattern |
|---|---|---|---|---|---|
| Acute, <1 wk (maximum healing potential) | Predynamic Dynamic | Congenital Traumatic | Radiocarpal Intercarpal | VISI DISI | CID CIND |
| Subacute, 1–6 wk (some healing potential) | | Inflammatory Arthritis Neoplastic | Midcarpal Carpometacarpal | Ulnar Radial | CIC CIA |
| Chronic, >6 wk (poor healing potential) | | Iatrogenic Miscellaneous | Specific bones/ ligaments | Ventral Rotatory | |

(CIA) refers to carpal malalignment in adaption to extracarpal changes (eg, carpal collapse in malunited distal radius fractures).

### Critical Imaging Studies

#### Plain film radiography
On the posteroanterior (PA) projection, 3 smooth arcs, termed Gilula lines,[6] can be traced (**Fig. 2**A). A disruption of any arc suggests the presence of carpal instability (**Fig. 2**B, C). Loss of carpal height indicates carpal instability with carpal collapse (**Fig. 2**D).

A well-taken lateral projection shows the axes of the radius and carpal bones (**Fig. 3**A–D), which form several important indices (**Fig. 3**E–G). Abnormal indices indicate static carpal malalignment and instability. The term, volar intercalated segmental instability (VISI), is used when the radiolunate angle exceeds 15° volarly (**Fig. 4**A) and typically is seen in lunotriquetral dissociation, whereas the term, dorsal intercalated segmental instability (DISI), is for when that angle exceeds 15° dorsally and most commonly is seen in scapholunate dissociation (**Fig. 4**B).

#### Stress radiography
Stress views are useful for diagnosing dynamic scapholunate instability. A PA clenched fist view with the wrist in neutral, ulnar deviation and radial deviation accentuates the gap/interval between the scaphoid and the lunate (**Fig. 5**).

#### Fluoroscopy
Fluoroscopy is useful to detect subtle dynamic scapholunate and lunotriquetral dissociations. This manifests as a step when axial traction is applied to the wrist (Video 1A). Traction views also are helpful in demonstrating the stage of a PLD and associated bony injuries (Video 1B). In midcarpal instability and other clunking wrist disorders, considerable information can be gleaned by observing the apex of motion at which clunking occurs as the wrist moves from radial to ulnar deviation (Video 2).

#### MRI
Powerful magnetic field (3T) MRIs with dedicated wrist coils, thin 1-mm slices, and advanced imaging software make MRI an invaluable noninvasive imaging adjunct for intercarpal ligament injuries and triangular fibrocartilage complex (TFCC) tears.

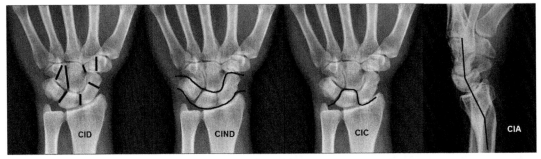

**Fig. 1.** Four patterns of carpal instability are demonstrated. The bold dark lines indicate potential sites where there is disruption in the continuity of the carpus either through fractures, ligament disruptions, or both. Left panel: Carpal instability dissociative. Left middle panel: Carpal instability non dissociative. Right middle panel: Carpal instability combined/complex. Right panel: Carpal instability adaptive.

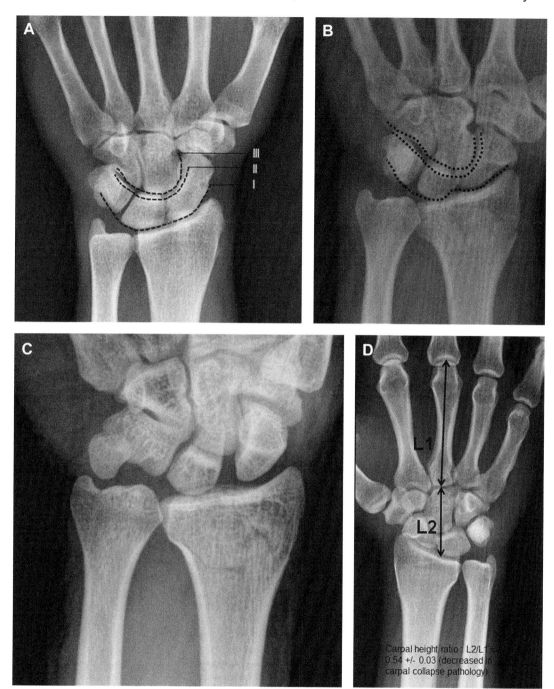

**Fig. 2.** (*A*) Gilula lines describe 3 smooth arcs that transcribe the proximal articular surfaces of the proximal carpal row (I), the distal articular surfaces of the proximal carpal row (II), and the proximal articular surface of the hamate and capitate (III). (*B*) In this minimally displaced distal radius fracture, Gilula first line is broken and is suspicious for a scapholunate ligament injury. (*C*) Clenched fist view demonstrates widening of the scapholunate interval consistent with a complete tear. (*D*) Carpal height (L2) and length of third metacarpal (L1). The carpal height ratio (0.54 $\pm$ 0.03) is derived from L2/L1.

## Clinical Conditions

### Scapholunate instability

Scapholunate instability is the most common form of carpal instability and represents a spectrum of disorders,[7] ranging from a predynamic state (radiographs normal) to a dynamic state (positive stress radiographs) to a static state (evident on plain film radiography). Left untreated, it may progress to arthritis.

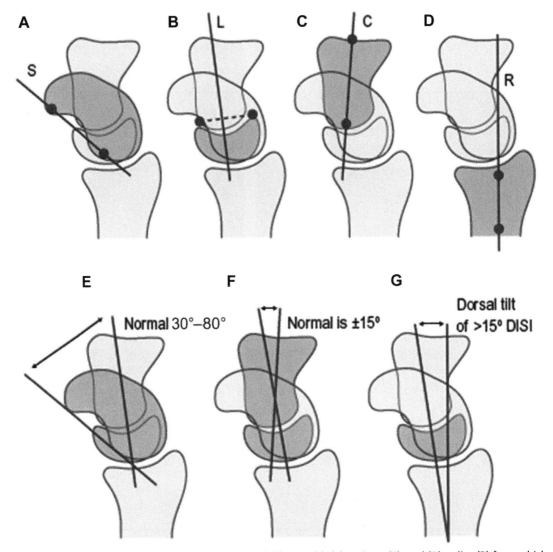

**Fig. 3.** Demonstrates the axes of the (*A*) scaphoid (S), (*B*) lunate (L), (*C*) capitate (C), and (*D*) radius (R) from which 3 important indices are determined: (*E*) scapholunate angle, (*F*) capitolunate angle, and (*G*) radiolunate angle. (*From* Chong AKS, Lim JX, Tan DMK. Diagnostic imaging of the hand and wrist In: Chang J, Neligan PC, eds. Plastic Surgery Volume 6 4th Ed. Philadelphia, PA: Elsevier; 2018: 71-95; with permission.)

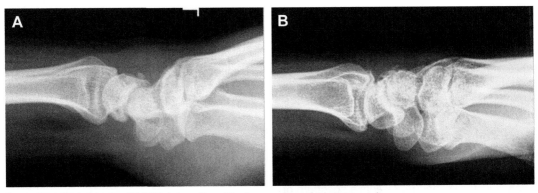

**Fig. 4.** (*A*) VISI deformity. (*B*) DISI deformity with abnormal scapholunate angle.

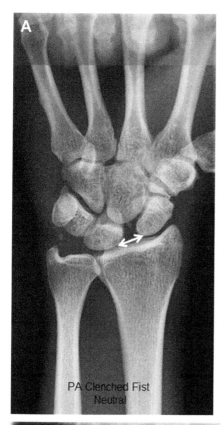

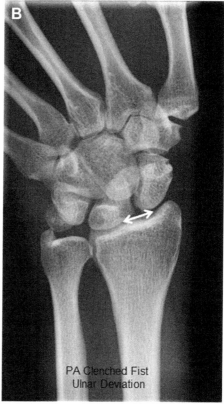

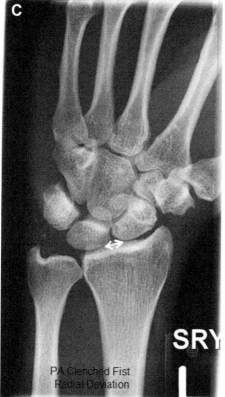

**Fig. 5.** There is widening of the scapholunate interval (A) in neutral position and when the wrist is (B) in ulnar deviation, which is reduced when the wrist is (C) radially deviated.

**Assessment** Pain is typically over the dorsum and dorsoradial aspect of the wrist, aggravated by loading the extended wrist or strenuous activity. This may be preceded by a fall, but a delayed presentation is not uncommon. Other symptoms include clicking of the wrist, weakness of grip, and limitation of motion.

Tenderness may be elicited over the dorsal scapholunate interval 1 cm distal to Lister tubercle as well as over the tip of the radial styloid, anatomic snuff box, and the scaphoid tubercle. Provocative tests include Watson scaphoid shift (**Fig.** 6A, B), the resisted finger extension test (**Fig.** 6C), and a positive scapholunate ballottement test.

**Imaging** Radiographs may show classic features of an increased scapholunate angle (>70°) and DISI deformity. These features (**Fig. 7**) are seen with a complete tear of the ligament and failure of the secondary stabilizers. When plain films are normal, stress views should be considered and an MRI may be indicated for further evaluation.

**Staging** The scapholunate ligament complex has a stout dorsal ligament, modest volar ligament, and weak proximal membranous component. The secondary stabilizers of the scapholunate joint are the dorsal intercarpal, scaphotrapezial-trapezoidal, and radioscaphocapitate ligaments. Disruption of the scapholunate ligament leads to progressive diastasis of the scapholunate interval whereas failure of secondary stabilizers leads to carpal malalignment. Garcia-Elias and colleagues[8] developed a staging system for scapholunate dissociation based on several factors (**Table 2**) and proposed treatment accordingly.

*Stage 1 (predynamic instability)* MRI sometimes may demonstrate a volar or membranous tear; however, arthroscopy is the standard in diagnosing these injuries and may be graded according to the system of Geissler and colleagues[9] (**Table 3**; Video 3).

Initial treatment consists of splinting to allow healing in acute and subacute injuries with subsequent proprioception training of the flexor carpi

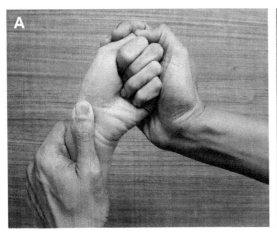
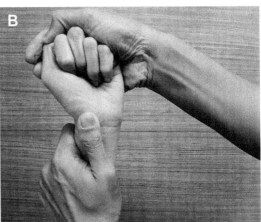
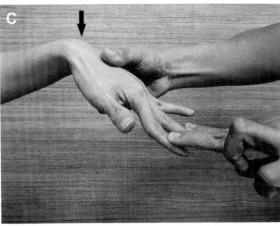

**Fig. 6.** The patient's wrist is positioned in slight dorsiflexion and the examiner places a thumb over the patient's scaphoid tuberosity and, while maintaining pressure, moves the wrist from a position of ulnar deviation (*A*) to radial deviation (*B*) and vice versa. Pain over the dorsal scapholunate interval and an associated clunk constitutes a positive test. Pain without clunking is considered a positive modified Watson scaphoid shift test. (*C*) The patient's wrist is held partially flexed and the index and middle fingers are extended against the examiner's resisting hand. Pain over the dorsal scapholunate interval (black arrow) is considered a positive test.

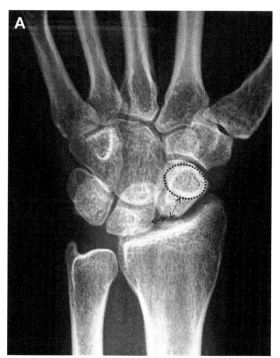 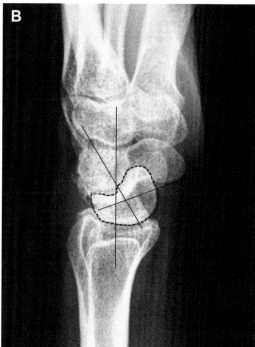

**Fig. 7.** (*A*) PA projection of the wrist shows widening of the scapholunate interval greater than 3 mm, a cortical ring sign (signet ring sign), a ring to proximal pole distance less than 7 mm. The lunate appears more rectangular. (*B*) Lateral projection of the wrist shows the scapholunate angle greater than 70° and abnormal radiolunate and capitolunate angles.

**Table 2**
**Staging of scapholunate dissociations**

| Scapholunate Dissociation Stage | 1 | 2 | 3 | 4 | 5 | 6 |
|---|---|---|---|---|---|---|
| Is there a partial rupture with a normal dorsal scapholunate ligament? | Yes | No | No | No | No | No |
| If ruptured, can the dorsal scapholunate ligament be repaired? | Yes | Yes | No | No | No | No |
| Is the scaphoid normally aligned (radioscaphoid angle ≤45°)? | Yes | Yes | Yes | No | No | No |
| Is the carpal malalignment easily reducible? | Yes | Yes | Yes | Yes | No | No |
| Are the cartilages at both radiocarpal and midcarpal joints normal? | Yes | Yes | Yes | Yes | Yes | No |

**Table 3**
**Arthroscopic grading of intercarpal ligament tears**

| Grade | Description |
|---|---|
| I | Attenuation/hemorrhage of interosseous ligament seen from the radiocarpal joint; no incongruency of carpal alignment in the midcarpal space |
| II | As in grade I, however, incongruency/step visible from the midcarpal joint, with a slight gap less than the width of a probe |
| III | As in grade II, there also is incongruency in the radiocarpal joint, and the probe may be passed between the carpal bones |
| IV | Obvious incongruency between the carpal bones and gross instability with manipulation, and the 2.7-mm scope may be passed through the gap between the carpal bones |

radialis and extensor carpi radialis muscles. Surgery for recalcitrant pain includes arthroscopic interventions, such as débridement alone or with thermal shrinkage and/or pinning, and has 80% to 90% success rates.

***Stages 2 and 3*** In acute complete tears, an open repair is indicated. This may be augmented by a capsulodesis, and the scapholunate and scaphocapitate joints should be pinned with Kirschner wires after reducing the scapholunate angle and scapholunate diastasis (**Fig. 8**) for 6 weeks. An all-arthroscopic technique of dorsal capsuloligamentous repair[10] for stages 2, 3, and 4 has been reported, with favorable results across all groups with minimal stiffness at an average of more than 2 years. Open techniques for stage 3 patients include capsulodesis[11] and bone ligament bone repairs. [12]

***Stage 4*** Garcia-Elias and colleagues[8] proposed their triligament reconstruction technique for the stage 4 group of patients using a distally based strip of the flexor carpi radialis tendon to augment the palmar distal connections of the scaphoid, reconstruct the dorsal scapholunate ligament, and reduce the ulnar translocation of the lunate

(**Fig. 9**). Although efficacious in pain relief and restoration of grip strength, stiffness in the flexion-extension and ulnar deviation plane is notable, and carpal malalignment could be seen to recur early in some instances and was associated with complications.[13] Other investigators have reported comparable success with capsulodesis[11] and different forms of tenodesis procedures, including the use of the extensor carpi radialis longus tendon.

***Stages 5 and 6*** When carpal malalignment is irreducible from chronic injury and scarring of extrinsic capsuloligamentous tissue, scaphotrapeziotrapezoid fusion,[14] and other forms of intercarpal fusion are indicated. With cartilage loss and arthritis (stage 6), a salvage procedure is indicated, most typically a proximal row carpectomy or a 4-corner fusion if arthritis involves the midcarpal joint.

### Lunotriquetral instability
Lunotriquetral instability remains frequently underdiagnosed, with a paucity of literature regarding its pathogenesis, diagnosis, and treatment. It may occur in isolation as an acute traumatic tear

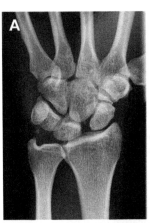
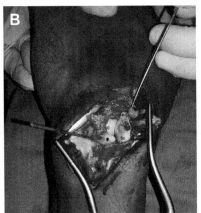
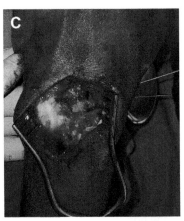
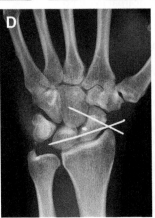
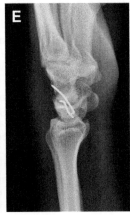

**Fig. 8.** (*A*) Acute presentation of a scapholunate ligament injury with a widened interval. (*B*) Intraoperative view demonstrating scapholunate ligament avulsion (*asterisk*) from the scaphoid (*Sc*). The proximal pole of the capitate (*C*) can be clearly seen. Kirschner wires are used as joysticks to reduce the scapholunate joint. (*C*) The scapholunate and scaphocapitate joint are pinned before the ligament is repaired to the scaphoid with a suture anchor (*black arrow*). (*D*) Radiograph demonstrates a reduced scapholunate interval, appropriate positioning of the wires, and suture anchor. (*E*) The lateral projection shows an adequately restored scapholunate angle.

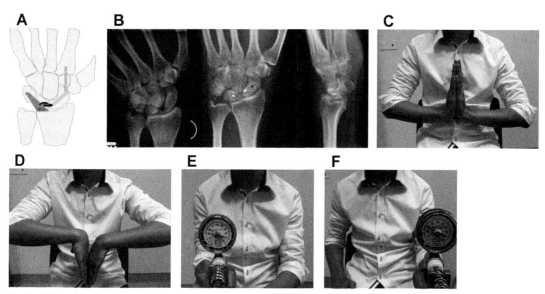

**Fig. 9.** (*A*) In this diagrammatic representation, a distally based strip of the flexor carpi radialis is passed from palmar to dorsal through a bone tunnel along the axis of the scaphoid to exit at the normal scaphoid insertion point of the ligament before it is secured to a bone trough on the dorsal lunate, woven into the dorsal radiotri-quetral ligament, and secured back to itself. (*B*) Preoperative films showing a static widened scapholunate interval (left panel) and closure of the gap after tenodesis has been done (centre panel). There still is an abnormal scapholunate angle (right panel). (*C–F*) Same patient with some stiffness in flexion and extension but satisfied and with good return of grip strength at 1-year follow-up.

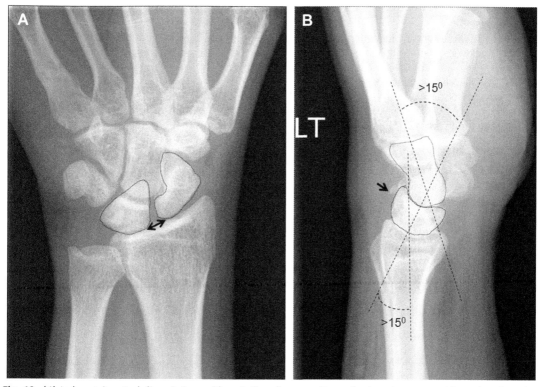

**Fig. 10.** (*A*) In lunotriquetral dissociation with a static collapse pattern, the lunate appears triangular, there is a pseudowidening of the scapholunate interval (*double-ended arrow*), and the scaphoid appears flexed on a PA projection. (*B*) Lateral views aside from a VISI pattern also may demonstrate an abnormal capitolunate angle as the carpus collapses. The small bony fleck at the dorsal aspect of the carpus (*arrow*) indicates a dorsal radio-triquetral ligament avulsion.

**Table 4**
**Staging of lunotriquetral instability (ulnar-sided perilunar instability) by Viegas and colleagues.[15]**

| Stage | Ligament Disruption | Radiologic Findings |
|---|---|---|
| I | Dorsal lunotriquetral and membranous component | Plain radiographs normal |
| II | Stage I as well as palmar lunotriquetral ligament | Dynamic VISI (when palmar translation force applied to dorsum of capitate with wrist in neutral or flexed position) |
| III | Stage II and dorsal radiotriquetral ligament | Static VISI deformity evident |

or in association with degenerative causes, such as ulnocarpal abutment and central TFCC tears, and as part of the perilunate complex injury, to name a few conditions.

**Assessment** Acute isolated injuries typically result from a backward fall with the hypothenar eminence striking the ground. Tenderness is localized to the lunotriquetral interval with the appearance of a volar sag, and the Reagan ballottement and Kleinman shear tests may be positive. The Reagan ballottement is performed by grasping the pisiotriquetral bones with the thumb and index finger of 1 hand and balloting/shearing them against the lunate, which is stabilized between the thumb and index finger of the examiner's other hand. Unfortunately, these tests, although sensitive, are not always specific.

**Imaging** Plain radiographs are normal with partial ligament injuries. With complete disruption of the lunotriquetral ligament complex as well as its extrinsic stabilizer the dorsal radiotriquetral ligament, classic VISI features can be seen on static films (**Fig. 10**). Traction videofluoroscopy may demonstrate positive findings in complete tears without failure of the extrinsic ligament (Video 4A). High-resolution MRIs may be helpful but the standard for diagnosis remains arthroscopy (Video 4B). Arthritis and a lunotriquetral step are late findings.

**Staging and treatment** Viegas and colleagues[15] proposed a staging system for lunotriquetral ligament instability based on biomechanical studies on cadavers, which had a pathomechanical and radiologic correlation (**Table 4**).

In acute partial injuries (stage I), above-elbow casting or splinting with a pad under the pisiform to boost the triquetrum into correct alignment is prescribed. Even in chronic situations, this should be the first line of treatment. Patients who remain symptomatic may benefit from arthroscopic débridement with or without pinning of the lunotriquetral joint. In some instances, thermal shrinkage may be an effective adjunct (**Fig. 11**; see Video 4B).

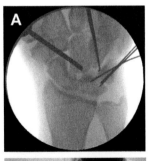
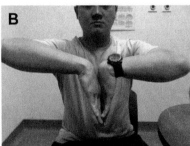
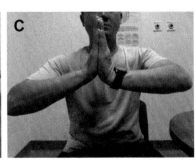
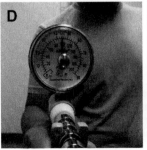
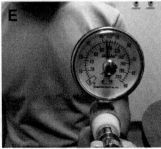

Fig. 11. (*A*) After thermal shrinkage, the lunotriquetral joint is pinned under direct arthroscopic visualization and reduction. (*B–E*) Six months postoperative result. There is satisfactory flexion and extension with full grip strength.

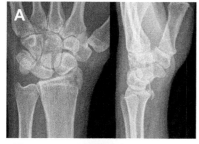
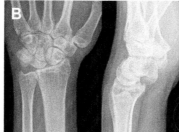
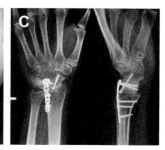
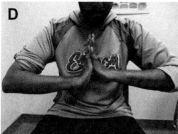
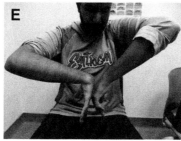

Fig. 12. (A) This patient was believed to have a radial styloid fracture after a motor vehicle accident. At time of presentation, there is already a VISI deformity. (B) Four months later there is progressive carpal collapse with a grossly abnormal capitolunate relationship. (C) Eighteen months status post-radioscapholunate fusion as well as a lunotriquetral fusion with wires and a distal scaphoidectomy. Cartilage loss of the scaphoid necessitated a radioscaphoid fusion. The patient has (D) fair wrist extension and (E) poor wrist flexion. Left panel: posteroanterior projection. Right panel: lateral projection.

In acute stage II injuries, surgical repair and pinning of the lunotriquetral joint for 6 weeks to 8 weeks are indicated. More commonly, diagnosis is delayed and patients may present after several months with chronic ulnar-sided wrist pain and an irreparable ligament. Treatment options then include ligament reconstruction using a distally based strip of the extensor carpi ulnaris[16], capsulodesis, or lunotriquetral joint fusion. Lunotriquetral fusions, although generally effective, are associated with problems of nonunion[16] as high as 40%.

In stage III, a global failure of intrinsic and extrinsic ligaments precludes local intercarpal surgical reconstruction strategies. In such uncommon situations, radiolunotriquetral fusion aligns the lunate appropriately with the radius, preserving midcarpal motion (**Fig. 12** and Video 5).

### Perilunate instability complex
Perilunate instability complex is the most common wrist dislocation and presents a spectrum of ligamentous and/or bony disruptions to the carpus in 4 enumerated stages (**Table 5**), as described by Mayfield.[17] The mechanism of injury is wrist axial loading and hyperextension, ulnar deviation, and intercarpal supination. Purely ligamentous injuries are termed lesser arc injuries (**Fig. 13**A) and those with a fracture greater arc injuries (**Fig. 13**B). These terms are synonymous with PLD and perilunate fracture dislocation (PLFD), with the most common fracture a scaphoid fracture.

In a multicenter study,[18] PLDs/PLFDs were associated with higher-energy injuries, frequently seen in polytrauma (26% of cases), and often were missed (25% of cases). PLFDs were twice as common as PLDs, with 97% of dislocations occurring dorsally (capitate dorsal to lunate) and the most common pattern of injury the dorsal transscaphoid PLFD. Scapholunate ligament tears are seen in a small percentage of transscaphoid PLFDs.

**Assessment** Aside from the acutely painful and swollen wrist, clinical findings may be subtle and there should be suspicion with a high-energy injury mechanism. Acute median neuropathy may be

**Table 5**
**Stages of perilunate dislocation (Mayfield)[17]**

| Stage | Ligament Injury | Bony Injury |
|---|---|---|
| I | Scapholunate ligament | Scaphoid fracture |
| II | Radioscaphocapitate ligament | Radial styloid fracture Capitate fracture |
| III | Lunotriquetral ligament | Triquetral fracture |
| IV | Dorsal radiotriquetral and radiolunate ligament | Lunate fracture |

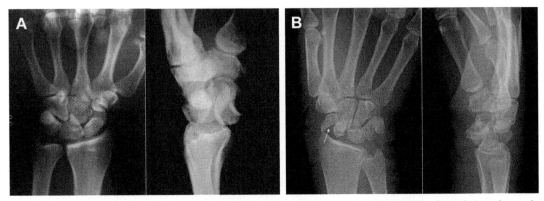

**Fig. 13.** (*A*) A lesser arc injury. The lunate appears triangular in shape on the PA view. The lateral view shows the capitate lying dorsally over the lunate, which has been displaced and demonstrates the spilt teacup sign (the teacup being the lunate). (*B*) A greater arc injury with a visible fracture of the scaphoid (*white arrow*). The overlapping carpal bones of the distal and proximal rows resemble a crowded carpus. Left panel: Posteroanterior projection trauma film. Right panel: Lateral projection trauma film.

present and was reported in 23% of cases in Herzberg and colleagues' series.[18]

PA wrist projections show the appearance of a crowded carpus and associated fractures, such as the scaphoid (see **Fig. 13**B) and radial styloid. The lateral projection demonstrates loss of collinearity between the axis of the radius, lunate, and capitate, with the capitate usually dorsal to the lunate. The displaced lunate may give the appearance of a spilt teacup (see **Fig. 13**A). CT scans are indicated when fractures are suspected.

**Treatment** Initially, closed reduction by Tavernier method should be attempted. When acute median neuropathy is present, emergent carpal tunnel release should be performed at the time of initial closed reduction in the operating room.

Definitive care is early open reduction and internal fixation of fractures, repair of the ligaments, and intercarpal pinning to maintain alignment and allow the ligamentous injury components to heal (**Fig. 14**). A single dorsal approach is commonly used, although a volar approach may be indicated, especially if the lunate is dislocated and/or enucleated and irreducible. The scaphoid screw can be inserted in antegrade fashion if a fracture is present and the dorsal scapholunate

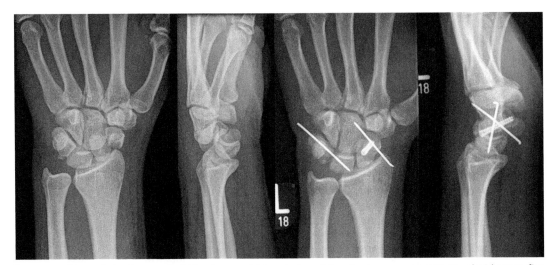

**Fig. 14.** In this PLFD, both a scaphoid fracture and triquetral avulsion fracture are present. Scaphoid screw fixation and reduction of the lunotriquetral step and pinning of the lunotriquetral joint addresses the lunotriquetral ligament avulsion fracture. Left panel: Posteroanterior projection trauma film. Left middle panel: Lateral projection trauma film. Right middle panel: Posteroanterior projection immediate postoperative film. Right: Lateral projection immediate postoperative film.

**Table 6**
**Causes of distal radioulnar joint instability**

| Nontraumatic | Traumatic | Postsurgical (Instability of Ulna Stump) |
|---|---|---|
| • Rheumatoid arthritis<br>• Connective tissue disorder (Ehlers-Danlos syndrome) | • Displaced distal radius fractures<br>• Basal ulnar styloid fractures<br>• TFCC injury<br>• Galeazzi fracture dislocation<br>• Essex-Lopresti injury<br>• Both bone forearm shaft fractures | • Ulna head resection<br>• Sauvé-Kapandji procedure |

and lunotriquetral ligament can be repaired if injured.

Beyond 6 weeks, the state of cartilage and reparability of the ligaments must be taken into consideration (intraoperative assessment) before performing definitive fixation and ligament repairs. If not possible, a salvage procedure typically in the form of a proximal row carpectomy or a midcarpal arthrodesis are options depending on where the cartilage injury has involved.

## DISTAL RADIOULNAR JOINT INSTABILITY

Distal radioulnar joint (DRUJ) instability can occur either from a variety of causes (**Table 6**). This review focuses on traumatic and nontraumatic causes, the evaluation, and treatment.

### Anatomy and Biomechanics

Primary stability of the DRUJ is contributed by the congruity of its articular surfaces and the TFCC.[19] The DRUJ is further reinforced by an osseocartilaginous lip[20] on the volar aspect of the radius. The secondary stabilizers include the joint capsule, extensor carpi ulnaris, pronator quadratus, and interosseous membrane.

### Pathology

DRUJ instability can be due to either alterations in the bony anatomy, resulting in altered sigmoid notch architecture or abnormal radioulnar relationship, and/or disruptions to the TFCC. DRUJ instability may accompany distal radius fractures due to TFCC disruption or basal ulnar styloid fractures. A fracture of the palmar lunate facet disrupts the buttress effect of the palmar lip and can cause instability. TFCC tears can be traumatic or degenerative[21] (**Table 7**). Synovitis in rheumatoid arthritis attrite the stabilizers of the DRUJ, causing instability.

### Evaluation

Patients may present with ulnar-sided wrist pain after a fall on outstretched hand that is usually exacerbated with loading of the wrist in extension, at the extremes of pronation or supination, or after lifting weights. Patients may report clicking and hypermobility.

There may be swelling over the ulnar side of the wrist with a dorsally subluxated ulna head

**Table 7**
**Triangular fibrocartilage complex abnormalities**

| | |
|---|---|
| Class 1—<br>traumatic | A. Central perforation<br>B. Ulnar avulsion with/without distal ulnar fracture<br>C. Distal avulsion<br>D. Radial avulsion with/without sigmoid notch fracture |
| Class 2—<br>degenerative<br>(ulnocarpal<br>abutment<br>syndrome) | A. TFCC wear<br>B. TFCC wear<br>  + lunate and/or ulnar chondromalacia<br>C. TFCC perforation<br>  + lunate and/or ulnar chondromalacia<br>D. TFCC perforation<br>  + Lunate and/or ulnar chondromalacia<br>  + Lunotriquetral ligament perforation<br>E. TFCC perforation<br>  + Lunate and/or ulnar chondromalacia<br>  + Lunotriquetral ligament perforation<br>  + Ulnocarpal arthritis |

*Data from* Palmer AK. Triangular fibrocartilage complex lesions: A classification. J Hand Surg Am 1989; 14: 594-606

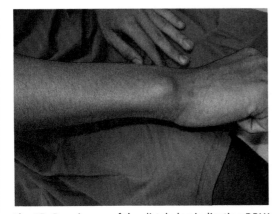

**Fig. 15.** Prominence of the distal ulna indicating DRUJ subluxation.

(**Fig. 15**). Pronation and supination are assessed with the elbows held close to the side of the body. The stability of the DRUJ is tested by first stabilizing the radius and carpus with 1 hand and then ballottement of the ulna volarly and dorsally with the wrist held in the neutral, supinated, and pronated position (Video 6) using the uninjured side as a control. Pain on compression of the DRUJ is indicative of synovitis or arthritis.

A true lateral radiograph of the wrist with greater than 50% uncovering of the ulna head (**Fig. 16**A) points toward DRUJ instability as does a widened DRUJ interval greater than 3 mm (**Fig. 16**B) on a PA projection. Dynamic DRUJ instability can be demonstrated on lateral weight-bearing

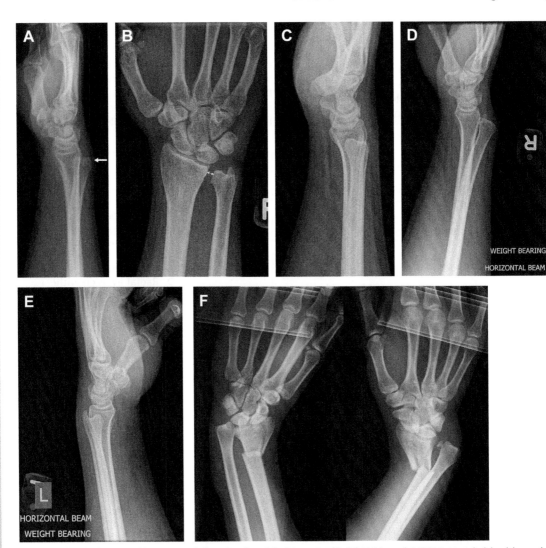

**Fig. 16.** (*A*) Significant subluxation of the ulna head (*white arrow*). (*B*) Widened DRUJ interval. (*double ended arrow*). (*C*) Non–weight-bearing films of symptomatic right DRUJ instability. (*D*) Lateral weight-bearing film demonstrates gross instability. (*E*) Opposite wrist lateral weight-bearing film for comparison. (*F*) Gross displacement of a distal radius fracture at risk of DRUJ instability.

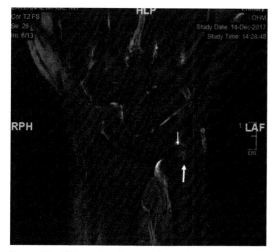

**Fig. 17.** MRI of the wrist demonstrates a complete TFCC tear (*slim arrow*) from the fovea (*broad arrow*).

projections of the wrist suspending 2.27 kg of weight (**Fig. 16**C, D) and always should be compared with the opposite side (**Fig. 16**E). DRUJ instability is an uncommon but important complication of distal radius fractures suggested by a combination of a widened distance between the distal radius and distal ulna, uncovering of the ulna head, and a basal ulna styloid fracture (**Fig. 16**F). MRIs can delineate foveal and peripheral tears of the TFCC (**Fig. 17**) as well as assess the state of cartilage in the DRUJ.

## *Treatment*

An algorithm for surgical options is presented in **Fig. 18**. Not all patients with DRUJ instability require surgical management, and progression to arthritis is uncommon.[22] TFCC injuries can occur with injuries to the extensor carpi ulnaris and fractures of the radius and/or ulna bone, and these must be addressed concurrently.

### *Acute distal radioulnar joint instability*

Nonoperative treatment of acute TFCC injury involves casting or splinting the patient in the position of stability for a period of 6 weeks. In patients with persistent DRUJ instability after fracture reduction or after a trial of nonsurgical treatment, TFCC repair is warranted. This can be done as an open procedure or arthroscopic-assisted or arthroscopic capsular repairs. An open repair can be done via an approach between the fifth and sixth extensor compartments. An inversed L-shaped capsulotomy is made (**Fig. 19**), preserving the dorsal radioulnar ligament. The TFCC is then anchored via bone tunnels or suture anchors.

Arthroscopic methods described include inside-out, outside-in, and all-arthroscopic techniques. Arthroscopy affords better visualization (Video 7) of the TFCC, less injury to surrounding structures, and better wrist motion after surgery. The standard outside-in technique, however, results in prominent suture knots in the subcutaneous layer of the skin, may cause injury

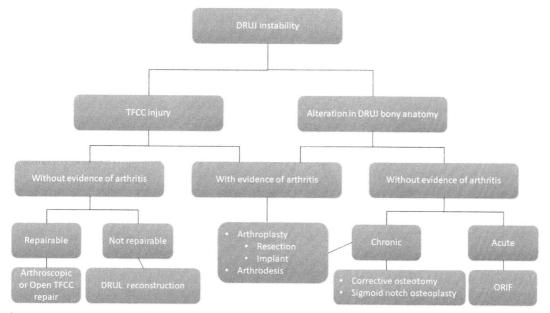

**Fig. 18.** Treatment algorithm for DRUJ instability. ORIF, Open reduction and internal fixation.

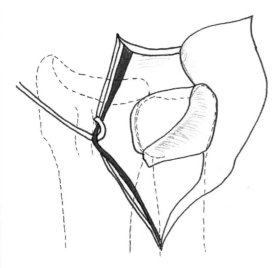

**Fig. 19.** Dorsal access to the ulnocarpal joint is via a dorsal curvilinear incision over the DRUJ and release of extensor digitiquinti minimi from its compartment before a capsulotomy is made to expose the ulna head and fovea.

to cutaneous nerves, and can be technically demanding. To date, there has been no difference shown in the outcomes between open and arthroscopic repairs.[23]

### Chronic distal radioulnar joint instability

A trial of splinting followed by strengthening of the secondary stabilizers should be attempted for chronic injuries, in addition to nonsteroidal anti-inflammatory medications and joint injections. If still symptomatic, TFCC repair can be performed as long as there is adequate substance for repair.[24] If the TFCC is irreparable, anatomic reconstruction of the distal radioulnar ligament is an option[25] (**Fig. 20**) with good long-term outcomes.[26] Instability secondary to radius or ulnar deformity requires corrective osteotomy with or without a distal radioulnar ligament reconstruction or TFCC repair.

With DRUJ arthritis, salvage procedures either in the form of resection arthroplasty, implant arthroplasty, or arthrodesis procedures are indicated. Resection arthroplasty includes hemiresection-interposition, matched ulna resection, and distal ulna resection. The Darrach procedure resects the distal ulna with a concurrent procedure to stabilize the ulna stump. The Sauvé-Kapandji procedure (**Fig. 21**) involves arthrodesis of the DRUJ, with creation of a proximal pseudoarthrosis that maintains the ulnar head in situ and provides support for the carpus.

Semiconstrained total joint prosthesis, such as the Aptis total DRUJ replacement (Aptis Medical, Louisville, KY), is ideal and allows proximal-distal migration of the radius during pronosupination but prevents anterior-posterior motion. Constrained prostheses are not used due to problems with implant loosening.

### SUMMARY

Carpal instability and DRUJ instability may arise from disruption of key ligamentous stabilizers as well as disrupted articular geometry from fractures. Crucial to the management and diagnosis is defining the structures injured and this in turn guides treatment. Radiographs, stress

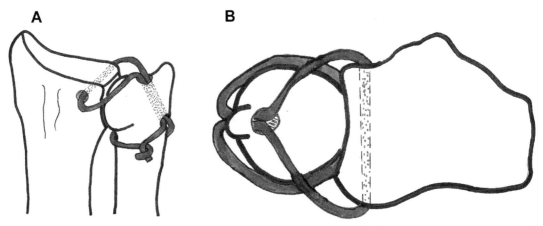

**Fig. 20.** (*A, B*) Schematic diagram of 2 described ligament reconstructions. (Adams BD, Berger RA. An anatomic reconstruction of the distal radioulnar ligaments for posttraumatic distal radioulnar joint instability. J Hand Surg Am 2002; 27: 243-251; and Teoh LC, Yam AK. Anatomic reconstruction of the distal radioulnar ligaments: Long-term results. J Hand Surg Br 2005; 30(2): 185-93.)

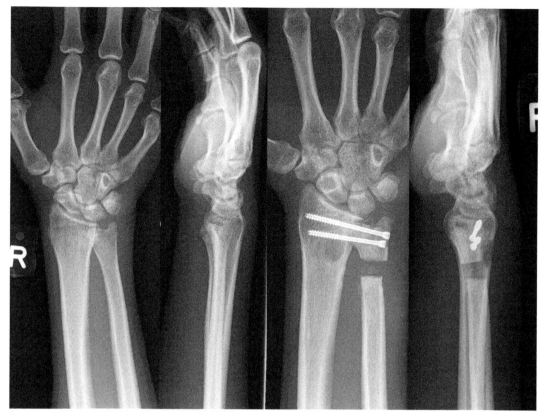

**Fig. 21.** DRUJ arthritis treated with a Sauvé-Kapandji procedure. Left panel: Posteroanterior film demonstrating DRUJ arthritis. Left middle panel: Lateral film demonstrating volar DRUJ instability. Right middle panel: Status post surgery, posteroanterior film. Right: Status post surgery, lateral film.

radiography, videofluoroscopy, and advanced imaging improve the acuity of diagnosis. Treatment also must be guided by etiology, chronicity of the injury, and severity of the instability.

## SUPPLEMENTARY DATA

Supplementary data related to this article can be found online at https://doi.org/10.1016/j.cps.2019.03.006.

## REFERENCES

1. Definition of carpal instability. The anatomy and biomechanics committee of the International Federation of Societies for surgery of the hand. J Hand Surg Am 1999;24(4):866–7.
2. Larsen CF, Amadio PC, Gilula LA, et al. Analysis of carpal instability: I. Description of the scheme [review]. J Hand Surg Am 1995;20(5):757–64.
3. Linscheid RL, Dobyns JH, Beabout JW, et al. Traumatic instability of the wrist. Diagnosis, classification, and pathomechanics. J Bone Joint Surg Am 1972;54(8):1612–32.
4. Wright TW, Dobyns JH, Linscheid RL, et al. Carpal instability non-dissociative. J Hand Surg Br 1994; 19(6):763–73.
5. Dobyns JH, Gabel GT. Gymnast's wrist. Hand Clin 1990;6:493–505.
6. Gilula LA. Carpal injuries: analytic approach and case exercises. Am J Roentgenol 1979;133(3):503–17.
7. Watson H, Ottoni L, Pitts EC, et al. Rotatory subluxation of the scaphoid: a spectrum of instability. J Hand Surg Br 1993;18:62–4.
8. Garcia-Elias M, Lluch AL, Stanley JK. Three-ligament tenodesis for the treatment of scapholunate dissociation: Indications and surgical technique. J Hand Surg Am 2006;31:125–34.
9. Geissler WB, Freeland AE, Savoie FH, et al. Intracarpal soft-tissue lesions associated with an intra-articular fracture of the distal end of the radius. J Bone Joint Surg Am 1996;78:357–65.
10. Wahegaonkar AL, Mathoulin CL. Arthroscopic dorsal capsule-ligamentous repair in the treatment of chronic scapho-lunate ligament tears. J Wrist Surg 2013;2:141–8.
11. Moran SL, Ford KS, Wulf CA, et al. Outcomes of dorsal capsulodesis and tenodesis for treatment of

scapholunate instability. J Hand Surg Am 2006;31: 1438–46.

12. Weiss AP. Scpaholunate ligament reconstruction using a bone-retinaculum-bone autograft. J Hand Surg Am 1998;23:205–15.

13. Pauchard N, Dederichs A, Segret J, et al. The role of three-ligament tenodesis in the treatment of chronic scapholunate instability. J Hand Surg Eur Vol 2012; 38:758–66.

14. Kleinman WB. Long term study of chronic scapholunate instability treated by scaphotrapeziotrapezoid arthrodesis. J Hand Surg Am 1989;14:429–45.

15. Viegas SF, Patterson RM, Peterson PD, et al. Ulnar-sided perilunate instability: an anatomic and biomechanic study. J Hand Surg Am 1990;15: 268–78.

16. Shin AY, Weinstein LP, Berger RA, et al. Treatment of isolated injuries of the lunotriquetral ligament. A comparison of arthrodesis, ligament reconstruction and ligament repair. J Bone Joint Surg Br 2001;83: 1023–8.

17. Mayfield JK. Patterns of injury to carpal ligaments. A spectrum. Clin Orthop Relat Res 1984;187: 36–42.

18. Herzberg G, Comtet JJ, Linscheid RL, et al. Perilunate dislocations and fracture-dislocations: a multicenter study. J Hand Surg Am 1993;18: 768–79.

19. Hagert E, Hagert CG. Understanding stability of the distal radioulnar joint through an understanding of its anatomy. Hand Clin 2010;26(4):459–66.

20. Tolat AR, Stanley JK, Trail IA. A cadaveric study of the anatomy and stability of the distal radioulnar joint in the coronal and transverse planes. J Hand Surg Br 1996;21(5):587–94.

21. Palmer AK. Triangular fibrocartilage complex lesions: a classification. J Hand Surg Am 1989;14: 594–606.

22. Mrkonjic A, Geijer M, Lindau T, et al. The natural course of traumatic fibrocartilage complex tears in distal radial fractures: a 13-15 year follow-up of arthroscopically diagnosed but untreated injuries. J Hand Surg Am 2012;37(8):1555–60.

23. Anderson ML, Larson AN, Moran SL, et al. Clinical comparison of arthroscopic versus open repair of triangular fibrocartilage complex tears. J Hand Surg Am 2008;33(5):675–82.

24. Hermansdorfer JD, Kleinman WB. Management of chronic peripheral tears of the triangular fibrocartilage complex. J Hand Surg Am 1991;16(2):340–6.

25. Adams BD, Berger RA. An anatomic reconstruction of the distal radioulnar ligaments for posttraumatic distal radioulnar joint instability. J Hand Surg Am 2002;27:243–51.

26. Teoh LC, Yam AK. Anatomic reconstruction of the distal radioulnar ligaments: long-term results. J Hand Surg Br 2005;30(2):185–93.

# Fractures of the Carpal Bones

Brian M. Christie, MD, MPH, Brett F. Michelotti, MD*

## KEYWORDS

• Scaphoid fracture • Fracture carpal bones • Wrist fractures

## KEY POINTS

- Carpal bone fractures may be missed on initial standard-view radiograph; therefore, a focused history and physical examination must be performed.
- Scaphoid and triquetrum fractures account for more than 80% of all carpal bone fractures.
- Scaphoid fracture management depends on anatomic location of fracture, displacement, patient activity level/occupation, and surrounding carpal stability (eg, perilunate dislocations, dorsal intercalated segment instability).
- Open reduction and internal fixation (ORIF) of scaphoid fractures can be accomplished with the use of headless compression screws. Depending on fracture location and displacement, open or percutaneous approaches from a volar or dorsal approach may be appropriate.
- Triquetral avulsion fractures may be managed conservatively with splinting or casting. Fragment excision is considered if pain persists. Displaced triquetral body fractures should be managed with ORIF.

## INTRODUCTION

Due to the tight articulations of the carpus, which maximize articular surface area and degrees of motion, vascularity is limited. With limited blood supply, fractures of the carpal bones may cause significant morbidity, both acutely and when injuries are missed. With early diagnosis and proper treatment, long-term morbidity may be avoided. Misdiagnosis or delay in diagnosis also limits our ability to determine the true incidence of carpal bone fractures. This article focuses on diagnosis and treatment of acute carpal bone fractures, emphasizing current management strategies and evidence-based care.

## CONTENT
### Scaphoid Fractures

Fractures of the scaphoid represent the most common carpal bone fracture, making up approximately 70% of carpal fractures,[1] and occurring predominantly in young men.[2] Diagnosis and proper management of scaphoid fractures is critical. The surface of the scaphoid is predominantly articular and thus has few areas for vascularization. The primary blood supply to the scaphoid is the dorsal carpal branch of the radial artery.[3] This distal to proximal pattern of blood flow limits vascularity to the proximal portion of the bone with displacement of a fracture.

Because approximately 15% to 25% of nondisplaced fractures may not appear immediately on plain radiograph,[4,5] one should be careful to prevent delay in diagnosis. Because the scaphoid is a key focus of carpal stability, the complications of nonunion, malunion, and avascular necrosis portend significant morbidity and lead to scaphoid-nonunion-advanced-collapse wrist, a predictable pattern of arthritis and instability.[6]

Most scaphoid fractures occur at the waist (70%), with 20% affecting the distal pole and 5% the proximal pole.[7] This injury is caused by forceful

Disclosure Statement: The authors have nothing to disclose.
Division of Plastic Surgery, Department of Surgery, University of Wisconsin Hospital and Clinics, 600 Highland Avenue, Madison, WI 53792-3236, USA
* Corresponding author.
E-mail address: michelotti@surgery.wisc.edu

Clin Plastic Surg 46 (2019) 469–477
https://doi.org/10.1016/j.cps.2019.03.007
0094-1298/19/Published by Elsevier Inc.

hyperextension due to a fall on an outstretched hand, or a direct blow to the wrist. Physical examination may elicit radial-sided wrist pain localized to the anatomic snuffbox or distal scaphoid tubercle, which is just distal to the distal wrist crease in line with flexor carpi radialis tendon. Imaging should first consist of plain radiographs in posteroanterior (PA), lateral, oblique, clenched fist, and scaphoid views (ulnar deviated view). Negative radiographs should prompt either short-arm casting with reexamination and radiographs in 10 to 12 days, or more advanced imaging, such as computed tomography (CT) or MRI.[4,5,8,9]

Once a scaphoid fracture is diagnosed, it may be classified by one of many systems that have been proposed. Herbert and Fisher[10] initially proposed a system based on stability (and thus, indications for surgery), consisting of Class A, or stable acute fractures; Class B, or unstable acute fractures; Class C, or delayed unions; and Class D, or nonunions. Cooney and colleagues[11] further refined this system by adding a number of findings indicative of unstable injuries, including the following:

- >1 mm displacement
- A lateral intra-scaphoid angle greater than 35°
- Bone loss or comminution
- Dorsal intercalated segment instability (DISI) alignment
- Perilunate fracture/dislocation
- Fracture of the proximal pole

Management of scaphoid fracture is determined by fracture pattern (Table 1). Nondisplaced distal pole fractures or incomplete fractures may be managed in a short-arm cast for 6 to 8 weeks. Displaced distal pole fractures are often radial-sided compression fractures, which may be managed with volar percutaneous or open screw fixation.

Stable fractures of the scaphoid waist (see previously discussed classification of Cooney and colleagues[11]) may be managed according to patient characteristics and preferences (Fig. 1). Bond and colleagues[15] demonstrated that, in a randomized military population, percutaneous cannulated screw fixation of nondisplaced scaphoid fractures resulted in faster radiographic union and return to military duty compared with cast immobilization. In 88 patients randomized to Herbert screw fixation or immobilization, Dias[16] noted no difference between groups apart from increased stiffness in the nonoperative group at 8 weeks that became equivocal by 12 weeks. For pediatric patients, sedentary individuals, or those who prefer nonoperative management, it is acceptable to place the patient in a long-arm thumb spica cast for 6 weeks, followed by short-arm thumb spica casting for 6 weeks. For young, active patients, those desiring return to work or athletic activities, or otherwise preferring early range of motion, a percutaneous or open dorsal approach with screw fixation is optimal.[12–16] Last, for any unstable fractures as mentioned previously (see Table 1), dorsal percutaneous or open screw fixation is required to optimize healing and to prevent nonunion or malunion. Combined scaphoid/distal radius fractures should prompt the surgeon to strongly consider operative fixation of the scaphoid fracture, as the prolonged immobilization required of a scaphoid fracture may result in unnecessary stiffness and loss of range of motion owing to the distal radius fracture.[17]

The evolution of headless screw design has largely replaced the use of Herbert screws, staples, and plates. Cannulated screws permit confirmation of screw placement, in which a Kirshner wire (K-wire) is used as guide to orient the screw along the long axis of the scaphoid. Approaches to the scaphoid fracture include open dorsal fixation

**Table 1**
**Scaphoid fracture location and corresponding treatment approach**

| Fracture Pattern | Displacement | Treatment | Approach |
|---|---|---|---|
| Distal pole | Nondisplaced | Casting | — |
| Distal pole | Displaced | ORIF vs percutaneous | Volar |
| Waist | Nondisplaced | Casting vs ORIF | Dorsal or volar |
| Waist | Displaced | ORIF | Dorsal of volar |
| Proximal pole | Displaced or nondisplaced | ORIF vs percutaneous | Dorsal |
| Other unstable (lateral intrascaphoid angle >35°, bone loss or comminution, DISI alignment, perilunate fracture/dislocation) | Displaced or nondisplaced | ORIF vs percutaneous | Volar and/or dorsal indicated based on injured structures |

Abbreviations: DISI, dorsal intercalated segment instability; ORIF, open reduction internal fixation.

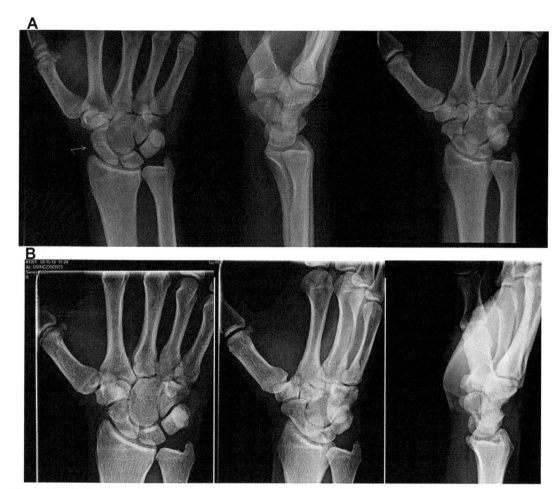

**Fig. 1.** Nondisplaced scaphoid waist fracture. Routine radiographs of a 42-year-old man with a fall onto his outstretched right wrist while playing bicycle polo, sustaining (*A*) a nondisplaced transverse fracture through the right scaphoid waist. (*B*) Repeat images 6 weeks later after casting and immobilization.

(**Fig. 2**), which lends itself to proximal pole fractures, or open volar fixation, for which both waist and distal pole fractures are amenable. Volar and dorsal percutaneous approaches have each been described.[18,19] The dorsal percutaneous approach permits more facile placement of a screw closer to the central axis of the scaphoid.[20,21] Arthroscopically assisted percutaneous scaphoid fixation, as advanced by Slade and colleagues,[22,23] has been described as a minimally invasive technique that permits direct visualization of reduction. This technique is particularly suited for unstable fractures and those with delayed presentation.[24]

Cost of scaphoid fracture diagnosis and management should be appreciated. In the setting of negative initial radiographs, numerous studies have suggested MRI as a cost-effective alternative owing to earlier mobilization and return to work.[25–27] Recently, Karl and colleagues[25] suggested that use of initial advanced imaging, such as CT or MRI, may prove less costly as compared

with immobilization and repeat radiographs at 2 weeks when considering patient productivity loss due to cast immobilization. This study has been questioned due to both low study cost estimates for advanced imaging and a presumption that advanced imaging would lead to an immediate return to work.[28] A comparison of cost of surgical and nonsurgical management suggests that nonoperative management may be costlier in terms of lost patient productivity and delayed return to work, although this may depend on patient occupation.[29–31]

## Triquetral Fractures

Fractures of the triquetrum are the second most common carpal bone fracture, making up approximately 18% of all carpal bone fractures.[1] Fractures of the triquetrum involve either the dorsal cortex of the bone or are fractures through the body of the triquetrum. Of the two,

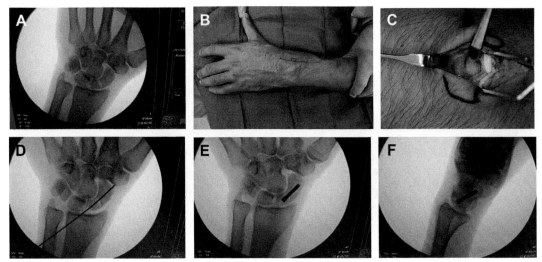

**Fig. 2.** Open dorsal approach to scaphoid waist fracture. A 23-year-old man 4 weeks after punching a heavy bag without immobilization. (*A*) Fluoroscopy demonstrates a left scaphoid waist fracture. (*B*) Preoperative markings of the Lister tubercle and planned dorsal incision over the third extensor compartment. (*C*) Dorsal approach with exposed proximal pole of scaphoid. (*D*) Guidewire placement down central axis of scaphoid. (*E, F*) Central placement of headless compression screw with anatomic reduction and compression of scaphoid.

dorsal cortical triquetral fractures are more common.[32]

The injury mechanism typically involves a fall onto either a flexed hand or an extended, ulnarly deviated hand. With dorsal cortical fractures, the ulnar styloid may act as a chisel that is driven into the cortex, causing the fracture.[33] Triquetral body fractures, however, are often the result of high-energy injuries, most commonly greater arc perilunate dislocations. In this scenario, the energy transmitted around the lunate generates a fracture through the triquetral body.[34]

Symptoms of triquetral fracture include ulnar-sided wrist pain, which localizes over the triquetrum, as well as pain with wrist flexion and extension. Diagnosis usually can be made with plain radiographs, best identified on a partial wrist pronation view.

Treatment of a dorsal cortical triquetral fracture is initially nonoperative, with casting and immobilization for 4 to 6 weeks (**Fig. 3**). Although the fragment may go on to fibrous nonunion and remain tender for several months, patients typically recover good motion and function long term.[35] If the fragment remains symptomatic after several months, it may be excised without significant functional consequence. As they are less common, there is limited evidence for the management of triquetral body fractures. Nondisplaced fractures, in isolation, may be managed similarly to dorsal cortical fractures, with casting and immobilization for 4 to 6 weeks. In the setting of a greater arc perilunate dislocation, the lunotriquetral joint

should be reduced and stabilized with K-wire fixation to immobilize the healing lunotriquetral interosseous ligament.[36] Displaced fractures should be managed with open reduction and internal fixation (ORIF).[12]

## Trapezium Fractures

Fractures of the trapezium make up approximately 4.3% of all carpal bone fractures.[1] These fractures are often associated with fractures of the thumb metacarpal or with fractures of the distal radius. The fracture pattern typically involves the body of the trapezium, or the trapezial ridge, which serves as the attachment for the transverse carpal ligament.

Patients typically present after a fall onto a radially abducted thumb, in which a vertical shear force results in a trapezial body fracture. A trapezial ridge fracture may be seen following a direct blow to the trapezium.[37] Tenderness is usually elicited dorsal and volar to the abductor pollicis longus tendon, and distal to the radial styloid. A diagnosis usually can be made by plain radiograph supplemented by a pronated anteroposterior (AP) view.

Treatment of nondisplaced fractures of the body of the trapezium can be managed with casting and immobilization, although close follow-up is recommended to assess for instability.[38,39] Displaced or unstable fractures require ORIF through a volar approach. As these fractures are often compressive in nature, they may require bone grafting to support the carpometacarpal articular surface.[40]

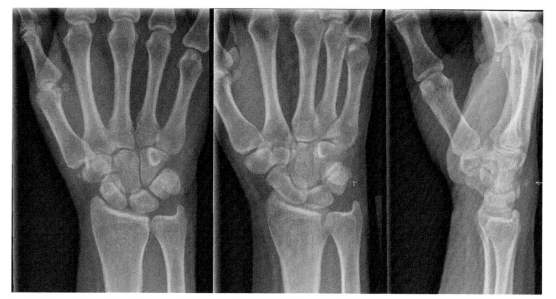

**Fig. 3.** Triquetral avulsion fracture. A 57-year-old woman following a fall on an outstretched wrist. Doral cortical avulsion fragment visualized in dorsoulnar soft tissue. This patient was managed with splinting for 6 weeks.

Fractures of the trapezial ridge are easily missed.[38,39,41] Patients with these fractures present with pain at the base of the thumb that is exacerbated by wrist flexion. Nondisplaced ridge fractures may be managed with casting and immobilization, whereas displaced fractures require ORIF.[41] Fractures of the tip of the ridge appear in the form of an avulsion fracture and are not amenable to ORIF. A trial of casting with the thumb in abduction may be attempted, although persistent symptoms should prompt excision of the fragment.[41]

### Lunate Fractures

Lunate fractures account for 3.9% of all carpal bone fractures.[1] Isolated fractures of the lunate are rare, and may be acute, as in the setting of trauma, or pathologic, following Kienbock disease. The mechanism of lunate fracture is direct axial compression of the capitate onto the lunate, and most commonly results in a transarticular fracture of the lunate body.[42] In pathologic Kienbock fractures, owing to avascular necrosis, the proximal articular surface separates from the lunate body. Patients typically present with pain and swelling over the dorsum of the wrist, deep to the fourth dorsal compartment extensor tendons. As plain radiographs often fail to demonstrate a fracture, CT or MRI may be necessary to confirm the diagnosis[43] (**Fig. 4**).

Proper treatment of lunate fractures is essential, as lunate nonunion may develop into Kienbock disease, especially those fractures that separate the volar surface from the rest of the bone.

Because 20% of lunates have only a palmar blood supply, fracture-disruption of the palmar surface in these patients may result in avascular necrosis.[44]

Nondisplaced fractures or small dorsal ridge fractures may be managed with casting and immobilization in which the flexed metacarpophalangeal joints are incorporated into the cast. Close follow-up with repeat imaging is required to assess progression to union. Displaced fractures require ORIF, especially in cases of volar subluxation of the capitate.[1] Dorsal fractures with avulsion of the scapholunate interosseous ligament require repair or reattachment of the ligament with bone tunnels or suture anchors. Last, fractures of the volar articular surface, although small, require operative fixation with a screw or K-wire, as the volar lip is critical to lunate vascularity.[12,44]

### Capitate Fractures

Capitate fractures represent 1.9% of carpal bone fractures.[1] These fractures may present in isolation or as a component of a greater arc perilunate fracture-dislocation. Patients typically present following a high-energy fall in which the wrist is hyperextended and radially deviated. In this injury, the neck of the capitate impacts the dorsal ridge of the radius and fractures.

Fractures of the capitate are often unstable, as the head and neck of the capitate are entirely covered in cartilage and are limited in limited blood supply, similar to the proximal pole of the scaphoid. Casting and immobilization is an option, but limited vascularity may result in delayed or

**A**

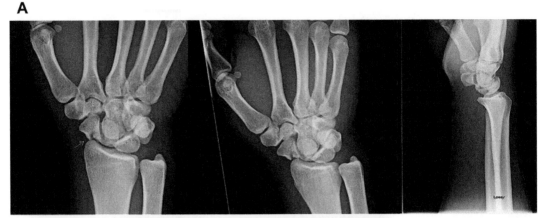

**B**

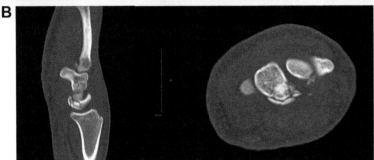

**Fig. 4.** Lunate fracture. A 23-year-old man presented following a fall onto an out-stretched hand. (*A*) Routine radiographs, while demon-strating a displaced scaphoid waist fracture, fail to demonstrate a lunate frac-ture. (*B*) CT demonstrating a comminuted fracture of the volar aspect of the lunate with an incongruent capito-lunate articular surface.

nonunion.[45] If fractures are inadequately immobilized, the capitate may collapse, requiring ORIF with bone grafting to prevent overloading of the scaphotrapeziotrapezoid and triquetrohamate joints.[46,47] Similarly, displaced fractures, delayed or collapsed fractures, and transcapitate/scaphocapitate perilunate fracture dislocations require ORIF through a dorsal approach to stabilize the capitate and reestablish carpal height.[48]

### Hamate Fractures

Fractures of the hamate represent 1.7% of all carpal bone fractures and may be divided into hook and body fractures.[1]

The hook of the hamate, which is located at the base of the hypothenar eminence, is palpated 2 cm distal and radial to the pisiform. It serves as the attachment for the transverse carpal ligament, the pisohamate ligament, the flexor digiti minimi, and the opponens digiti minimi. It also acts as a pulley for the flexor tendons of the fingers.

Injuries to the hook are most common in athletes who play in racquet, club, or bat sports, in which the object gripped can transmit a direct blow.[49–51] Fractures of the hook of the hamate often present late, and may result in persistent tenderness, ulnar nerve (or occasionally, median nerve) paresthesias,

and weakened grip.[52] Occasionally these fractures present as pain with active grasping that is worsened with ulnar deviation (due to flexor tendon irritation) or as flexor tendon rupture.[53] Plain radiographs are often unremarkable, and CT is usually required to permit diagnosis.[54]

Acute nondisplaced hook fractures may be managed with casting and immobilization. Should the fracture remain symptomatic or present with pain in a delayed fashion, excision of the hook may be performed.[50] Unfortunately, persistent pain and weakness of finger flexion have been described; as a result, internal fixation has been reported in an attempt to avoid late complications.[55,56] Due to the rarity of the fracture, long-term results are largely unknown.

Fractures of the body of the hamate are significant in that the ring and small finger carpometacarpal (CMC) joints articulate with the hamate, and their motion is important for power grip. Body fractures often occur with CMC dislocations following axial loading of a clenched fist. Nondisplaced fractures may be managed with casting and immobilization, but displaced or articular fractures involving the CMC joint should be managed with percutaneous pinning or ORIF using an H-plate or compression screws.[57]

## Pisiform Fractures

Fractures of the pisiform, a sesamoid bone in the flexor carpi ulnaris, are rare, consisting of only 1.3% of all carpal bone fractures.[1] Patients typically present following a hyperextension injury or direct blow to the hypothenar region.[58] Patients complain of ulnar-sided wrist pain, which localizes directly over the pisiform, or they may complain of ulnar neuropraxia. Diagnosis of pisiform fractures may be confirmed with plain radiograph. An oblique film, with the wrist supinated at 45° in slight extension, or as an AP with the fist clenched and in ulnar deviation will permit visualization of the pisiform.[58]

Treatment of an acute nondisplaced pisiform fracture consists of casting and immobilization for 4 to 6 weeks. Fractures that are comminuted, or progress to symptomatic nonunions, may be managed with excision.[59]

## Trapezoid Fractures

The trapezoid, in its protected position in the wrist, is very rarely fractured, and accounts for only 0.4% of all carpal bone fractures.[1] Patients present with pain over the proximal index metacarpal following a mechanism of high-energy axial loading through the index metacarpal. Plain radiograph is sufficient to confirm the diagnosis. Nondisplaced fractures are managed with casting and immobilization, whereas displaced fractures should be managed with ORIF using K-wires or screws.[60]

## SUMMARY

Fractures of the carpus are often missed initially and this oversight may result in significant morbidity due to the critical role of the wrist and interdependence of the carpal bones. Scaphoid fractures represent approximately 70% of all fractures; advanced imaging may be indicated to confirm a diagnosis if routine radiographs are negative. In cases of >1 mm displacement, lateral intrascaphoid angle greater than 35°, bone loss or comminution, DISI alignment, perilunate fracture/dislocation, or fracture of the proximal pole, ORIF is warranted. Approach and subsequent fixation depends on the location of fracture. The triquetrum represents the second most common carpal bone fracture, commonly identified as an avulsion of the dorsal cortex, which may be managed initially with immobilization and later with fragment excision if persistently symptomatic. Other carpal bone fractures are much rarer; fractures of the lunate, hamate, and pisiform are often difficult to detect on routine radiograph and require additional imaging for prompt diagnosis.

## REFERENCES

1. Papp S. Carpal bone fractures. Hand Clin 2010; 26(1):119–27.
2. Hove LM. Epidemiology of scaphoid fractures in Bergen, Norway. Scand J Plast Reconstr Surg Hand Surg 1999;33(4):423–6.
3. Gelberman RH, Menon J. The vascularity of the scaphoid bone. J Hand Surg Am 1980;5(5):508–13.
4. Gaebler C, Kukla C, Breitenseher M, et al. Magnetic resonance imaging of occult scaphoid fractures. J Trauma Acute Care Surg 1996;41(1):73.
5. Hunter JC, Escobedo EM, Wilson AJ, et al. MR imaging of clinically suspected scaphoid fractures. AJR Am J Roentgenol 1997;168(5):1287–93.
6. Shah CM, Stern PJ. Scapholunate advanced collapse (SLAC) and scaphoid nonunion advanced collapse (SNAC) wrist arthritis. Curr Rev Musculoskelet Med 2013;6(1):9–17.
7. Dias J, Kantharuban S. Treatment of scaphoid fractures. Hand Clin 2017;33(3):501–9.
8. Mallee W, Doornberg JN, Ring D, et al. Comparison of CT and MRI for diagnosis of suspected scaphoid fractures. J Bone Joint Surg Am 2011;93(1):20.
9. Brydie A, Raby N. Early MRI in the management of clinical scaphoid fracture. Br J Radiol 2003; 76(905):296–300.
10. Herbert T, Fisher W. Management of the fractured scaphoid using a new bone screw. J Bone Joint Surg Br 1984;66-B(1):114–23.
11. Cooney WP, Dobyns JH, Linscheid RL. Fractures of the scaphoid: a rational approach to management. Clin Orthop 1980;149:90–7.
12. Wolfe SW, Hotchkiss RN, Pederson WC, et al. Green's operative hand surgery. 2017. Available at: https://www.clinicalkey.com/dura/browse/bookChapter/3-s2.0-C20121066969. Accessed August 17, 2018.
13. Modi CS, Nancoo T, Powers D, et al. Operative versus nonoperative treatment of acute undisplaced and minimally displaced scaphoid waist fractures—a systematic review. Injury 2009;40(3):268–73.
14. Adolfsson L, Lindau T, Arner M. Acutrak screw fixation versus cast immobilisation for undisplaced scaphoid waist fractures. J Hand Surg Br 2001; 26(3):192–5.
15. Bond CD, Shin AY, McBride MT, et al. Percutaneous screw fixation or cast immobilization for nondisplaced scaphoid fractures. J Bone Joint Surg Am 2001;83(4):483.
16. Dias JJ, Wildin CJ, Bhowal B, et al. Should acute scaphoid fractures be fixed? A randomized controlled trial. J Bone Joint Surg Am 2005;87(10):2160.
17. Trumble TE, Benirschke SK, Vedder NB. Ipsilateral fractures of the scaphoid and radius. J Hand Surg 1993;18(1):8–14.
18. Slade JF, Jaskwhich D. Percutaneous fixation of scaphoid fractures. Hand Clin 2001;17(4):553–74.

19. Haddad FS, Goddard NJ. Acute percutaneous scaphoid fixation. A pilot study. J Bone Joint Surg Br 1998;80(1):95–9.

20. Jeon I-H, Micic ID, Oh C-W, et al. Percutaneous screw fixation for scaphoid fracture: a comparison between the dorsal and the volar approaches. J Hand Surg Am 2009;34(2):228–36.e1.

21. Chan KW, McAdams TR. Central screw placement in percutaneous screw scaphoid fixation: a cadaveric comparison of proximal and distal techniques. J Hand Surg Am 2004;29(1):74–9.

22. Slade JFI, Gutow AP, Geissler WB. Percutaneous internal fixation of scaphoid fractures via an arthroscopically assisted dorsal approach. J Bone Joint Surg Am 2002;84(suppl_2):S21.

23. Slade JF, Gillon T. Retrospective review of 234 scaphoid fractures and nonunions treated with arthroscopy for union and complications. Scand J Surg 2008;97(4):280–9.

24. Slade JFI, Geissler WB, Gutow AP, et al. Percutaneous internal fixation of selected scaphoid nonunions with an arthroscopically assisted dorsal approach. J Bone Joint Surg Am 2003; 85(suppl_4):20.

25. Karl JW, Swart E, Strauch RJ. Diagnosis of occult scaphoid fractures: a cost-effectiveness analysis. J Bone Joint Surg Am 2015;97(22):1860.

26. Brooks S, Cicuttini FM, Lim S, et al. Cost effectiveness of adding magnetic resonance imaging to the usual management of suspected scaphoid fractures. Br J Sports Med 2005;39(2):75–9.

27. Dorsay TA, Major NM, Helms CA. Cost-effectiveness of immediate MR imaging versus traditional follow-up for revealing radiographically occult scaphoid fractures. Am J Roentgenol 2001;177(6):1257–63.

28. Michelotti BF, Sanchez RJ, Christie B, et al. A deeper dive into cost 2017.

29. Davis EN, Chung KC, Kotsis SV, et al. A cost/utility analysis of open reduction and internal fixation versus cast immobilization for acute nondisplaced mid-waist scaphoid fractures. Plast Reconstr Surg 2006;117(4):1223–35.

30. Vinnars B, Ekenstam FA, Gerdin B. Comparison of direct and indirect costs of internal fixation and cast treatment in acute scaphoid fractures: a randomized trial involving 52 patients. Acta Orthop 2007;78(5):672–9.

31. Arora R, Gschwentner M, Krappinger D, et al. Fixation of nondisplaced scaphoid fractures: making treatment cost effective. Arch Orthop Trauma Surg 2007;127(1):39–46.

32. van Onselen EBH, Karim RB, Hage JJ, et al. Prevalence and distribution of hand fractures. J Hand Surg Br 2003;28(5):491–5.

33. Garcia-Elias M. Dorsal fractures of the triquetrum-avulsion or compression fractures? J Hand Surg Am 1987;12(2):266–8.

34. Levy M, Fischel RE, Stern GM, et al. Chip fractures of the os triquetrum: the mechanism of injury. J Bone Joint Surg Br 1979;61-B(3):355–7.

35. Höcker K, Menschik A. Chip fractures of the triquetrum. Mechanism, classification and results. J Hand Surg Br 1994;19(5):584–8.

36. Stanbury SJ, Elfar JC. Perilunate dislocation and perilunate fracture-dislocation. J Am Acad Orthop Surg 2011;19(9):554.

37. Pointu J, Schwenck JP, Destree G, et al. Fractures of the trapezium. Mechanisms. Anatomopathology and therapeutic indications. Rev Chir Orthop Reparatrice Appar Mot 1988;74(5): 454–65 [in French].

38. McGuigan FX, Culp RW. Surgical treatment of intra-articular fractures of the trapezium. J Hand Surg Am 2002;27(4):697–703.

39. Walker JL, Greene TL, Lunseth PA. Fractures of the body of the trapezium. J Orthop Trauma 1988;2(1):22–8.

40. Matzon JL, Reb CW, Danowski RM, et al. Single-incision open reduction and internal fixation of comminuted trapezium fractures with distal radius cancellous autograft. Tech Hand Up Extrem Surg 2015;19(1):40–5.

41. Palmer AK. Trapezial ridge fractures. J Hand Surg Am 1981;6(6):561–4.

42. Teisen H, Hjarbaek J. Classification of fresh fractures of the lunate. J Hand Surg Br 1988;13(4):458–62.

43. Arnaiz J, Piedra T, Cerezal L, et al. Imaging of Kienböck disease. Am J Roentgenol 2014;203(1):131–9.

44. Gelberman RH, Bauman TD, Menon J, et al. The vascularity of the lunate bone and Kienböck's disease. J Hand Surg Am 1980;5(3):272–8.

45. Vander Grend R, Dell PC, Glowczewskie F, et al. Intraosseous blood supply of the capitate and its correlation with aseptic necrosis. J Hand Surg Am 1984;9(5):677–80.

46. Minami M, Yamazaki J, Chisaka N, et al. Nonunion of the capitate. J Hand Surg Am 1987;12(6):1089–91.

47. Yoshihara M, Sakai A, Toba N, et al. Nonunion of the isolated capitate waist fracture. J Orthop Sci 2002; 7(5):578–80.

48. Herzberg G, Forissier D. Acute dorsal trans-scaphoid perilunate fracture-dislocations: medium-term results. J Hand Surg Br 2002;27(6):498–502.

49. Weiland AJ. Treatment of fracture of hook of the hamate in baseball players. Hand Clin 2012; 28(3):301.

50. Devers BN, Douglas KC, Naik RD, et al. Outcomes of hook of hamate fracture excision in high-level amateur athletes. J Hand Surg Am 2013;38(1): 72–6.

51. Stark HH, Jobe FW, Boyes JH, et al. Fracture of the hook of the hamate in athletes. J Bone Joint Surg Am 1977;59(5):575–82.

52. Bishop AT, Beckenbaugh RD. Fracture of the hamate hook. J Hand Surg Am 1988;13(1):135–9.

53. Milek MA, Boulas HJ. Flexor tendon ruptures secondary to hamate hook fractures. J Hand Surg Am 1990;15(5):740–4.

54. Andresen R, Radmer S, Sparmann M, et al. Imaging of hamate bone fractures in conventional X-rays and high-resolution computed tomography. An in vitro study. Invest Radiol 1999;34(1):46–50.

55. Watson HK, Rogers WD. Nonunion of the hook of the hamate: an argument for bone grafting the nonunion. J Hand Surg Am 1989;14(3):486–90.

56. Scheufler O, Radmer S, Andresen R. Dorsal percutaneous cannulated mini-screw fixation for fractures of the hamate hook. Hand Surg 2012; 17(2):287–93.

57. Hirano K, Inoue G. Classification and treatment of hamate fractures. Hand Surg 2005;10(2–3): 151–7.

58. Fleege MA, Jebson PJ, Renfrew DL, et al. Pisiform fractures. Skeletal Radiol 1991;20(3):169–72.

59. Palmieri TJ. Pisiform area pain treatment by pisiform excision. J Hand Surg Am 1982;7(5):477–80.

60. Yasuwaki Y, Nagata Y, Yamamoto T, et al. Fracture of the trapezoid bone: a case report. J Hand Surg Am 1994;19(3):457–9.

# Joint Fusion and Arthroplasty in the Hand

Michiro Yamamoto, MD, PhD[a],*, Kevin C. Chung, MD, MS[b]

## KEYWORDS

- Joint fusion • Arthroplasty • Implant • Osteochondral graft

## KEY POINTS

- Joint fusion and arthroplasty of the hand are important techniques for restoring hand function. Surgeons must appropriately judge indications and select surgical procedures.
- Because there are currently no available disease-modifying osteoarthritis drugs, reconstructive surgery has an important role in restoring hand function.
- Continuous efforts to develop novel implants and surgical techniques are required to ensure better outcomes.

## INTRODUCTION

There are several options for osteoarthritis or inflammatory arthritis of the hand. Surgical procedures can be divided into joint fusion and arthroplasty. Arthroplasty is further divided into implant arthroplasty, arthroplasty with an autologous osteochondral graft, and vascularized joint transfer to reconstruct the injured joint. The best option depends on the condition of the hand. The indication for each procedure is critical to outcome success (**Table 1**).

## PREOPERATIVE ASSESSMENT

Surgical management is considered for patients with painful, deformed, unstable, or stiff joints after nonsurgical treatment failure. Symptom cause and patient age are important factors in surgical procedure selection. Arthrodesis can be indicated for patients of all ages when joint reconstruction is not indicated. Arthroplasty with an autologous graft is indicated for young patients with posttraumatic arthritis, whereas implant arthroplasty is

indicated for an elderly patient with degenerative or inflammatory arthritis because implants will require revision several years later. Inflammatory arthritis includes not only rheumatoid arthritis (RA) but also psoriatic arthritis and systemic lupus erythematosus. Surgeons must carefully check each patient's medications, general condition, disease momentum, and treatment expectations.

Once finger surgery is scheduled, joint active and passive range of motion (ROM), grip and pinch strength, a pain scale such as the visual analog scale (VAS), and patient-reported outcome measures (PROMs) should be recorded for comparison with further assessments. Various PROMs are used to evaluate outcomes after arthroplasty or arthrodesis of the hand. Disability of the Arm, Shoulder, and Hand (DASH) is the most frequently used outcome measure,[1,2] followed by the quick DASH,[3,4] Michigan Hand Questionnaire (MHQ),[5,6] Canadian Occupational Performance Measure,[7] and Patient Evaluation Measure (PEM).[8,9]

Preoperative radiography is necessary to evaluate joint condition. A plain radiograph is taken to assess joint deformity, bone stock, and cavity

Disclosure Statement: The authors have nothing to disclose.
a Department of Hand Surgery, Nagoya University Graduate School of Medicine, 65 Tsurumai-cho, Showa-ku, Nagoya, Aichi 466-8550, Japan; b Section of Plastic Surgery, Department of Surgery, Michigan Medicine, Comprehensive Hand Center, Michigan Medicine, University of Michigan, 2130 Taubman Center, SPC 5340, 1500 East Medical Center Drive, Ann Arbor, MI 48109-5340, USA
* Corresponding author.
*E-mail address:* michi-ya@med.nagoya-u.ac.jp

Clin Plastic Surg 46 (2019) 479–488
https://doi.org/10.1016/j.cps.2019.03.008

**Table 1**
**Summary of surgical indication**

| Surgery | Indication | Contraindication |
| --- | --- | --- |
| Joint fusion | Painful DIP, PIP, and MCP joint arthritis with or without poor soft tissue condition<br>Post failed arthroplasty | Joint with possible arthroplasty |
| Silicone implant arthroplasty | MCP joint arthritis with moderate to severe deformity<br>Painful PIP joint arthritis | Young patient |
| Surface replacement arthroplasty | MCP and PIP joint arthritis with minimal to moderate deformity<br><br>Painful PIP joint arthritis | MCP and PIP joint arthritis with severe deformity<br>Young patient |
| Arthroplasty with autologous osteochondral cartilage graft | MCP and PIP joint (posttraumatic) osteoarthritis with age <50 y | Elderly patients |
| Vascularized joint transfer | MCP and PIP joint disorder of young patients | Elderly patients |

*Abbreviations:* DIP, distal interphalangeal; MCP, metacarpophalangeal; PIP, proximal interphalangeal.

size. Computed tomography and MRI are sometimes used to visualize both bone quality and soft tissue condition. Ultrasonography has been used more widely for inflammatory arthritis to evaluate synovitis with or without Doppler ultrasonography.[10–12]

## ARTHRODESIS

Arthrodesis of the metacarpophalangeal (MCP) and interphalangeal joints of the hand is indicated for patients with severe pain, deformity, instability, or primary arthroplasty failure, although MCP joint fusion is seldom performed because the arc of finger motions starts at the MCP joint. Fusion of the MCP joint limits motion; therefore, arthroplasty is the preferred choice. Arthrodesis of the MCP joint can be performed after bone tumor resection (**Fig. 1**). The most common indication is Heberden nodules (**Fig. 2**). Pain and instability restoration are expected to improve hand function, appearance, and patient satisfaction.

Finger position, angle, and length can be designed by arthrodesis. The surgeon must carefully evaluate the patient's needs. The most appropriate joint position should be selected. Increasing flexion angle is generally applied for MCP or proximal interphalangeal (PIP) joints of the ulnar finger, which is important for grasping. For example, the index finger MCP joint is fixed at 25°, the middle finger at 30°, the ring finger at 35°, and the small finger at 40°. Amount of flexion for the PIP joint is recommended to be 30° to 40°; however, these positions are changed according to patient needs.[13,14]

Various surgical techniques are reported using Kirshner wire, tension band wiring, screws, and plates.[15–18] Autologous and/or artificial bone grafts are used according to bone quality and stock. Rigid fixation is necessary to achieve early bony fusion. Infection and delayed or nonunion are reported complications.[14]

## ARTHROPLASTY

Numerous types of finger arthroplasties have been reported: implant arthroplasty, arthroplasty with an autologous osteochondral graft, and vascularized joint transfer.

## HINGED METAL IMPLANT ARTHROPLASTY

Hinged metal implants for the MCP and PIP joints were introduced by Brannon and Klein in 1959.[19] This was thought to be the first report on finger total joint arthroplasty with an implant. However, their results were unsatisfactory because hinged metal implants have common problems of bone absorption, implant loosening, and osteophyte formation. Hinged metal implants are used much less often than silicone implants and surface replacement (SR) arthroplasty.

## SILICONE ARTHROPLASTY

Since Swanson[20] introduced the silicone implant to treat PIP and MCP joint arthritis, these implants have been widely used for more than half a century. Silicone implants have been used to treat both MCP joint RA and PIP joint

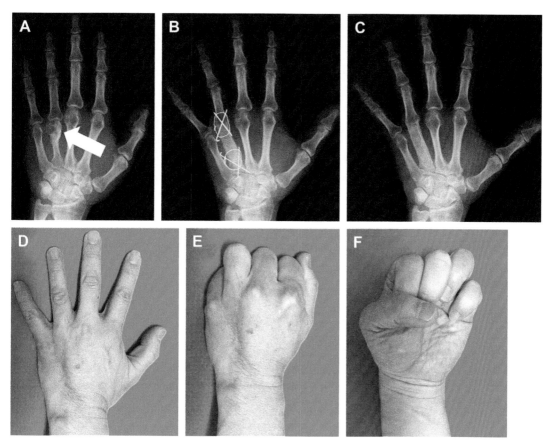

**Fig. 1.** Metacarpophalangeal joint fusion after bone tumor resection. Preoperative radiograph of the hand (*A*). The white arrow indicates a recurrent giant cell tumor of the fourth metacarpal head. Metacarpophalangeal joint fusion with autologous iliac bone grafting was performed using tension band wiring (*B*). A radiograph reveals bony fusion and no evidence of disease at 7-year follow-up (*C*). Finger motion after fourth metacarpophalangeal joint fusion (*D–F*).

osteoarthritis.[21] Most surgeons have favored a dorsal approach for silicone implants because of easier joint exposure. A volar approach for the PIP joint was introduced by Schneider in 1991.[22] He emphasized the merit of a volar approach, as the extensor system was not violated and immediate motion was feasible (**Fig. 3**). He also stated that the combination use with local anesthesia enabled complete evaluation during surgery.

In a systematic review, the revision surgery rate after silicone arthroplasty for the PIP joint using a dorsal approach was higher than that of a volar approach.[23] More than a few patients required secondary tenolysis or revision surgery for stiffness after dorsal-approach silicone arthroplasty, but none required the same after volar-approach silicone arthroplasty. The complication rates of silicone implants for the PIP joint using a volar or dorsal approach were 6% at the mean 41-month follow-up and 11% at the mean 17-month follow-up, respectively.[24]

## SILICONE IMPLANT TYPES

Swanson flexible finger joint implants (Wright Medical Technology Inc, Arlington, TN) have traditionally been used the most frequently.[1] The NeuFlex silicone implant (Depuy, Warsaw, IN) and the Avanta silicone implant (Avanta Orthopaedice, San Diego, CA) were recently introduced with favorable outcomes. The NeuFlex silicone implant has a 15° prebend at the PIP hinge to improve postoperative flexion and durability against implant fracture.[6] The Avanta silicone implant has a volarly shifted center of flexion compared with the Swanson implant to improve the postoperative flexion angle.[3] There are not significant differences between silicone implant types in terms of postoperative flexion or implant fracture rates in treatment of the PIP joint. However, a prospective randomized controlled study comparing NeuFlex and Swanson implants for RA showed that the NeuFlex group demonstrated superior postoperative arc of motion (AOM) of the MCP joint.[25]

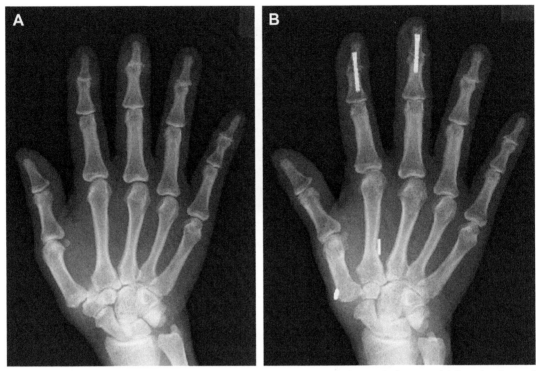

**Fig. 2.** Distal interphalangeal joint fusion using a screw. Preoperative radiograph shows multiple Heberden nodules and thumb carpometacarpal (CM) joint osteoarthritis (A). Index and middle finger distal interphalangeal joint fusion with screws and thumb CM joint suspension arthroplasty using a suture button (B).

MCP joints are frequently affected in rheumatoid patients. Silicone metacarpophalangeal joint arthroplasty (SMPA) can be a good option for patients with RA with severe deformities of the MCP joints. Chung and colleagues[26] conducted a prospective cohort study of SMPA for patients with RA. At 3 years, the mean overall MHQ score showed significant improvement in the surgical versus nonsurgical group. At 7 years, SMPA did not improve in grip and pinch strength; however, MHQ scores showed large improvements postoperatively with low rates of implant fracture or

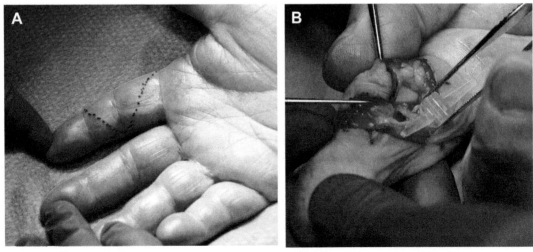

**Fig. 3.** Silicone implant using the volar approach for the index PIP joint osteoarthritis. A zigzag incision is made at the volar side of the index finger PIP joint (A). A silicone implant is inserted into the PIP joint (B).

deformity.[27] Trail and colleagues[28] reported on a 17-year survivorship analysis of silastic MCP joint replacement, as two-thirds of the implants were verified as broken on radiographs. Surgeons must inform patients about possible implant failure (**Fig. 4**).

## SURFACE REPLACEMENT ARTHROPLASTY
### Surface Replacement–Proximal Interphalangeal and Surface Replacement–Metacarpophalangeal Implant

The first anatomic surface replacement arthroplasty was reported by Linscheid and colleagues in 1979.[29] The initial Mayo-type surface replacement arthroplasty was a mated internally constrained prosthesis; therefore, progressive erosions of the cortical bone occurred. The results of the initial constrained prosthesis were unsatisfactory like those of hinged metal implants. In 1997, Linscheid and colleagues[30] reported on an unconstrained surface replacement arthroplasty for the PIP joint with better outcomes. Because of several improvements in material, design, and technique, SR-PIP and SR-MCP are still available (**Fig. 5**). Current SR-PIP prostheses have a titanium alloy stem that is intended to integrate with bony surfaces.[30] SR-MCP has a semiconstrained design and is manufactured from cobalt chrome and polyethylene. The current SR-PIP has a cementless design, whereas the SR-MCP is implanted with cement. Unconstrained surface replacement arthroplasty for the MCP joint is indicated for patients with good bone stock and fewer deformities. Osteoarthritis rather than RA of the MCP joint can be a candidate for surface replacement arthroplasty.[31]

### PyroCarbon Implant

The PyroCarbon implant has an iso-elasticity to cortical bone with higher durability and biocompatibility. PyroCarbon has been introduced for artificial heart valve and used in more than 4 million heart valves annually.[32] In the field of hand surgery, the first MCP joint surface replacement using PyroCarbon was developed and reported by Beckenbaugh in 1983.[33] Since then, PyroCarbon implants have been used in various forms, such as hemi, total, and interposition arthroplasty with approximately 15 currently available types.[34] The PyroCarbon implant has a microporous structure that enhances bone fixation and is used without cement. However, loosening and subsidence of the PyroCarbon implant have been reported frequently at longer follow-up. An experimental study showed that the PyroCarbon has poorer implant–bone contact

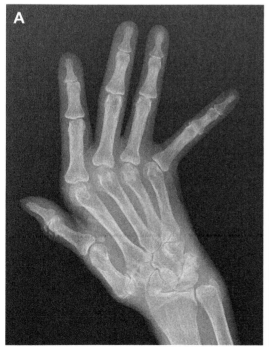
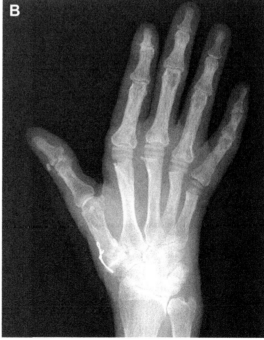

**Fig. 4.** SMPA. Preoperative radiograph showing a metacarpophalangeal (MCP) joint deformity of all fingers and thumb carpometacarpal (CM) joint dislocation (*A*). This patient has systemic lupus erythematosus, not RA. Note the mild MCP joint erosion in all fingers as well as severe ulnar deviations. Thumb CM joint fusion and SMPA of all fingers were performed. After surgery, the alignment of all fingers was improved (*B*).

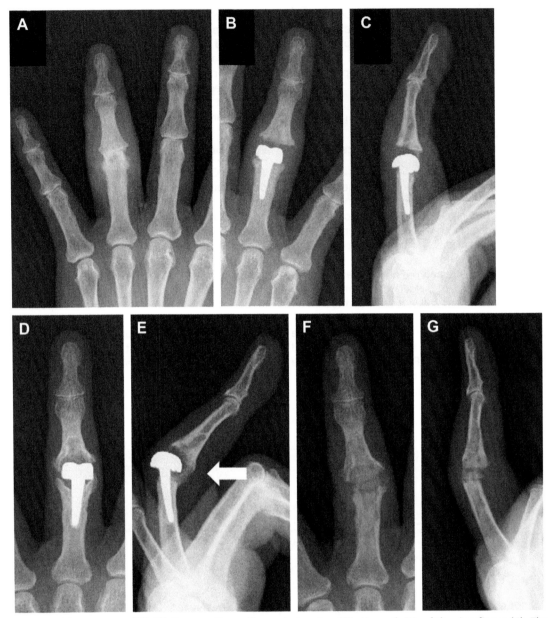

**Fig. 5.** Revision surgery of SR-PIP. Preoperative radiograph showing PIP osteoarthritis of the ring finger (*A*). The SR-PIP prosthesis was inserted with cement through the dorsal approach (*B, C*). At 10 years, the PIP joint of the ring finger developed bony ankylosis (*D, E*). The white arrow shows bony ankylosis at the volar side. The implant was removed and converted to a silicone implant with a volar approach (*F, G*).

than titanium in vivo. PyroCarbon PIP and MCP arthroplasty has the potential to achieve pain relief, a good AOM, and deformity correction. The implant survival rate after MCP arthroplasty in noninflammatory arthritis was reportedly 88% at 10 years.[35] Osteoarthritis of the MCP joint is a good indication for PyroCarbon arthroplasty. However, the results in PIP joints were unpredictable because of a high migration rate and not better than other arthroplasties.[36]

## CapFlex-Proximal Interphalangeal

An implant's surface is important because it affects osteointegration. The Capflex-PIP (KLS Martin Group, Tuttlingen, Germany) has a titanium pore base for cement-free osteointegration similar to that of another recent version of the SR-PIP implant. Schindele and colleagues[37] reported favorable results with a 1-year follow-up of 50 patients. The AOM improved from 43.4 to 55.9 and only 5 patients required revision surgery. A painful PIP joint due to degenerative or posttraumatic osteoarthritis is a good indication. For patients with inflammatory arthritis, PIP joints with low inflammatory activity and good bone preservation are also indicated for surgery.

### MatOrtho Proximal Interphalangeal Replacement

In 2016, Flannery and colleagues[9] reported on MatOrtho proximal interphalangeal replacement (PIPR) (Mole Business Park, Leatherhead, UK) arthroplasties with a minimum 2-year follow-up. The MatOrtho PIPR is a cementless surface replacement prosthesis with a hydroxyapatite coating to enhance osteointegration. A total of 109 implants were inserted in 56 patients using a dorsal approach. Significant postoperative improvements in functional scores using the MHQ and PEM were noted. A radiograph revealed no evidence of loosening or subsidence of implant at the final follow-up. A Kaplan-Meier survival analysis showed an 85% overall survival rate at 77 months if implant removal was considered the end point. They cautioned against its use for a stiff or severely deformed or unstable joint.

### TACTYS

The TACTYS (Stryker-Memometal, Bruz, France) is also an unconstrained total PIP joint prosthesis; its proximal and distal stems are created of an anatomic titanium alloy with a hydroxyapatite coating on the epiphyseal-metaphyseal portion.[38] Degeorge and colleagues[39] reported on a minimum 1-year follow-up study of the TACTYS implant with a dorsal approach. Pain, AOM, grip strength, and quick DASH scores were significantly improved after surgery. Four patients required reoperation: dorsal tenoarthrolysis in 3 and correction of swan neck deformity in 1. These results were comparable to those of other PIP arthroplasties.

### SURFACE REPLACEMENT ARTHROPLASTY WITH A VOLAR APPROACH

Although favorable results of silicone implant for the PIP joint using a volar approach were reported, such an approach for surface replacement arthroplasty does not always provide satisfactory results. Shirakawa and Shirota[40] reported on postoperative contracture of the PIP joint using the Ishizuki Total Finger System (Nakashima Medical, Okayama, Japan) in 12 cases and the Self-Locking Finger Joint System (Nakashima Medical) in 3. Eight of 15 fingers required revision surgery

due to contracture during the average 73 months of follow-up. The mean AOM decreased from 46° preoperatively to 40° at the final follow-up.

Better surgical outcomes of SR-PIP arthroplasty were recently reported. Trumble and Heaton[41] implanted SR-PIP in 21 patients with primary osteoarthritis using a volar approach. Although 4 patients (21%) required extensor tenolysis, the average AOM significantly improved from 29° to 87°, whereas the mean DASH score significantly improved from 43 to 14. They concluded that SR-PIP arthroplasty with a volar approach enables early exercise and greater improvements in AOM and DASH scores.[41] Swan neck deformity and flexor tendon adhesion might be concerns with the volar approach. However, there was no incidence of swan neck deformity with repair of the volar plate and postoperative use of a dorsal blocking orthosis. Furthermore, flexor tendon adhesions were not encountered because of the early ROM exercise.[41]

Appropriate implant design selection, surgical approach, and patient condition are all essential factors for successful arthroplasty. Unlike hinged implants, these unconstrained surface replacement arthroplasties have a risk of joint dislocation or instability. Careful soft tissue rebalancing and the reconstruction of good finger alignment are necessary to ensure promising results.

### ARTHROPLASTY WITH AUTOLOGOUS OSTEOCHONDRAL CARTILAGE GRAFT

Hemi-hamate replacement arthroplasty and volar plate arthroplasty are used to treat chronic fracture dislocation of the PIP joint.[42–44] Hemi-hamate arthroplasty reconstructs the injured volar to proximal surface of the middle phalanx to avoid dorsal subluxation. Although volar plate arthroplasty does not repair bone defects of the joint surface, it can help avoid dorsal subluxation of the PIP joint. Hemi-hamate and volar plate arthroplasties can be combined to augment PIP joint stability, even in chronic cases.[45]

Osteochondral grafting from the costo-osteochondral junction for posttraumatic osteoarthritis of the finger has been reported.[46,47] This technique has been used as hemi-arthroplasty. However, total joint reconstruction with costal osteochondral graft for posttraumatic MCP joint ankylosis was reported recently with a good result at 2-year follow-up.[48] This technique may be an option for a young patient with posttraumatic osteoarthritis of the finger.

More recently, Kodama and colleagues[49] reported on arthroplasty with osteochondral grafting from the knee for posttraumatic or degenerative osteoarthritis of the fingers. Ten patients underwent reconstruction of MCP joint (4 cases) and PIP joint (6 cases). Total arthroplasty was performed in 4 cases (1 MCP, 3 PIP), and hemiarthroplasty was performed in 6 cases (3 MCP, 3 PIP). The mean patient age was 35 years (range, 15–52) and the mean follow-up period was 48 months (range, 16–89). The osteochondral graft healed in all cases without resorption or necrosis noted on radiograph. The mean AOM of the affected joint was significantly improved from 21 to 61, whereas the mean VAS for pain improved significantly from 7.0 to 1.5. There were no cases of donor-site morbidity. Revision surgeries were required for tenolysis in 2 patients and screw removal in 2 patients. The investigators reported that the indications for this technique are age younger than 50 years and no osteoarthritis of the knee, which begins to develop at approximately 50 years of age.[49]

## VASCULARIZED JOINT TRANSFER

Vascularized toe joint transfer is another treatment option for posttraumatic osteoarthritis of the finger. This procedure enables simultaneous soft tissue reconstruction, and bony growth of the joint can be expected for patients with premature bones. Therefore, vascularized toe joint transfer is indicated for young and active patients with finger joint disorders[50–52]; however, its poor outcome demonstrated in a systematic review does not justify its wide application for reconstructing posttraumatic finger joints. Vascularized toe joint transfer has a worse AOM and higher complication rate than silicone implant arthroplasty for PIP and MCP joints.[53]

In summary, numerous options for posttraumatic, degenerative, or inflammatory arthritis of the hand have been introduced. Patient condition, appropriate indications, and surgeon skill are essential to successful management. Every technique has advantages and disadvantages. Because there are no currently available disease-modifying osteoarthritis drugs, reconstructive surgery has an important role in restoring hand function. Continuous efforts to develop novel implants and surgical techniques are required to ensure better outcomes.

## REFERENCES

1. Daecke W, Kaszap B, Martini AK, et al. A prospective, randomized comparison of 3 types of proximal interphalangeal joint arthroplasty. J Hand Surg 2012;37(9):1770–9.e1-3.

2. Dickson DR, Nuttall D, Watts AC, et al. Pyrocarbon proximal interphalangeal joint arthroplasty: minimum five-year follow-up. J Hand Surg 2015;40(11):2142–8.e4.

3. Proubasta IR, Lamas CG, Natera L, et al. Silicone proximal interphalangeal joint arthroplasty for primary osteoarthritis using a volar approach. J Hand Surg 2014;39(6):1075–81.

4. Merle M, Villani F, Lallemand B, et al. Proximal interphalangeal joint arthroplasty with silicone implants (NeuFlex) by a lateral approach: a series of 51 cases. J Hand Surg Eur Vol 2012;37(1):50–5.

5. Ono S, Shauver MJ, Chang KW, et al. Outcomes of pyrolytic carbon arthroplasty for the proximal interphalangeal joint at 44 months' mean follow-up. Plast Reconstr Surg 2012;129(5):1139–50.

6. Namdari S, Weiss AP. Anatomically neutral silicone small joint arthroplasty for osteoarthritis. J Hand Surg 2009;34(2):292–300.

7. Pettersson K, Wagnsjo P, Hulin E. Replacement of proximal interphalangeal joints with new ceramic arthroplasty: a prospective series of 20 proximal interphalangeal joint replacements. Scand J Plast Reconstr Surg Hand Surg 2006;40(5):291–6.

8. Schindele SF, Hensler S, Audigé L, et al. A modular surface gliding implant (CapFlex-PIP) for proximal interphalangeal joint osteoarthritis: a prospective case series. J Hand Surg 2015;40(2):334–40.

9. Flannery O, Harley O, Badge R, et al. MatOrtho proximal interphalangeal joint arthroplasty: minimum 2-year follow-up. J Hand Surg Eur Vol 2016;41(9):910–6.

10. Fournié B, Margarit-Coll N, de Ribes TLC, et al. Extrasynovial ultrasound abnormalities in the psoriatic finger. Prospective comparative power-Doppler study versus rheumatoid arthritis. Joint Bone Spine 2006;73(5):527–31.

11. Scheel AK, Hermann KGA, Kahler E, et al. A novel ultrasonographic synovitis scoring system suitable for analyzing finger joint inflammation in rheumatoid arthritis. Arthritis Rheum 2005;52(3):733–43.

12. Scheel AK, Hermann KA, Ohrndorf S, et al. Prospective 7 year follow up imaging study comparing radiography, ultrasonography, and magnetic resonance imaging in rheumatoid arthritis finger joints. Ann Rheum Dis 2006;65(5):595–600.

13. Carroll RE, Hill NA. Small joint arthrodesis in hand reconstruction. J Bone Joint Surg Am 1969;51(6):1219–21.

14. Burton RI, Margles SW, Lunseth PA. Small-joint arthrodesis in the hand. J Hand Surg Am 1986;11(5):678–82.

15. Engel J, Tsur H, Farin I. A comparison between K-wire and compression screw fixation after arthodesis of the distal interphalangeal joint. Plast Reconstr Surg 1977;60(4):611–4.

16. Allende BT, Engelem JC. Tension-band arthrodesis in the finger joints. J Hand Surg 1980;5(3):269–71.

17. Faithfull DK, Herbert TJ. Small joint fusions of the hand using the Herbert Bone Screw. J Hand Surg Br 1984;9(2):167–8.

18. Leibovic SJ, Strickland JW. Arthrodesis of the proximal interphalangeal joint of the finger: comparison of the use of the Herbert screw with other fixation methods. J Hand Surg 1994;19(2):181–8.

19. Brannon EW, Klein G. Experiences with a finger-joint prosthesis. J Bone Joint Surg Am 1959;41-a(1): 87–102.

20. Swanson AB. Silicone rubber implants for replacement of arthritis or destroyed joints in the hand. Surg Clin North Am 1968;48(5):1113–27.

21. Swanson AB, Maupin BK, Gajjar NV, et al. Flexible implant arthroplasty in the proximal interphalangeal joint of the hand. J Hand Surg 1985;10(6 I):796–805.

22. Schneider LH. Proximal interphalangeal joint arthroplasty: the volar approach. Semin Arthroplasty 1991; 2(2):139–47.

23. Yamamoto M, Malay S, Fujihara Y, et al. A systematic review of different implants and approaches for proximal interphalangeal joint arthroplasty. Plast Reconstr Surg 2017;139(5):1139e–51e.

24. Yamamoto M, Chung KC. Implant arthroplasty: selection of exposure and implant. Hand Clin 2018; 34(2):195–205.

25. Escott BG, Ronald K, Judd MG, et al. NeuFlex and Swanson metacarpophalangeal implants for rheumatoid arthritis: prospective randomized, controlled clinical trial. J Hand Surg 2010;35(1):44–51.

26. Chung KC, Burns PB, Kim HM, et al. Long-term followup for rheumatoid arthritis patients in a multicenter outcomes study of silicone metacarpophalangeal joint arthroplasty. Arthritis Care Res (Hoboken) 2012;64(9):1292–300.

27. Chung KC, Kotsis SV, Burns PB, et al. Seven-year outcomes of the silicone arthroplasty in rheumatoid arthritis prospective cohort study. Arthritis Care Res (Hoboken) 2017;69(7):973–81.

28. Trail IA, Martin JA, Nuttall D, et al. Seventeen-year survivorship analysis of silastic metacarpophalangeal joint replacement. J Bone Joint Surg Br 2004; 86(7):1002–6.

29. Linscheid RL, Dobyns JH, Beckenbaugh RD, et al. Proximal interphalangeal joint arthroplasty with a total joint design. Mayo Clin Proc 1979;54(4): 227–40.

30. Linscheid RL, Murray PM, Vidal MA, et al. Development of a surface replacement arthroplasty for proximal interphalangeal joints. J Hand Surg 1997;22(2): 286–98.

31. Rizzo M. Metacarpophalangeal joint arthritis. J Hand Surg 2011;36(2):345–53.

32. Slaughter MS, Pederson B, Graham JD, et al. Evaluation of new Forcefield technology: reducing platelet adhesion and cell coverage of pyrolytic carbon surfaces. J Thorac Cardiovasc Surg 2011;142(4): 921–5.

33. Beckenbaugh RD. Preliminary experience with a noncemented nonconstrained total joint arthroplasty for the metacarpophalangeal joints. Orthopedics 1983;6(8):962–5.

34. Bellemere P. Pyrocarbon implants for the hand and wrist. Hand Surg Rehabil 2018;37(3):129–54.

35. Dickson DR, Badge R, Nuttall D, et al. Pyrocarbon metacarpophalangeal joint arthroplasty in noninflammatory arthritis: minimum 5-year follow-up. J Hand Surg 2015;40(10):1956–62.

36. Reissner L, Schindele S, Hensler S, et al. Ten year follow-up of pyrocarbon implants for proximal interphalangeal joint replacement. J Hand Surg Eur Vol 2014;39(6):582–6.

37. Schindele SF, Altwegg A, Hensler S. Surface replacement of proximal interphalangeal joints using CapFlex-PIP. Oper Orthop Traumatol 2017;29(1): 86–96 [in German].

38. Athlani L, Gaisne E, Bellemere P. Arthroplasty of the proximal interphalangeal joint with the TACTYS((R)) prosthesis: preliminary results after a minimum follow-up of 2 years. Hand Surg Rehabil 2016; 35(3):168–78.

39. Degeorge B, Athlani L, Dap F, et al. Proximal interphalangeal joint arthroplasty with Tactys((R)): clinical and radiographic results with a minimum follow-up of 12 months. Hand Surg Rehabil 2018; 37(4):218–24.

40. Shirakawa K, Shirota M. Post-operative contracture of the proximal interphalangeal joint after surface replacement arthroplasty using a volar approach. J Hand Surg Asian Pac Vol 2016; 21(3):345–51.

41. Trumble TE, Heaton DJ. Outcomes of surface replacement proximal interphalangeal joint arthroplasty through a volar approach: a prospective study. Hand (N Y) 2017;12(3):290–6.

42. Williams RM, Hastings H 2nd, Kiefhaber TR. PIP fracture/dislocation treatment technique: use of a hemi-hamate resurfacing arthroplasty. Tech Hand Up Extrem Surg 2002;6(4):185–92.

43. Williams RM, Kiefhaber TR, Sommerkamp TG, et al. Treatment of unstable dorsal proximal interphalangeal fracture/dislocations using a hemi-hamate autograft. J Hand Surg 2003;28(5):856–65.

44. Eaton RG, Malerich MM. Volar plate arthroplasty of the proximal interphalangeal joint: a review of ten years' experience. J Hand Surg 1980;5(3): 260–8.

45. Thomas BP, Raveendran S, Pallapati SR, et al. Augmented hamate replacement arthroplasty for fracture-dislocations of the proximal interphalangeal joints in 12 patients. J Hand Surg Eur Vol 2017;42(8): 799–802.

46. Hasegawa T, Yamano Y. Arthroplasty of the proximal interphalangeal joint using costal cartilage grafts. J Hand Surg Br 1992;17(5):583–5.

47. Sato K, Sasaki T, Nakamura T, et al. Clinical outcome and histologic findings of costal osteochondral grafts for cartilage defects in finger joints. J Hand Surg 2008;33(4):511–5.

48. Okuyama N, Sato K, Nakamura T, et al. Re: total joint reconstruction for MP joint ankylosis using costal osteochondral graft: a case report. J Hand Surg Eur Vol 2009;34(1):132–3.

49. Kodama N, Ueba H, Takemura Y, et al. Joint arthroplasty with osteochondral grafting from the knee for posttraumatic or degenerative hand joint disorders. J Hand Surg 2015;40(8):1638–45.

50. Ishida O, Tsai TM. Free vascularized whole joint transfer in children. Microsurgery 1991;12(3):196–206.

51. Tsai TM, Wang WZ. Vascularized joint transfers. Indications and results. Hand Clin 1992;8(3):525–36.

52. Kimori K, Ikuta Y, Ishida O, et al. Free vascularized toe joint transfer to the hand. A technique for simultaneous reconstruction of the soft tissue. J Hand Surg Eur Vol 2001;26(4):314–20.

53. Squitieri L, Chung KC. A systematic review of outcomes and complications of vascularized toe joint transfer, silicone arthroplasty, and PyroCarbon arthroplasty for posttraumatic joint reconstruction of the finger. Plast Reconstr Surg 2008;121(5):1697–707.

# Treatment of Common Congenital Hand Conditions

Bin Wang, MD, PhD[a],*, Xiaofei Tian, MD[b], Yong Hu, MD[c]

## KEYWORDS

- Congenital • Hand • Difference • Surgical • Treatment

## KEY POINTS

- The treatment principle for congenital hand differences is to achieve functional and aesthetic reconstructions.
- Surgery should be performed before joint deformity occurs, ideally at approximately age 2 years when hand dexterity is developed.
- Postsurgery management is critical for prevention of scarring and recurrence.

## INTRODUCTION

Congenital hand difference refers to anomaly of the hand structure at birth that is caused by abnormal embryonic development of the limb. According to the appearance, it can be classified into malformations, deformations, and dysplasias and syndromes. Thumb duplication and syndactyly are the most common congenital hand differences. The treatment objective is to reconstruct the anatomic structures and to restore the normal functions and appearance. However, treatment success is not always guaranteed due to the variability in phenotypes.

## THUMB DUPLICATION
### Clinical Manifestations

Thumb duplication or radial polydactyly refers to extra digit(s) or excrescence of the phalanges, soft tissue, or metacarpal bone of the thumb. It is caused by abnormal development of the anterior-posterior axis, due to either genetic or environmental factors. The incidence of thumb duplication is approximately 0.08% to 0.18%. The deformity usually includes the thumb only and can sometimes manifest itself in a syndrome such as Beckwith-Wiedemann syndrome, Bloom syndrome, or Holt-Oram syndrome.

The clinical manifestation of nonsyndromic thumb duplication can vary. The presence of the extra digit can be at either the radial or ulnar side of the thumb, or both. The size, shape, structure, and function of the extra thumb often differs from the normal thumb with different degrees of dysplasia and deformity, or occurs as a triphalangeal thumb. When 2 thumbs are similar in shape, they are considered as mirror thumbs. When 2 thumbs duplicate with the lateral flexion, palmar flexion, or angulation malformation of the interphalangeal joint and the metacarpophalangeal joint, it is called crablike thumb duplication.

The most popular anatomic classification of thumb duplication is Flatt classification (**Fig. 1**), which is based on the position of separation and

Disclosure Statement: This study was supported by National Natural Science Foundation of China No. 81772115, 81571930 to Bin Wang.

[a] Department of Plastic and Reconstructive Surgery, Shanghai 9th People's Hospital, Shanghai Jiaotong University School of Medicine, 639 Zhizaoju Road, Shanghai 200011, People's Republic of China; [b] Department of Burns and Plastic Surgery, Children's Hospital, Chongqing Medical University, 136 Zhongshan 2nd Road, Chongqing 400014, People's Republic of China; [c] Department of Hand and Foot Surgery, The Second Hospital of Shandong University, 247 Beiyuan Street, Shandong Province, Jinan 250033, People's Republic of China
* Corresponding author.
E-mail address: wangbin1766@163.com

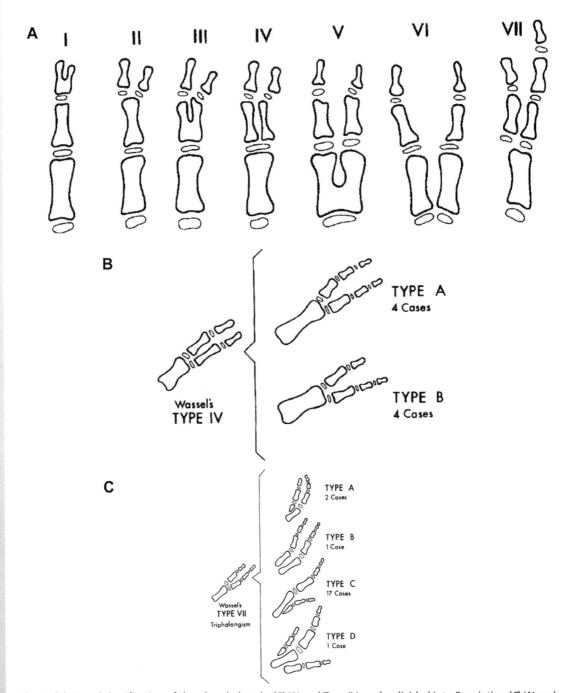

**Fig. 1.** (*A*) Wassel classification of thumb polydactyly. (*B*) Wassel Type IV can be divided into 2 varieties. (*C*) Wassel type VII can be divided into 4 varieties. (*Reprinted from* The Journal of Hand Surgery Volume 3 Issue 5, Wood VE. Polydactyly and the triphalangeal thumb, pages 436–444, Copyright 1978, with permission from Elsevier.)

involvement of joints, plus the type of triphalangia.[1] The 3 most common types are type IV (approximately 47%), type VII (approximately 23%), and type II (approximately 15%). Wood[2] subcategorized type IV to form a more completed classification (see **Fig. 1**).

## Treatment

### Principles of treatment for thumb duplication

In principle, the thumb with normal appearance and better function is kept. If the digit to be resected is accompanied with major neurovascular bundles, it should be carefully separated and protected. If there are insertions of major tendons or intrinsic muscles, they also should be shifted to the corresponding position of the thumb retained. The joint capsule and ligament tissue of the polydactyly should be retained to repair the joint capsule of the thumb and to maintain the stability of the joint at the metacarpophalangeal or interphalangeal joint capsule. When the preserved thumb is severely deformed, arthrodesis or corrective osteotomy is necessary after physeal growth has ceased. Mirror thumbs can be combined to create a new thumb.

### Timing of surgery

In general, surgery should be performed before the formation of clearly skewed joint and the development of pinch and grasp force, usually at 10 to 12 months after birth. For a superfluous digit with a narrow pedicle connected to the normal digit, simple excision can be performed immediately after birth. For those with other congenital conditions, the timing of surgery is usually 8 to 15 months after birth. For those with severe malformations that need digit resection, tissue transfer and transposition using microsurgical techniques are necessary. Surgery can be performed after the age of 1 year. The patients should be followed up after surgery and treatment of secondary deformities should be performed before the preschool age.

### Surgical methods

Surgical treatment requires comprehensive application of plastic surgery, microsurgery, orthopedics, and hand surgery.[3] The surgical method should be chosen according to individual cases.

**Simple removal of extra digit** For thumb duplication with clear primary thumb, the redundant digit can be simply removed (**Fig. 2**).

**Ablation of extra thumb and reconstruction of lateral collateral ligament** For thumb duplication with clear primary thumb, the redundant digit can be removed and the main thumb can be centralized. The lateral collateral ligament should be sutured to the side of the main thumb to stabilize the joint (**Fig. 3**).

**Bilhaut-Cloquet method** This method can be used for mirror thumbs with similar appearance and shape of the phalanges.[4] Half of the soft tissue, phalanges, and nails of the 2 thumbs are removed and the halves are combined to form a new thumb. In this operation, attention should be paid to the smoothness of the articular surface, the retention of the insertion of tendon, the alignment of the bone surface, and the nail bed to minimize the protuberance or depression of the nail at a later stage (**Fig. 4**).

**Osteotomy and bone grafting** When there is a radial or ulnar deviation of the phalange and metacarpal bone, a wedge osteotomy is needed to correct the angular deformity. A K-wire fixation might be necessary. An open osteotomy is occasionally required, together with the cancellous bone grafting of the supernumerary thumb (**Fig. 5**).

**Dynamic balance of the tendon** The abnormal flexor, extensor tendons, and pulley system are often found in thumb duplication. Rebalancing of the tendon to functional position is conducive to the correction of joint deformity and maintenance of the developmental alignment. For this reason, the extensor tendon and flexor tendon of the excised thumb should be retained for reconstruction of the extension and flexion function of the retained thumb or correction of lateral deformity of the joint (**Fig. 6**).

**Repair with local island flaps** When the preserved thumb lacks tissue or is too small, a local island

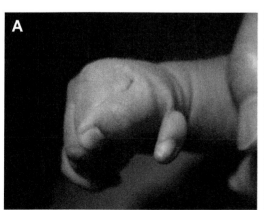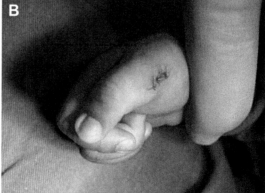

**Fig. 2.** Excision of the floating thumb. (*A*) Presurgery view. (*B*) Postsurgery view.

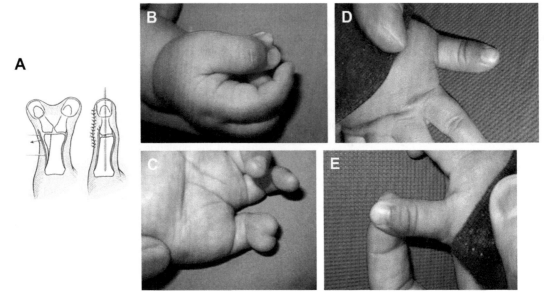

**Fig. 3.** Ablation of the supernumerary thumb and reconstruction of lateral collateral ligament. (*A*) Schematic of the surgical operation. (*B, C*) Presurgery view. (*D, E*) Postsurgery view.

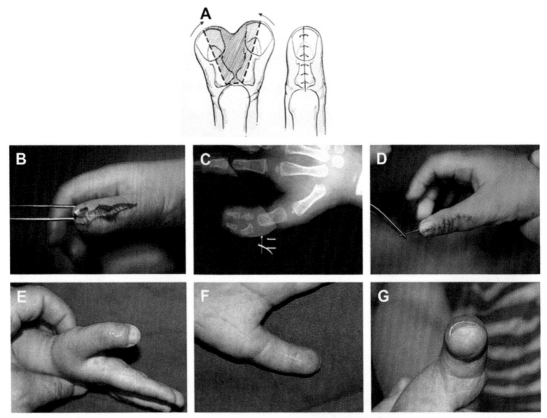

**Fig. 4.** Correction of bifid thumb by using Bilhaut-Cloquet procedure. (*A*) Schematic of the surgical operation. (*B, C*) Presurgery view. (*D*) Immediately postsurgery view. (*E–G*). Follow-up view.

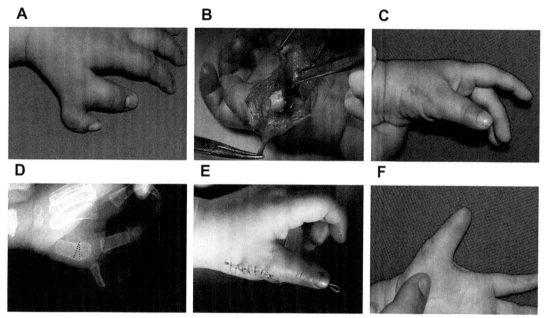

**Fig. 5.** Correction of the angular deformity of the metacarpophalangeal joint by osteotomy under the physis. (*A, D*) Presurgery view. (*B*) Intraoperative view. (*E*) Immediately postsurgery view. (*C, F*) Follow-up view.

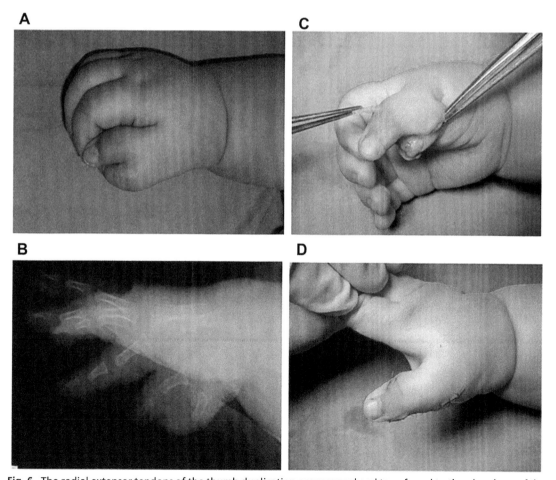

**Fig. 6.** The radial extensor tendons of the thumb duplication are reserved and transferred to the ulnar base of the ulnar side of the distal phalanx to balance the tendon and correct the developmental alignment. (*A, B*) Presurgery view. (*C*) Intraoperative view. (*D*) Immediately postsurgery view.

flap with neurovascular pedicle can be transferred from the thumb to be removed to augment the tissue deficit. The flap can also carry partial phalanges and nails to enlarge the surface area and improve the appearance of the preserved thumb (**Fig. 7**).

**On-top plasty** Indications for this procedure include clinical scenarios in which one thumb was not clearly dominant over the other based on physical examination and radiographs, with one having a better proximal portion whereas the other had a better distal portion. Thus, the distally well-developed thumb that preserves the neurovascular pedicle is transferred to the base of the thumb with a well-developed metacarpal bone. Which metacarpophalangeal joint and osteotomy plane to keep should be decided according to the development of the metacarpophalangeal joint of the thumb (**Fig. 8**).

### Correction of the triangular thumb

The triangular redundant phalange often causes skewed deformity, which can be corrected by the central osteotomy and the wedge bone grafting.[5] It is also possible to use a reverse wedge osteotomy.[6] We perform a wedge osteotomy on the long side of the interface of the triangular phalange and transplant it to the short side of the interface to correct the angulation deformity of the digits. For a triphalangeal thumb without angulation deformity, we can choose to fuse one of the joints based on the development of the proximal or distal interphalangeal joint. When necessary, we can perform the osteotomy to shorten the phalange or to remove the triangular phalange (**Fig. 9**).

### Repair of postoperative secondary deformity

Simple resection of duplicated thumb often leads to secondary deformities, such as deviation of the digit, adduction of the thumb, instability of the joints, weakness of the muscle, and dysplasia of the thumb. It is necessary to analyze the anatomic anomalies and do corresponding measures for comprehensive repair, including revision and osteotomy of the articular surface, reconstruction of the lateral collateral ligaments, refixation of the muscle insertions, and transplantation of the tendons. Partial reconstruction of the dysplastic thumb can be performed if needed.

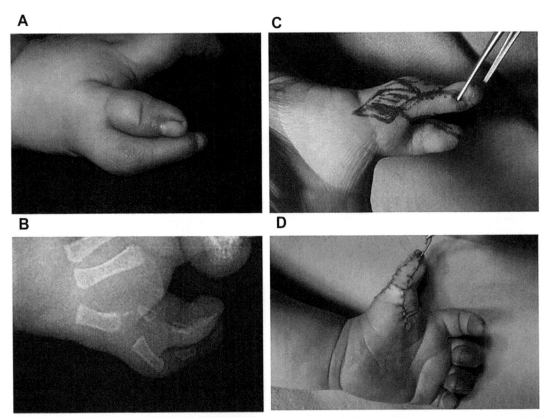

**Fig. 7.** By transferring the island flap to supplement the insufficient soft tissue of the reconstructed thumb. (*A, B*) Presurgery view. (*C*) Intraoperative view. (*D*) Immediately postsurgery view.

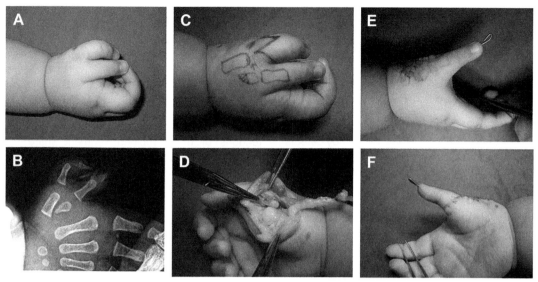

**Fig. 8.** On-top plasty surgery of duplicated thumb. (*A, B*) Presurgery view. (*C, D*). Intraoperative view. (*E, F*) Immediately postsurgery view.

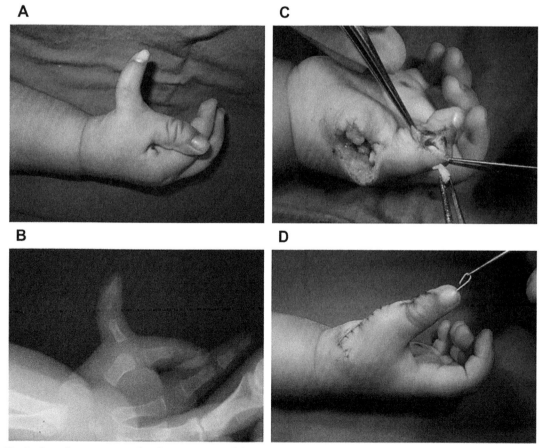

**Fig. 9.** A wedge osteotomy for the correction of the skewed deformity of phalange in Wassel type IV. (*A, B*) Presurgery view. (*C*) Intraoperative view. (*D*) Immediately postsurgery view.

### Postoperative management

Early brace fixation is necessary to maintain the relative position. Reasonable and moderate rehabilitation exercise is conducive to better functional recovery.

## SYNDACTYLY

Syndactyly is characterized by cutaneous or bony fusion between adjacent digits, caused by defects in the embryonic hand-plate differentiation due to genetic mutations or environmental factors. It can occur separately or appear with other malformations including polydactyly, camptodactyly, brachydactyly, symphalangism, and synostosis. The incidence of syndactyly is approximately 1 in 2000, of which 50% are bilateral. Approximately 10% to 40% of children have a family history, showing autosomal dominant inheritance, variable phenotype, and incomplete penetrance. In isolated syndactyly, the third-fourth finger web space is most frequently affected, followed by the fourth-little fingers. In syndromic forms, the other web space maybe affected.

### Clinical Manifestations

Syndactyly can be simple cutaneous or complex bony fusion. Bony syndactyly can be categorized into 3 classes: (1) osseous fusion of 2 phalanges at proximal or distal end; (2) transverse bony bridge connecting 2 phalanges; (3) synpolydactyly with the connection through the phalange of the polydactyly in the middle (**Fig. 10**).[7]

Bony syndactyly has unique characteristics in skin tension, blood vessels, nerves, tendons, and joint abnormality. The skin tension of the fused segment of the bone is tight in osseous fusion, but may be loose in transverse bony bridge and synpolydactyly. For blood vessels and nerves, 2 fingers each have 2 vessels and nerves, but one side may be stunted, which is often seen in the middle and distal bony syndactyly. It is common in proximal bony syndactyly that 2 fingers share a blood vessel or nerve in the middle. Tendons are often normal in the middle and distal bony syndactyly. In proximal bony syndactyly, the tendons are merged proximally, separated distally, and the tendons of the combined segment share the tendon sheaths and pulleys. The bone deformity includes bone widening, bending, bracket epiphysis, and osteodystrophy. Joint stiffness can appear as joint fusion, cartilaginous junction, and joint stenosis. Of note, the joints may deviate after syndactyly separation.

### Treatment

#### Reconstruction of the web space

Rebuilding functional and well-formed web spaces is the key of syndactyly separation. Normal second, third, and fourth webs are characterized by the hourglass shape and a 45° slope from proximal-dorsal to distal-palmar. They add to the proximal transverse digital stria at the level of the midpoint of the metacarpal head to the proximal phalanx (**Fig. 11**). The second and fourth web spaces are wider than the third one, which makes the index finger and the little finger capable of more abduction. The first web space is a broad, diamond-shaped skin consisting of the hairless skin on the palmar side and the thinner one with greater motility on the dorsal side.

For incomplete syndactyly limited to the proximal phalanx, Z-plasty, 4 flap-plasty, rectangle flaps, and butterfly flaps can be applied to deepen or extend existing web spaces. Other methods use combination of local flaps, such as triangular flap

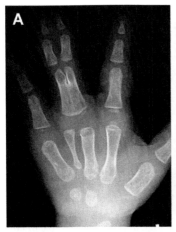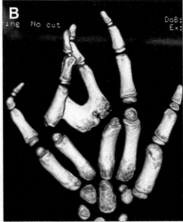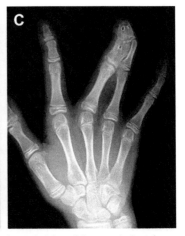

**Fig. 10.** Classification of bony syndactyly. (*A*) Osseous fusion. (*B*) Transverse bony bridge. (*C*) Synpolydactyly.

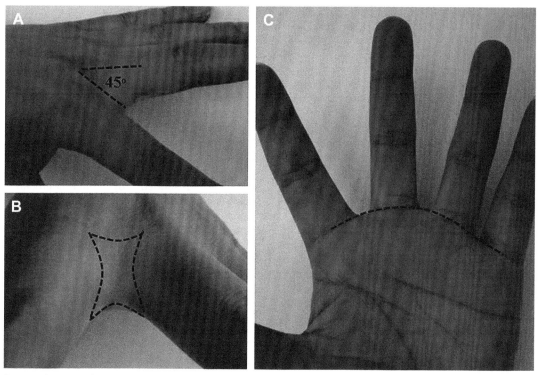

**Fig. 11.** The normal second, third, and fourth webs are characterized by an hourglass shape and a 45° slope from proximal-dorsal to distal-palmar. They add to the proximal transverse digital stria at the level of the midpoint of the metacarpal head to the proximal phalanx. (*A–C*) Operational design.

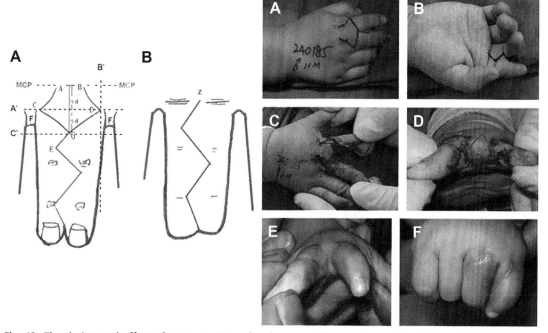

**Fig. 12.** The design and effect of reconstruction of web space with a pentagonal local flap. (*Left: A, B*) Operational design. (*Right: A, B*) Presurgery view. (*C*) Intraoperative view. (*D*) Immediately postsurgery view. (*E, F*) Follow-up view. (*From* Gao W, Yan H, Zhang F, et al. Dorsal pentagonal local flap: a new technique of web reconstruction for syndactyly without skin graft. Aesthetic plastic surgery. 2011; 35:530-537 with permission.)

web plasty, and V-M web plasty. Reconstruction of web space by dorsal advancement flaps can mobilize more skin to rebuild the web spaces. Gao and colleagues[8] designed a pentagonal local flap to reconstruct the web, which can fully cover the sidewalls of the webs (**Fig. 12**). To maintain the structural integrity and the physiologic inclination, Ni and colleagues[9] used hourglass dorsal advancement flaps to directly reconstruct the finger webs (**Fig. 13**). Tian and colleagues[10] proposed that the use of modified double-wing flaps can effectively improve the flap advancement and avoid excessive tension (**Fig. 14**).

### Reconstruction of the nail fold

The nail fold is a transition from the nail bed and nail to normal skin. As an important part of the distal segment of the finger, the reconstruction of the nail fold is crucial for the aesthetics of the nail. The following principles should be kept in nail fold reconstruction: (1) keep the symmetry with the contralateral nail fold of the finger and the symmetry with the nail fold of the corresponding finger in the contralateral hand; (2) apply local flap to reduce scars on the reconstructed nail folds and make the reconstructed nail folds plumper; (3) form the nail groove and the smooth transition from the nail bed to the nail fold during reconstruction; (4) the lower edge should be smooth in radian to avoid deflection or herringbone deformity.

The distal phalanx can be treated with the technique described by Buck-Gramcko.[11] Cross-lingual flaps at the distal ends of the syndactylous digits can be designed and folded to recreate the bilateral nail folds. A dorsal lingual rotation flap and a lingual flap on the fingertip can be used to reconstruct the nail folds (**Figs. 15** and **16**). It is also possible to reconstruct a nail fold with a flap at the connected finger

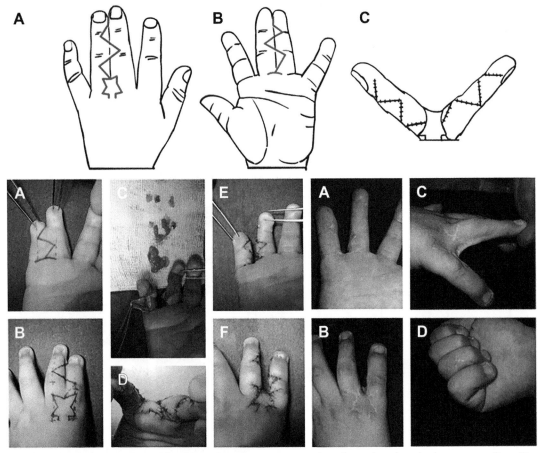

**Fig. 13.** The design and effect of reconstruction of web space with an hourglass dorsal advancement flap. (*Top: A–C*) Operational design. (*Lower left: A, B*) Presurgery view. (*C*) Intraoperative view. (*D–F*) Immediately postsurgery view. (*Lower right: A–D*). Follow-up view. (*From* Ni F, Mao H, Yang X, et al. The use of an hourglass dorsal advancement flap without skin graft for congenital syndactyly. The Journal of hand surgery. 2015; 40:1748-1754 e1741 with permission.)

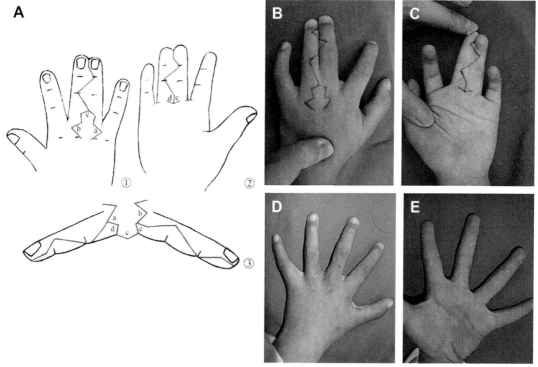

**Fig. 14.** The design and effect of reconstruction of web space with a modified double-wing flap. (*A*) Operational design. (*B, C*) Presurgery view. (*D, E*) Follow-up view. (*From* Tian X, Xiao J, Li T, et al. Single-stage separation of 3- and 4-finger incomplete simple syndactyly with contiguous gull wing flaps: a technique to minimize or avoid skin grafting. The Journal of hand surgery. 2017; 42:257-264 with permission.)

pulp. The subcutaneous fat flap and skin graft can then be used to reconstruct the nail fold of the other finger. It is also desirable to use pedicle flaps such as thenar flap, or transplanting skins and subcutaneous tissue from the toe to reconstruct the nail fold.

*Treatment for complex (bony) syndactyly*
Specific treatments can be used to deal with different aspects of bony syndactyly. The difficulty in covering bone wounds can be solved by the

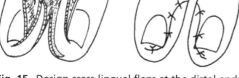

**Fig. 15.** Design cross-lingual flaps at the distal ends of the syndactylies to repair the defect of the fingers and reconstruct the nail folds.

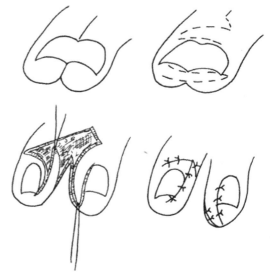

**Fig. 16.** Design a dorsal lingual rotation flap and a lingual flap on the fingertip to repair the defect of the fingers and reconstruct the nail folds.

following methods: (1) expanded flap: expanded flap is transferred after stretching with mini expander and external stent; (2) local gyral flap: local flaps can be adjusted to cover small bone wounds; (3) island flap: palmar or dorsal retrograde flap can cover proximal bone wound. For distal bony syndactyly, the flap can cover one side and the other can be covered with fascial flap.[12]

For patients with 2 fingers sharing the same tendon, flexor digitorum profundus (FDP) should be separated to the middle of the palm. After the proximal separation, the pulley should be rebuilt. The distal insertion should then be placed to the middle. For patients with tendon dysplasia or even absence, tendon-diverted transplantation is needed at second stage. To achieve joint stability, the joint capsule defect after separation can be repaired by adjacent periosteal flap or the free fascia flap. To maintain blood supply, at least one well-developed finger intrinsic vessel should be retained.

Other difficulties to separate joint malformations, such as bone bending, articular surface inclination, bracket epiphysis, joint adhesion, stenosis, and fusion-skeletal dysplasia, can be corrected by open or wedge osteotomy. Joint adhesions and stenosis should be early released (**Fig. 17**).

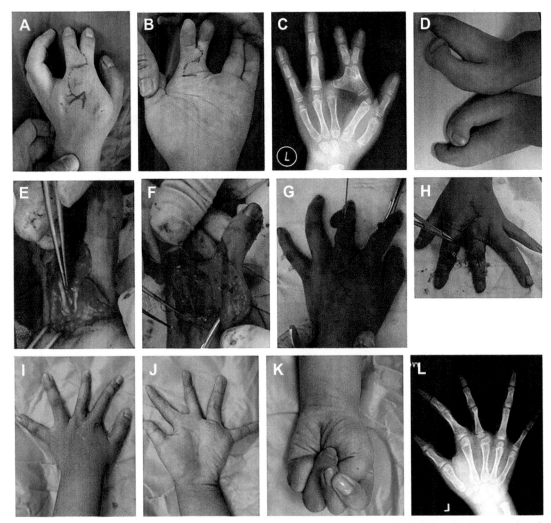

**Fig. 17.** Girl, 6 years and 9 months old, two-thirds of the proximal phalanx in the left hand is bony syndactyly, osseous fusion, no family history, accompanied by cleft foot deformity. Proximal flexion and extensor tendon merged. Remove bone bridges and cover the bone wounds with palmar and dorsal skin flaps respectively. The remaining wounds were given skin graft. Reset the metacarpophalangeal joint and correct the proximal phalanx by wedge osteotomy. The shape and function improved significantly 2 years postoperatively. (*A–D*) Presurgery view. (*E–G*) Intraoperative view. (*H*) Immediately postsurgery view. (*I–L*) Follow-up view.

## Separation and reconstruction of toe syndactyly

The differences between the toes and fingers should be considered in treatment of toe syndactyly. The mobility of the dorsal and metatarsal skin of feet is poorer than that of the hands. Therefore, when toe-web is reconstructed, the range of skin movement is not as good as that of the fingers. The web spaces and lateral wounds of toe deformity can be treated by island flap or cutaneous branch flap with toe artery. The distal toe pulp can be used to repair the nail folds or lateral part of the toe.

Dorsal rectangular, pentagonal flaps and metatarsal advancement flaps can be used to reconstruct the toe-web. An island flap can be obtained from the distal part of toe pulp with toe artery on one side to reconstruct the toe-web. Toe artery flaps can be taken from the syndactylous digits or adjacent toes. The soft tissue of the toe-web should be debulked so that the flaps will not appear bloated postoperatively. Linear stitches should be avoided on flaps and lateral sides to prevent linear scar contracture (**Fig. 18**).

For lateral coverage of the toe, a zigzag incision should be used to avoid scar contracture. The toe skin is generally looser than the finger. Therefore, distal toe pulp can be sutured directly after cutting off the flap. The pedicle flap also can be obtained from the middle and proximal toe pulp, web space, and the side of the middle and proximal part of the adjacent toes. If it cannot be completely covered, a small defect can be covered by skin graft from the medial malleolus or medial plantar area. The toe pulp can be used to reconstruct the nail folds with a cross-triangular flap. However, prevention of acronyx should be noticed.

After toe separation, it is necessary to observe whether the toe is deviated in the weight-bearing position. If it is caused by tendons, reconstruction of the tendon insertion is required. Tenolysis of extensor and flexor tendon can be considered if necessary. If it is caused by phalanx deviation, osteotomy is required. Make sure the row line is good.

When toe syndactyly is associated with polydactyly, trimming the enlarged articular surface and reconstruct the collateral ligament of joint capsule is usually required.

## Management of postoperative keloids

Keloid is a dermal fibrosis disease caused by skin injury, characterized by excessive deposition of collagen, invasive growth beyond the initial lesion with persistent and powerful proliferation that was clinically known as benign dermal tumors. Keloids usually occur on the chest, shoulders, ear lobes, upper arms, and cheeks. The clinical manifestations often include itchiness, pain, and tingling, as well as the unlikable appearance. Although rare after syndactyly separation, keloids in hands often lead to significant dysfunction.

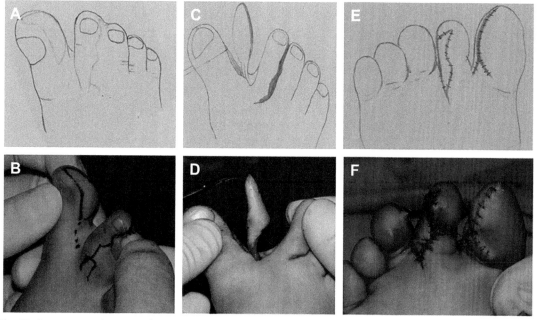

**Fig. 18.** Reconstruct the toe-webs or cover the soft tissue defect using island flaps from the lateral side of the toe pulp. (*A, C,* and *E*) Schematics of the operation. (*B, D,* and *F*) Operational view.

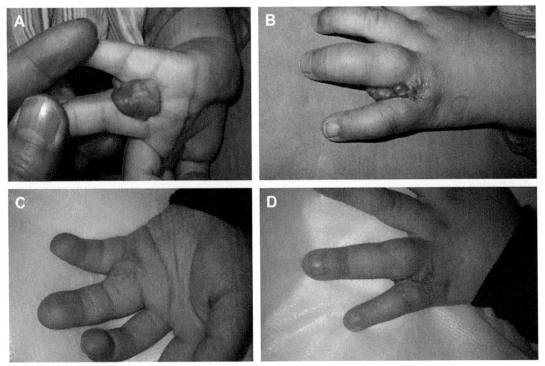

**Fig. 19.** (*A,B*) Keloid formation after syndactly separation. (*C,D*) Spontaneous regression after 2 years.

Due to the high rate of recurrence, there are many controversies about the timing of intervention and the choice of treatments. With the increasing understanding of the mechanism of keloids, early postoperative intervention is advisable.

Early intervention methods include the following: (1) Scar injection therapy. The standard method involves local injection of 5-fluorouracil and steroids into scar tissue. It was found that the injection of low-dose methotrexate combined with folic acid

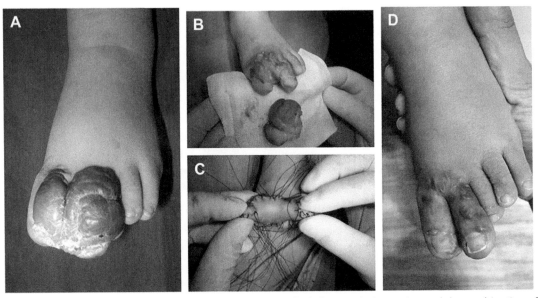

**Fig. 20.** Keloid formed after syndactyly separation was controlled after surgical resection and the combination of intense pulse laser and hormone injection. (*A*) Presurgery view. (*B, C*) Intraoperative view. (*D*) Postsurgery view.

can inhibit the growth of scar tissue, which needs to be performed as early signs of scar hyperplasia appear.[13-15] (2) Photoelectric treatment. This method is currently a hot topic in clinical research, including laser and other related treatments.[16] Intense pulse laser and pulsed dye laser with a wavelength of 595 nm match the absorption peak of hemoglobin, so they can reduce blood supply and eliminate the red color of scars, which is suitable for hyperplastic scars or keloids. (3) Optical fiber therapy. When an optical fiber was introduced inside the scars, direct photothermal interaction can promote the scars to subside. (4) Radiotherapy. The use of postoperative radiotherapy for children with keloids is still debatable, because it may induce malignant tumors and inhibits bone development. Therefore, it is necessary to weigh the pros and cons in clinical practice. (5) Pressure therapy. Pressure therapy on the webs should be started early after the operation. It uses a brace that can exert axial pressure on the webs and can effectively reduce the formation of keloids.[17]

In some cases, the keloids regress spontaneously after 2 years. Therefore, treatment in the regression period can reduce the pain (**Fig. 19**). Surgery combined with comprehensive treatment of scars is still the most important measure for severe keloids. The wounds often require skin grafting to achieve tension-free coverage (**Fig. 20**).

Prevention is the most important in controlling keloid formation. Aseptic operation during surgery and prevention of infection after surgery are the first key steps. The use of silicone and pressure therapy has become routine management after surgery. In the event of scar hyperplasia, early intervention should be taken to control the progression of the disease in time.

## SUMMARY

Congenital hand difference poses a big challenge for hand surgeons. New surgical operation advances in recent years achieved good restoration of hand function and appearance. By combinatorial use of the principles, timing, surgical techniques, and postsurgery management, good outcome can be achieved in thumb duplication and syndactyly treatment.

## REFERENCES

1. Wassel HD. The results of surgery for polydactyly of the thumb. A review. Clin Orthop Relat Res 1969;64: 175-93.
2. Wood VE. Polydactyly and the triphalangeal thumb. J Hand Surg 1978;3:436-44.
3. Tonkin MA. Thumb duplication: concepts and techniques. Clin Orthop Surg 2012;4:1-17.
4. Baek GH, Gong HS, Chung MS, et al. Modified Bilhaut-Cloquet procedure for Wassel type-II and III polydactyly of the thumb. J Bone Joint Surg Am 2007;89:534-41.
5. Kozin SH. Reconstruction of Wassel type IV thumb duplication. Tech Hand Up Extrem Surg 2010;14: 58-62.
6. Chew EM, Yong FC, Teoh LC. The oblique wedge osteotomy of the metacarpal condyle for reconstructing Wassel type IV thumb duplication in older children and adults. J Hand Surg Eur Vol 2010;35: 669-75.
7. Malik S. Syndactyly: phenotypes, genetics and current classification. Eur J Hum Genet 2012;20: 817-24.
8. Gao W, Yan H, Zhang F, et al. Dorsal pentagonal local flap: a new technique of web reconstruction for syndactyly without skin graft. Aesthetic Plast Surg 2011;35:530-7.
9. Ni F, Mao H, Yang X, et al. The use of an hourglass dorsal advancement flap without skin graft for congenital syndactyly. J Hand Surg 2015;40: 1748-54.e1.
10. Tian X, Xiao J, Li T, et al. Single-stage separation of 3- and 4-finger incomplete simple syndactyly with contiguous Gull wing flaps: a technique to minimize or avoid skin grafting. J Hand Surg 2017;42:257-64.
11. Buck-Gramcko D. Progress in the treatment of congenital malformations of the hand. World journal of surgery 1990;14(6):715-24.
12. Goldfarb CA, Steffen JA, Stutz CM. Complex syndactyly: aesthetic and objective outcomes. J Hand Surg 2012;37:2068-73.
13. Kong BY, Baek GH, Gong HS. Treatment of keloid formation following syndactyly division: surgical technique. Hand Surg 2012;17:433-7.
14. Muzaffar AR, Rafols F, Masson J, et al. Keloid formation after syndactyly reconstruction: associated conditions, prevalence, and preliminary report of a treatment method. J Hand Surg 2004;29:201-8.
15. Tolerton SK, Tonkin MA. Keloid formation after syndactyly release in patients with associated macrodactyly: management with methotrexate therapy. J Hand Surg Eur Vol 2011;36:490-7.
16. Tonkin MA, Willis KR, Lawson RD. Keloid formation resulting in acquired syndactyly of an initially normal web space following syndactyly release of an adjacent web space. J Hand Surg Eur Vol 2008;33: 29-31.
17. Son D, Harijan A. Overview of surgical scar prevention and management. J Korean Med Sci 2014;29: 751-7.

# Moving?

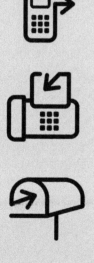

## Make sure your subscription moves with you!

To notify us of your new address, find your **Clinics Account Number** (located on your mailing label above your name), and contact customer service at:

**Email: journalscustomerservice-usa@elsevier.com**

**800-654-2452** (subscribers in the U.S. & Canada)
**314-447-8871** (subscribers outside of the U.S. & Canada)

**Fax number: 314-447-8029**

**Elsevier Health Sciences Division**
**Subscription Customer Service**
**3251 Riverport Lane**
**Maryland Heights, MO 63043**

Printed and bound by CPI Group (UK) Ltd, Croydon, CR0 4YY

08/05/2025

01864746-0010